The
Seven
Deadly
Whites

Evolution to Devolution – The Rise of The
Diseases Of Civilization

The
Seven
Deadly
Whites

Evolution to Devolution – The Rise of The
Diseases Of Civilization

Karl Elliot-Gough

EARTH

BOOKS

Winchester, UK
Washington, USA

First published by Earth Books, 2016
Earth Books is an imprint of John Hunt Publishing Ltd., Laurel House, Station Approach,
Alresford, Hants, SO24 9JH, UK
office1@jhpbooks.net
www.johnhuntpublishing.com
www.earth-books.net

For distributor details and how to order please visit the 'Ordering' section on our website.

Text copyright: Karl Elliot-Gough 2015

ISBN: 978 1 78535 179 2
Library of Congress Control Number: 2015946049

A CIP catalogue record for this book is available from the British Library.

Design: Stuart Davies

Printed and bound by CPI Group (UK) Ltd, Croydon, CR0 4YY, UK

We operate a distinctive and ethical publishing philosophy in all
areas of our business, from our global network of authors to
production and worldwide distribution.

CONTENTS

elements from?; Unimental — all of time and space in a grain; 5 elemental chemicals; From unimental to the really mental: The cell; Where health begins and refined salt ends.

Inspiration and motivation for this book has been a life long journey; from the friends, conversations, places visited, books read, music listened to, films watched and too much more, all has gone into the melting pot. For those who have helped me specifically with this book, I'd like to thank Paul Kellett and John Nunn, for their faith, encouragement and patience, as well as of course all those at John Hunt Publishing. Lastly and always first, my wife Sara and our lovely children, Maya, Khymer, Wolfie and Aurora – please accept my humblest apologies for sharing with you this most stressful path, as I weekly uncovered a never-ending trail of deceit and an incredible lack of ethics and morals amongst so many industries. I selfishly made you live the book, instead of you having the choice to read it when it was finished, sorry.

Introduction

"We may find in the long run, that tinned food is a deadlier weapon than the machine gun."
(George Orwell)

The seed for this book was initially planted over a quarter of a century ago, whilst on a field trip in Indonesia studying archaeology and anthropology. There I was, completely lost and disorientated, somewhere in the depths of the lush Indonesian rainforest. It had only been thirty seconds since my flip-flopped guide and his bare-footed young son had disappeared through the trees, walking silently, effortlessly and gracefully, as if floating just above the ground. I was admiring their natural physique, as well as being somewhat jealous of the way they blended into the environment as they slipped away; there was no question they and the forest were in unison. The same could not be said for myself, sweating, covered in bites and sores, I stuck out like the proverbial sore thumb. Bemused at my frailty, I asked myself a question that planted the seed, which has finally blossomed into this book: "If the caveman or present day hunter-gatherers very rarely died from cancer or heart disease, why should we?"

Diseases of Civilization

Today, well over 80% of deaths in the industrialised world are as a result of heart disease, cancer and iatrogeny. Iatrogeny is the third biggest individual killer in the developed world, only beaten by heart disease and cancer. Amazingly, the vast majority of the population have never even heard of this word and nor had I before researching this book. An illness or death caused by medical intervention, prescription or surgical, is known as an iatrogenic disease, where *iatro* means 'physician or medicine' and *genic* means 'caused by'. These three diseases (heart disease, cancer and iatrogeny), as well as diabetes, obesity, depression, Alzheimer's, Parkinson's, Crohn's, Autistic Spectrum Disorders (ASD), Attention Deficit Disorders (ADD) and many more, are all collectively known as diseases of civilization. A phrase that is unlikely to be brandished about by the BMA (British Medical Association) or the government. There is no way that these institutions would want to draw public attention to any potential association between these two words, disease and civilization, as it appears derogatory, implying that in some shape or form these diseases have been caused by, or have something to do with, civilization.

Which is indeed where the real root of the problem lurks and indeed where the answer resides for these diseases of civilization. The human organism is not at ease with civilization, it is at disease. This alone should start the alarm bells ringing. So why is it so quiet? Especially as there is something so seriously amiss with civilization that it now names the very diseases we are dying from.

We believe we are living in a privileged position, at the pinnacle of human evolution, with humans always purposefully striving to evolve, to ultimately become what we are today, supposed superior beings of the twenty first century. Undeniably, there have been many modern advancements; in science, space exploration, the study of atoms, medicine, surgery, computers and technology, all of which has given us the potential to guarantee health, wealth and longevity, far outstretching the dreams and aspirations of our great-grandparents a hundred years ago. So why are so few actualizing this potential? And if we are so advanced and evolved, why do so few people die from simply old age? The truth is, we in the industrialised world, are dying and falling sick from an ever-increasing list of diseases. With a society that is dysfunctional in youth, depressed in middle age, with dementia and uncared for in old age, whilst suffering a never-ending catalogue of illnesses throughout life. Is that civilized?

We are dying and being afflicted by all these diseases of civilization at an ever-increasing rate. These diseases are also afflicting a forever younger demographic, with little discrimination between race, class or age. Often death from cancer or heart disease is brushed aside, claimed to be simply a consequence of our 'modern lifestyle' or 'we are living to a greater age today', although getting old, does not, and it most certainly should not equate, to immobility of the mind and body, whilst a degenerative disease strips all life away. This disparity in deaths between the present day hunter-gatherers and us, of the civilized world, rubs against the grain of evolution. Why would we have evolved as the species, *Homo*, over millions of years, just to have within each and every one of us a self-destruct button that can end life?

A button that is being switched on-and-off at an ever-increasing rate in the West.

Is it Mankind or Mother Nature flicking this switch?

The 7 Deadly Whites is a look at seven different variables to do with food and diet and any associations these may have with the diseases of civilization. The 7 Deadly Whites are a direct reference to the processed foods made from white flour, white sugar, white rice, milk, salt and fats/oils, with the seventh being white lies. The actual colour of the six deadly food whites is immaterial, although pallid white to grey does prevail. Termed 'white' because they are all processed and as such contain considerably less nutritious content than their whole food compatriots, often providing only calories. A stupendous 80% of the modern diet is made from these six deadly food whites, by both weight and calorific content.

Supermarkets have a deliberately laid out floor plan, where

the fresh produce (fruit and vegetables) is found at the front of store, greeting the customer, giving the impression of fresh whole foods being the norm from your shopping experience around the whole store, when in fact this fresh produce section is less than 5% of total shelf space; all those other food aisles, these are where the processed foods live, the vast majority of which are made from endless combinations of the six deadly food whites. There is reputedly somewhere in the region of five hundred million different varieties of processed food worldwide. Most of the processed food varieties were developed in the 1950s, achieving global dominance by the 1980s, with absolute supremacy by the 1990s. With the modern diet becoming overwhelmed in products, the very things food was supposed to deliver, those vitamins, minerals and amino acids, have been replaced with carbohydrates (calories) and very little else (apart from the whole heap of problems introduced throughout this book).

The food industry has boosted what is erroneously called economy. This word 'economy' holds a key in explaining the poor state of our health and food today, needing to look no further than that old chestnut, money. Coupled with the unquenchable, insatiable desire to possess as much of it as possible, often pursued via unethical, unhealthy and un-environmental avenues of short-term profit. It is the by-products of this profiteering that is starting to have such drastic and dire consequences. The factory produced and processed foods, the 30 billion tonnes of carbon dioxide emitted from industry, or the 500 million tonnes of highly toxic chemicals used every year to produce and sustain our present capitalist, consumerist lifestyle. All this pollution has been created so someone can make a profit.

Oikonomia

Very little of this profit, if any, finds its way to contributing to our survival and continuity on this wonderful planet. This profit is even used as a form of justification for the pollution created in obtaining the profit. This is what we erroneously call economics, or the economy, and it is our current economy, dominated by money, which is causing so much disequilibrium. This might appear obvious, but the real meaning of the word 'economy', is a word derived from the Greek, for 'good household-management': *oikonomia*. Today, it cannot be denied, our household-management has been severely compromised. This also applies to the sayings, *keeping your house in order* and *shipshape*, phrases that apply to all day-to-day-dealings from the individual to the societal. Money commands all notions of economics today, having completely replaced this household-management. Thankfully the present economic model does not give the impression that it will last much longer. A return to *oikonomia* is long overdue.

The economy of the food industry has stretched profits considerably from any given raw material, be that a coconut, corn, milk or wheat. With corn for instance, it is quite staggering how far its uses have been stretched, making money from every conceivable industry. When once it was used to exclusively make foods direct from the flour, eating the corn from the cob or pressed for fresh oil, now it finds its way into the manufacture of plastics, bio-fuel, sweeteners, toothpastes, animal feeds, human foods and much more. When corn is processed for bio-fuel, the waste gets a good price, sold on to be further processed to make high fructose corn syrup (HFCS), often labelled as glucose-fructose. Corn's versatility just within the food industry is quite astonishing, with all the following being derived from corn: Ascorbic acid (which many assume is the technical biological name for vitamin C, it isn't), amino acids, calcium lactate, calcium stearoyl, citric acid (this is also not vitamin C), dextrose, ethyl maltol, fructose (not just HFCS), lactic acid, hydrolyzed vegetable protein, maltodextrin, maltol, mannitol, polydextrose, polysorbates, potassium glucomate, propylene glycol monostearate, tocopherol and xanthan gum and hundreds if not thousands more. These are ingredients that have been arrived at after considerable toxic chemical extraction, as well as being heated to immense temperatures with all sorts of other adulterations taking place. The food industry is not doing you a favour with all this processing, all it is doing is squeezing as much profit as it possibly can out of everything natural. The fact that this often results in ingredients with only negative effects is immaterial, they are legal and they have made some money, so job done, in our skewed definition of an economic world.

Food Is Your Medicine

Everyone knows food is important, that we are what we eat and as Hippocrates said 'food is your medicine'. Hippocrates is the Father of modern medicine, with all doctors once taking a Hippocratic Oath when they qualified, (two versions are in the appendices, although less in Britain and Europe now take it). Hippocrates himself lived to the ripe age of 83, living from 460BC to 377BC, although it seems that not many people, and worryingly not many doctors, actually understand what this truly means. It's as if the truth about the healthiness of food has been deliberately covered up, if not deep-fried, sugar coated and dyed blue!

This covering-up of the truth about food has of course been done deliberately, paid for by the producers of processed foods and the pharmaceutical corporations, with the help of the sinisterly subtle advertising and marketing agencies, lawyers and lobbyists, who all continuously tell us their version of the truth, which very conveniently also sells them the most units. The industries of food processing, pharmaceuticals and advertising were relatively new with little power or prestige in the 1950s; since then, their power has grown, and hand-in-hand, they have managed to create and maintain a large proportion of the global market share for their new, brightly-packaged-heavy-in-slogans-no-nutrient-processed-foods and the no-curative-make-me-sicker-processed-pills.

This alliance of business with advertisers made it possible to swerve the inconvenient scientific truth and create a new illusory truth about food. All scientific reports from the 1930s to 1980s painted a very negative picture with regards to consumption of processed foods, especially if this consumption became perpetual and not occasional. Sadly, the independent scientists were in no position to spend vast sums of money in advertising their findings and research, guaranteeing every citizen knew of the consequences of consumption of these processed foods. The scientists were also in no position to lobby governments to create legislation, guaranteeing that such foods can never be readily available. The government should have listened and acted upon these scientific results before processed foods became the staple of the diet and economy.

The negative findings of the scientific research about processed food consumption was published in many scientific journals, with a few newspapers running articles, indicating that these new processed foods should be avoided. To counter these reports, the food industry spent vast sums of money, repeatedly, again and again, making it inevitable their message was the one that sank into the consciousness of the public. The government only heard the cash registers ringing from all this new processed food being sold. Whilst the marketing gurus easily managed to make this processed, 'convenient' food, appear the perfect embodiment of what food should be in the modern world. The food producers and advertisers, increasingly armed with psychological bullets, have managed to distort our perception of the food we are eating. Often to such an extent that we believe our diets to be healthy and the best for us, even when the opposite is true. The repetitious advertising and the endless 2-for-1 offers of multi-bags of crisps, sweets, biscuits, fizzy sweetened coloured water, sugared cereals and ice-creams, has firmly entrenched the consumer in a rut of malnutrition. Why is the whole-wheat pasta or tofu never on a BOGOF promotion?

A dietary paradox

The daily poisoning from erroneous diets not only feeds degenerative diseases, in many instances the diet will have been the causative agent of the disease. The health industry, which benefits hugely from a never-ending and increasing amount of sick customers, for some reason forgot to mention that it was the food that was to blame, until it was too late. Today, we are just surviving on the food being eaten, as well as living in what appears to be a dietary paradox, where more food is being consumed than ever before, with accompanying increases in overweight and obese people, whilst at the same time, many of these very people are suffering from malnutrition. The paradox only arises as we assume the word, malnutrition, means a *lack* of food, when in fact it means, *bad* nutrition.

This book will attempt to separate the truth from the marketing speak, as well as prising the real science away from the industrially financed pseudo-science. The result of industrially financed research has been to deliberately cause confusion amongst the general public, whether about health, pharmaceuticals, chemicals, food or so much more. I just hope that I manage to get this very important point of view across (it could be viewed as a theory) in a memorable and clear way. Much of what I have read whilst researching this book has been written in such a dry and formulaic manner, it made the digestion of the information comparable to being force-fed sandpaper. My aim had to be to present this theory as if it were a delicious, sweet, juicy mango, oozing with facts, just craving to be lapped up.

With an answer to the question of why we are getting the diseases of civilization and how they can be best avoided, this book (and the planned series of four books) could be a critical link in the marriage of modern science and complimentary, or alternative therapies. Attempting to reconnect mankind with nature, or as Jean-Jacques Rousseau stated as long ago as 1754: "The greater part of our ills are of our own making, and we might have avoided them, nearly all, by adhering to that simple manner of life that nature prescribed."

Recently, my 11 year-old son asked me what my least loved animal is. I answered the mosquito, because of the more than million deaths malaria causes every year and the billions since the caveman, 30,000 or so years ago. He was very surprised, as he thought I'd answer 'mankind', for all the destruction and extinctions we have caused. Clever kid.

Next he asked what my least loved plant is. After a little hesitation, I answered that it was the sugarcane, as it is sugar that is a major risk factor for so many of the diseases of civilization, as well as being responsible for the majority of the slave trade, where well over 60% of African slaves who survived the horrendous transportation, went to work in the sugar plantations of the New World. These sugar plantations also caused massive upheavals and exterminations of many indigenous peoples in South and Central America, as well as financing the Industrial Revolution. He had no comeback to this as an answer.

So let's begin with sugar.

The First Deadly White

Sugar

"I love to eat Kit Kats or cookies-and-cream ice cream. I need sugar like five times a day"
(Kim Kardashian)

The initial intention was to come out with all guns blazing, proclaiming sugar as the scourge of the human race, saturating your head with an endless stream of statistics, facts, diseases and problems, all caused by sugar. Such a start would have put sugar firmly where it deserves to be, being a toxic, omnipresent ingredient in the food chain. However, such an approach would have distorted the reality, as sugar is not alone in the devolution of our species, a devolution that involves all of the deadly whites found within this book. With no need to rush into the negativity, let's begin at a slower pace, with a little history and information about sugar.

Was Buddha a misogynist?

The etymology (that's the study of the origins of words) of sugar derives from the Arabic, *sukkar*, which in turn finds its root in the Sanskrit, *shakkara*, referring to a 'granular material'. The granulated sugar we are familiar with today was probably first processed in India around 1,500 years ago, although the original homeland of the sugar cane is almost certainly Papua New Guinea, many millennia before this.

One of the earliest written references to sugar, or at least the cane, comes from the words of the Buddha, Siddhartha Guatama, who likened women's involvement in religion to that of a fungal infection that affects sugar canes, known as red-rot. This indicates that at the time of the Buddha, around 550BC, sugar canes must have been growing fairly extensively in India, whether it indicates that Mr Guatama was a misogynist is another matter. Admiral Nearchus, sailing under Alexander the Great in 325BC, described 'Indian canes, dripping in honey', which surely has to be referring to sugar cane. It was from India that the granulated crystal form was first processed by at least 500AD, if not considerably earlier. This technique had been passed onto the Persians and the Chinese some time soon after, having spread west to all Arabic lands by 800AD, where the first factories and refineries were established. It was first introduced to Europe by either the crusaders in the eleventh or twelfth centuries, or the Arabs and Berbers from the Iberian Peninsula, sometime in the tenth or eleventh centuries.

Atlantic Europe's Slave Age

The Portuguese were the first Europeans to establish sugar exportation from their plantations in Madeira by about 1450, with refineries soon being established in Antwerp, Bologna and Venice as well. The Portuguese were also the first to use slaves for sugar production, when they settled Sao Tome in 1486 (an island off the coast of present day Equatorial Guinea and Gabon), initially using expelled Spanish Jews, switching to African slaves soon after. By 1500, Madeira had about 80 sugar mills and was exporting 1,700 tons of sugar to Venice, England and elsewhere. It was proving to be a very lucrative trade, although the main hurdles to expansion were that large quantities of land and water were required to grow the canes, as well as being extremely labour intensive. It is here that the real legacy left by Columbus comes into play, as it was no coincidence that on his second voyage in 1493, he took with him sugar cane from the Canaries to Hispaniola (the island split between Haiti and the Dominican Republic today). This single import was to change the course of history, facilitating European global economic dominance. From this time on, sugar cane spread throughout the West Indies like wildfire and with it the awful slave trade, transporting Africans to the West Indies.

Sugar became far more readily available with the colonial expansion of the seafaring European nations, where the British yearly sugar consumption in 1700 was no more than 2kg per person, almost exclusively at this time due to its price, consumed by the rich until well into the nineteenth century. The slave trade saw supply vastly increased, with an estimated 13 of the 20 million African slaves who survived the horrendous crossing to America put to work in the new sugar plantations, all in order to feed the spreading addiction amongst the upper classes in Europe for this sugar-rush.

Many writers and social commentators of the day expressed grief at the blood and misery that the sugar industry had brought, to both the African slaves and the Central and South American populations, who were exterminated to make room for the sugar plantations and the slaves. The local populations had already been decimated by as much as 95%, after the initial European contact, spreading smallpox, diphtheria, influenza and other contagious diseases amongst the Native Americans, who unfortunately had a total lack of any form of immunity to these diseases, whilst the Europeans had built up an immunity over the preceding several thousand years; as these are zoonotic diseases, brought about by humans close proximity to cattle and avian species during our domestication of such animals. Yellow Fever further escalated this death-count with the introduction of the Africans to the continent, a disease that also wiped out many Europeans. The sugar also went towards the production of a considerable quantity of rum, which was traded with the Indians for fur, further adding to the general subjugation and overthrow of the Native Americans. The karmic payback for all this slavery and sugar, if you tread such boards of spirituality, is the rise of the diseases of civilization. Karma or not, there are some very real physical ailments that this sugar has been responsible for, or significantly contributed towards, as seen in a few pages.

More mention needs to be made of the fact that it was slavery and sugar that financed the whole Industrial Revolution, alas this book is not the place to discuss this. A brief mention will suffice for now to merely arouse the appetite of curiosity (and anti-establishmentarianism). The monies directly made from sugar and the subsequent reparations paid to slave owners when slavery was abolished significantly helped to finance and expand the various industries that had been invented since the 1740s, as well as paying for the construction of many stately homes. The industrialisation of the sugar industry and its associated technology was for some time the most significant leap in machinery use, until the Luddites turned against the mechanized looms in the 1810s. Britain may well have led the way in inventions that enabled the Industrial Revolution to finally flourish from the 1820s, but it only became seriously viable and profitable once the saying "its takes money to make money" became a reality. Without slavery or sugar, this financial clout would not have been accessible to Britain, and Britain would not have been in the position it found itself in, where it undeniably was at the forefront of this new machine age and the economic possibilities this created. Without sugar and slavery the Industrial Revolution would have been very different and not centred in Britain.

The emergence of European sugar beet enormously added to the steady growth in the supply of sugar cane from the colonies. Helped in no small way by Napoleon, as the French had lost out in the control of sugar from the West Indies, the expansion of European sugar beet secured a steady supply for them. The first beet-processing factories were established in Eastern Europe at the very beginning of the nineteenth century. The resultant competition between cane and beet sugar began a price war which saw the price drop considerably, becoming even cheaper after the abolition of the sugar taxes in 1874. By 1915, the average annual consumption in Britain had risen to about 8 to 10kg per person, with its consumption no longer the preserve of the wealthiest. Today, the average sugar consumption is over 50kg, with many people eating more than their own body weight in refined sugar each and every year, making consumption of 130kg to 200kg per year increasingly common.

Widespread sugar use, addiction and increasing health problems

Many physicians from the end of the seventeenth century observed the detrimental health affects caused by the rise in the popularity of sugar, coining the phrase 'sugar-blues', which manifested itself in any number of symptoms, from nervousness, depression, insomnia and mental instability. In most instances, it was intolerance to such large inputs of refined sugar, causing havoc with digestion, hormones and mind. This was the first time that sugar had been introduced into the general population's diet and it was clear to see, to those observers at the time, that the before-and-after effects of refined sugar becoming readily available were extremely varied, albeit predominately negative and certainly most worrying. The spread of early sugar addiction was on a comparable level to observing a whole city today getting addicted to crystal-meth or crack cocaine. The effects of sugar were truly monumental. Incredibly, there is very little mention or thought given to this today, hardly even warranting a historic footnote, although the reasoning for this exclusion is answered below. A deadly poison in sheep's clothing had surreptitiously joined the flock.

It was because of this surge in refined sugar consumption that the establishment of a number of 'mental institutions' was made necessary to take care of those who had been too damaged by this initial flow and public consumption of sugar at the end of the eighteenth and beginning of (and throughout) the nineteenth century. Just as with any other drug, for the first few hits the negative effects had an enormous range of symptoms, then after a month of consumption it became tolerated for the majority, as addiction settled in. For the minority, this addiction was the catalyst to many further psychological problems, hence the requirement of the institutions. (Although I'm not implicating sugar as being the only factor involved in mental disorders, it certainly made the situation far worse). When it was a minority of the rich going off their rockers from sugar, they could afford to live with it, as well as them being able to afford a more varied diet; when it affected the minority of the general public, this numbered easily into the tens of thousands, if not much more, it became much more of a problem.

Hardly anyone calls it an addiction, but an addiction it is for the vast majority. Just try to cut out all sugar from your diet for a day, and see if you have any cravings for this sugar drug-rush. That is an addiction, both physical and mental. And so it has continued for over two centuries, only now we have sweeteners ten thousand times sweeter than nature has. We have unwittingly assimilated sugar addiction into our culture, weaning children onto it from as young as six to twelve months old, if not before. However, as with any addiction, there is always going to be quite a few contra-indications and these are the very diseases of civilization that title this series of books.

Sugar has absolutely no health benefits or nutritional content whatsoever. It is actually a poison. If you only had refined sugar and water to survive on, you would die much quicker if you consumed both the sugar and the water, as opposed to just the water. A fact that was noticed as long ago as 1793, when five shipwreck survivors, who only had sugar and rum for sustenance, had in only the nine days till they were rescued, become thoroughly ravaged. It was clear to see, they were in a much worse condition than if just water had been consumed for those nine days. Tests were subsequently carried out on dogs and rats, all of which died in a surprisingly short time when fed just sugar. Unsurprisingly, this alerted the sugar industry to beware of any future scientific meddling in their affairs. Since then, numerous animal experiments, scientific medical evidence as well as anthropological and ethnological comparative analysis, all overwhelmingly show sugar plays a detrimental role on the human organism. There is nothing positive to read about sugar from any independent sources. This is the reason why the detrimental sociological affects of the introduction of sugar don't even warrant a historical footnote, because the sugar industry has incessantly undermined the truth with their propaganda, editing and tippexing out the inconvenient truth about their industry, writing in their own version of the truth, exactly as with the case of the Nutrition Society below.

Industrial manipulation

In 1939, dental researcher Dr Weston Price published his 'Nutrition and Physical Degeneration: A Comparison of Primitive and Modern Diets and their Effects'. He travelled around the world to make his observations and took over 15,000 photographs to further substantiate his claims. The results of his research must have come as a bit of a shock to the establishment, as it clearly identified that the general health and wellbeing of some of the most primitive cultures far exceeded that of Europe and America. Indeed, his stunning photographs all show what can only be described as perfect specimens of the human race. Dr Price further noted that when the healthy 'primitives' became acculturated (changed from their traditional culture to a 'civilized' culture), the physical degeneration was very evident after only a few years. He recorded that the tooth decay rates of those living by eating only wild foods was as low as 0.1% of the population. Amongst some Canadian Inuit who were predominately hunters at this time, the rate was 0.16%, when only a few miles away, the white settlers enjoyed a rate of 25.5%. This makes tooth decay 160 times more prevalent amongst the eaters of a western diet, compared to those eating a wild diet. If our teeth and diet had improved since 1939, this comparison would be irrelevant, however, our teeth have not got better and our diets have deteriorated, along with our health, as clearly signified by the emergence of the diseases of civilization. Needless to say, Price's meticulous and amazing work found many adversaries in the food industry. His impressive and studious book was superseded amongst much fanfare in 1957 by Prof McCollum's 'A History of Nutrition'. The media buzz surrounding this book stated McCollum was apparently one of America's greatest nutritionists, drawing from over 200,000 published scientific papers to substantiate and corroborate his work. Within this vast tome, there is not one single mention of any possible deleterious effect that sugar may play upon the human, or even rat for that matter. There certainly had been loads of experiments with rats before 1957, all clearly showing sugar's negative health impacts, although apparently none in the 200,000 McCollum used, which is extremely unlikely, if not impossible. This 'History of Nutrition' was a standard reference book in libraries for decades, with the book only being made possible by the generosity of The Nutrition Society, whom the author and publishers thanked accordingly. This all appears perfectly in order, as an informative book about nutrition should, after all, be helped along its way into the public consciousness by an organization with such a name as The Nutrition Society.

Until that is, one realises that The Nutrition Society was a ruse, used and paid for by Coca-Cola, Pepsi-Cola, Nestle, General Mills and a few other conscious and caring companies, keen and eager to get their point of view across. It seems logical to suggest that the first draft of McCollum's book would have mentioned the dangers of sugar, only to be removed at the insistence of The Nutrition Society before allowing publication to take place. A manoeuvre that is standard practice for all sectors of industry, hence why McDonalds, Coca-Cola et al. are always involved with nutritional agencies, institutions and conferences, in the same light that petroleum corporations head environmental and climate change agencies. It's not because they genuinely care about the considerable negative impacts of their industries, it's just their lofty academic persona allows for better control and censure of the information that gets filtered down to the public about their nefarious, clandestine, money-making activities.

What is sugar?

When we think of sugar, the mind's eye conjures up a picture of a bowl or packet of white refined sugar, or even a cube, although who uses these today? This is not the only sugar, nor is it the only meaning of the word 'sugar'. Somewhat confusingly, the word sugar now refers to this refined sugar in the same breath as blood sugar, artificial and natural sweeteners and foods that sugar, when in reality all these are totally different, though all share a negative outcome if left unchecked. This chapter is more concerned with the sugar used in the food industry, as it is this variety that constitutes the majority of the sugar consumed by the general population. Although sugar, which would have until only the past couple of decades been virtually exclusively white refined cane or beet sugar, the term today applies to a whole plethora of sweeteners, with refined cane and beet sugar still having the largest market share. This lead has been eaten away with the recent rise of highly refined vegetable fructose extract, mostly from corn, known as high fructose corn syrup (HFCS) and the artificial sweeteners, notably aspartame, sucralose and acesulfame K, all of which will get a mention throughout this chapter, although the focus will remain on the popular view of sugar being the white refined, granulated version.

The sugar used in the food industry and that found in your cupboard will be of this refined white variety. Unless it states it is unrefined, such as Muscovado; even if brown, it will have begun as refined white, with a little molasses (raw, sweet, sticky syrup produced from sugar refining) added to make it brown; a 3%

molasses content goes into light brown sugar and up to 15% in dark brown sugar. This molasses content does give the sugar some nutrition, but overall it is only marginally less detrimental than refined white sugar, especially when excessively consumed. It all requires insulin to convert it to glucose and then it is utilised as either expended energy via exercise, or more commonly these days, deposited as fat around the body. Processed white sugar is most definitely not to be considered as an item of food, it is an unnecessary, detrimental and a highly addictive additive.

Refined sugar is initially produced by shredding and pressing all the juice out of either sugar cane or sugar beet, then this pressed juice is boiled, with chemical solvents added to remove any impurities, which also pretty much kills off any remaining nutritious content (for impurities read nutrients, which have the inconvenience to 'go off'). It is then boiled again, bleached with other chemicals and filtered through bone char, a powder made from cow and pig bones, then centrifuged to form crystals. If a brown sugar is required, molasses are added and it is re-spun. After all this, the product bears absolutely no resemblance to its natural form as a cane or beet. Annoyingly, considering the millions of tons used, the unprocessed sugar cane is very hard to find and much more expensive than the same weight of heavily processed white sugar.

The human body has to bio-assimilate every microgram of sugar ingested, because something has to be done with it, as it can't be left to flow around the blood. It isn't just eaten and then excreted if not needed, as none of it is 'needed' for any normal, healthy biological processes. The human body has had no time to adapt to this constant, excessive, unnecessary addition to the diet. The rise in consumption over the past two centuries of refined sugar has been so rapid, sufficient time has not elapsed for the biological mechanisms of the human body to adapt, let alone adjust to the massive surge in HFCS which has compounded the problem in the past few years. All the body can do is deal with the sugar in the same way that it would have dealt with any excessive sugar, carbohydrate or fat consumption in the past. This was achieved by converting the excessive energy into adipose tissue (fat) for future use, a method that had proven to be extremely effective, allowing ingested food, in times of surplus, to not only provide for immediate sustenance, but also as an internal larder for later use. This is a perfect survival backup for the times when food cannot be found by either hunting or foraging, particularly essential in areas with extremes of weather, such as desert or polar regions, as well as being especially important for women in the weeks before and after childbirth. Obviously not such a useful survival strategy today, with 24hr supermarkets, fast food and grocery stores on every corner.

The evolutionary or genetic changes required to bio-assimilate sugar have not only lacked the time to deal with this perpetual and global epidemic of vast dietary excesses of sugar, the human biological system has been completely obliterated by the sudden rise of all the seven deadly whites together. The body is having serious difficulties in dealing with these excesses in the same old ways, especially when it is confronted every day with these unrestrained harmful dietary inputs. Insulin tries its hardest to keep up with the constantly elevated blood sugar levels, always working overtime, but it often lags behind, leaving sugar coursing around the blood until it can be dealt with. Whilst in the blood, this sugar creates an acidic bodily environment that has to be neutralized as quickly as possible if it is to avoid inflammation and other aggravating ailments, with heartburn or acid reflux being the least of these. To alkalinize itself the body removes calcium from the bones and teeth, as well as other minerals, a direct way that sugar consumption is a risk-factor in the development of osteoporosis and dental cavities.

Sugared water and who's in control

To make matters worse, many meals are accompanied by a sugar solution of squash, juice, alcohol or even milkshake. This fluid, instead of helping to dilute the excess sugars from the food, exasperates the problem, as this liquid also needs to be neutralised, metabolised and eliminated. Whilst all this is going on, the body still has to perform its constant duties of cellular maintenance and production, duties already being seriously hampered by the diet not providing the required nutrients in either quantity or balance. This dietary deficiency is further compounded by the daily exposure to a multitude of pollutants, most of which are carcinogenic, mutagenic (changing DNA and chromosomes) and endocrine (hormone system) disrupting, all of which also have to be dealt with, whilst all the harmful fat-soluble pollutants find their way to the ever-expanding deposits of human fat tissue.

It is the ignorant consumption of litres of heavily sugared water, especially those sweetened with HFCS (or any fructose) and the artificial sweeteners, that are at the centre of the present obesity and diabetes crisis. It recently shook me to the core that a government recommendation for the removal of sugar from soft drinks was to be replaced with low calorie sweeteners (as it is currently calories that are incorrectly being solely blamed for obesity), such as aspartame, sucralose and the new stevioside. This switch will allow the drink manufacturers to label their product as 'new', 'healthier' and 'diet', although in reality it will heighten the problem that the human system is currently experiencing with the consumption of these sweeteners; it will be nothing short of catastrophic to replace sugars with sweeteners, as will be shown later in this chapter. It cannot be the consumers fault when the food producers and government agencies have little idea of what they are trying to do, aimlessly implementing such dangerous measures, no doubt done so under the guidance of the producers of the artificial sweeteners themselves.

The word 'government', provides an interesting etymological aside, as *govern,* means to control, regulate, by force if necessary, derived from the Greek root, 'to steer'; *ment* – as in mental, the mind, whose root is the word 'man'. Therefore, the actual meaning of the word government is 'to steer man' and indeed the aim of any government has always been to control your mind. Nothing's been concealed, it's just that no one seems to be looking in the right places, especially as it's been hidden in plain view. Or as Paul Valery said, "Politics is the art of preventing people from taking part in affairs which properly concern them". As much as I'd love to have a rant about unnecessary politicians, big business and the need for a more egalitarian society, this is not the place, beyond this interval.

A Little bit of pseudoscience

The sugar industry has been feeding us their version of the truth about their product for over 220 years now, ever since the shipwreck survivor story of 1793 got negative international news coverage. Anything that is supposedly understood about sugar being energy, or how sugar is a vital source of this energy, has come from the sugar producers themselves, and what began as marketing and propaganda has now become embedded as 'cultural knowledge'. There have been many decades worth of misinformation from the food industry, some of which has seeped into health and medical literature. For instance, the supposed fact that carbohydrates provide all the energy for the human organism. The actual biological way energy is obtained in nature has little to do with carbohydrates, this is just the myth spread by the sugar industry. This definition of an energy source was lifted from the biological sciences, creating a marketing buzzword for the sugar-pushers around the use of the words 'energy' and 'carbohydrate', thus bedding sugar firmly into our consciousness as being an essential part of our diets, as well as being particularly beneficial during exercise. In reality, a carbohydrate is merely any substance that contains carbon, oxygen and hydrogen, which accounts for most things. The body can obtain energy far more effectively and efficiently from a host of other substances, such as fruit, proteins or stored fats. As the refined sugars exclusively have these three elements (carbon, oxygen and hydrogen) in varying proportions there is the proclamation of their 'pureness', and with sugar being pure carbohydrate, in the distorted medical view of the food industry, this must equal pure energy. With the emphasis on 'pure' conjuring up an angelic image, when all it has ever been is pure bullshit.

It would be a fruitless search to try to find any scientific evidence that proves that sugar consumption is translated as energy when the body assimilates it. It might be pure carbohydrate and act a certain way in a test-tube under laboratory conditions but when it's eaten, as a cake or cereals, this sucrose may well be turned into glucose but the net biological effect will not be a potential for greater exercise. There is a very brief sugar high, as the insulin spikes and glucose is produced, although this is followed by a much longer low, when the body feels the effect of having been nutritionally depleted.

A classic example is comparing children at a birthday party: in those fed high sugar content food the activity levels are lower (apart from those behaving weird from the colourings and sweeteners) than in those where the main food was wholesome and savoury. Discounting the children's general excitement at being at a party, double-blind tests have proved the above apparent contradiction to our erroneous cultural assumption of sugar producing energy. Real energy that can be translated into physical energy would be far better sourced from a starch or nuts, it is once again only the sugar-pushers incessantly informing us about sugar equalling energy that has altered our perception of reality. A recent ad for Ferrero's Kinder eggs claimed it 'helps you grow', failing to add '...fatter and unhealthier', in much the same way that a Mars Bar "Helps you work, rest and play". According to who? By Mars of course, definitely not by independent doctors, nutritionists or scientists. Adverts from the 1950s in America clearly stated that scientific evidence had proven that sugar was in fact non-fattening, that it could be used as a dieting aid because it was so pure it was utilized immediately (just like the cigarette adverts from the 1930s and 1940s claiming smoking was an essential digestion aid). 'Facts' we might laugh at now, without realising we are still being brainwashed by the advertisers.

Raw cane sugar, Sir Banting and Semantics

The basic ingredient of sugar, raw sugar cane, rather ironically has beneficial dietary attributes. It has excellent quantities of chromium, a superb mineral used to prevent, of all things, the craving for sugar, a natural inbuilt protection for the plant so it doesn't get overeaten. This chromium is nearly all lost by the time sugar has been refined, processed and used as an ingredient in the food industry. Sugar cane also contains calcium (which alkalinizes the system, whereas processed sugar only acidifies) and vitamins A, B1, B2 and B3, with some magnesium and iron thrown in as well. The chewing of the cane has no effect on the prevalence of teeth cavities, as it is actually alkalinizing, whilst the chewing of the woody pulp cleans the teeth and gums better than a nylon brush ever can. It is the acidity of refined sugars that depletes the teeth of calcium, making them weaker, as calcium is robbed from the teeth and bones to dilute the acidity caused by the sugar (and all the other deadly whites, which as we will see, all behave in a similar, negative way, by also increasing acidity, blood sugar levels and promoting inflammation).

It was through questioning the difference in consumption of raw cane sugar and refined sugar that led Sir Frederick Banting to become the co-discoverer of insulin with Charles Best, (both being awarded the 1923 Nobel Prize in Medicine for their endeavours). The initial observation was that plantation workers cutting the sugar cane also consumed a large amount of it, although only very rarely, if ever, suffered from diabetes or teeth cavities, whereas, those working in the refineries, consuming refined sugar, suffered quite commonly from diabetes and cavities. In actual fact, the work he and Best conducted was far more scientific than simply observational comparison, involving isolating and removing the pancreas of dogs and noticing this induced diabetes. Correctly deducing there was something specific within the pancreas that was the key to curing, or at least controlling diabetes, as indeed it is, as the islets of Langerhans are the production centre for insulin which are located in the pancreas. Insulin is instrumental in converting the sucrose and fructose of refined sugar into glucose, providing energy for the cells and muscles, and as already mentioned, it is only very recently that the energy requirement derived from food has come from predominately highly refined carbohydrates, requiring insulin to convert this erroneous food to energy.

It has long been known (although kept rather quiet) that the removal of sugar from the diet is a likely prevention and cure for cancer, diabetes and heart disease, depending on how well advanced the diseases are. So, working backwards, would it be true to say that sugar was the cause of the ailments in the first place? Well, certainly not if the sugar industry was to get its way, having been left to its own devices, regulations and pseudoscientific analysis and disinformation, almost unquestioned since the 1950s (if not since 1793). The impression given by the sugar manufacturing companies is that sugar is part of a healthy balanced diet. It isn't. What they fail to mention is that a healthy balance is only achieved by all the other foods eaten that *don't* contain sugar, therefore balancing out the sugar. What their statement actually provides is a legal loophole warning the consumer that their product could kill you if other foods of a recognised healthy nature are not eaten with it. This shows how much pressure is exerted by food producers, (via lobbyists and lawyers), with such a weak disclaimer persisting. Today this phrase 'as part of a healthy balanced diet' is not even seen as a warning, often the exact opposite impression is formulated.

Staying with semantics, check out this play-on-words, which can only have been conjured up to cause consumer confusion. If a product states on the packaging that it is 'Sugar Free', this could still mean it contains plenty of HFCS, just no refined white sugar, and almost certainly any number of sweeteners. If the packaging states there is 'No Added Sugar', this almost guarantees that it does actually contain sugar, all the claim of no added sugar means is that the end producer added no extra sugar, although earlier in the production chain any amount of sugar could have been added to the ingredients used by the end-producer (this is actually illegal according to Trading Standards but it doesn't stop most of the food corporations making false claims on their packaging). It also probably has sugar, although the use of the sugar alcohols, such as erythritol and xylitol, which are clearly sweet and a sugar of sort, although for labelling purposes, not sugar at all. How bewildering is that? This is also the case when the packaging claims there is no added preservatives or colourings. Now you know.

What's sugar been implicated in?

There is no question that white refined sugar has played a major role in the demise of our diets since the 1950s, leading to far more worries than just tooth decay or calories. It strips the nutrients within the body, acidifies the blood, causes inflammation and is a significant contributor to the downward spiral of the general public's health. The list of ruinous ailments and ill-effects that sugar has been shown to significantly increase the risk of being afflicted by is an ever-growing list, including amongst many others: cancers. All that needs to be said here is that the cancer cells' favourite food is sugar (glucose). Excessive sugar consumption is already seen as a major risk factor with cancers of the throat, breast, ovaries, prostrate and intestines, if not most cancers. Cancer has a definite correlation with sugar consumption, demonstrated by Otto Warburg as long ago as the late 1920s, for which he was awarded the Nobel Prize in 1930, showing that glucose was the preferred food of cancer cells, where his Petri-dish cancer cells perished when denied glucose. This is why glucose dyes are drunk or injected to detect cancer, as the dyed glucose appears to disappear on scans when it comes into contact with cancer, having been eaten by the cancer cells. Surely this demonstrates that the medical profession is well aware of this association of glucose and cancer, as this technique has been used for decades and is becoming more advanced, although always using glucose. In the same way that tooth cavities are deliberately caused in experimental animals by making them eat sticky sweets, it is crazy to refute the suggestion that sugar causes caries, just as it's nonsense to state there is no association between sugar and cancer. Cancer also favours an acidic environment (created by all the dietary deadly whites) and it is probably triggered by other mechanisms other than sugar, be they growth factors in dairy to the multifarious carcinogens in intimate and continual personal contact with us, from plastics to paints, clothing to air and even foods and additives. Sugar has not as of yet been officially recognised as a carcinogen, so until that time, I will contend that it merely feeds cancer cells (which is surely bad enough). Although it must be added, cancers in females have been linked to oestrogen and bowel cancers with insulin, two hormones definitely affected by sugar consumption, and we'll see throughout this book how disruptive to overall health the altering of one hormone can be, let alone multiple.

Atherosclerosis is a reduction in tissue elasticity, an increase in the stickiness of the blood platelets and an accumulation of plaque-like deposits on the arteries. Atherosclerosis significantly increases the risk-factor of suffering from high blood pressure, heart attack, other cardiovascular diseases and stroke. The nutritional assumption that it is fat consumption which directly leads to cholesterol and heart disease is no more than an incorrect dogma, first postulated by Ancel Keys in the 1950s, perpetuated ever since, even as more and more evidence disproves this or at least exonerates certain fats, (fully covered in the Fats/Oils chapter). At the same time as Keys' dodgy 'scientific' observations, there was evidence emerging from Professor Yudkin that it was in fact sugar that was the main culprit. We will return to Professor Yudkin throughout the next few pages, as he was one of the most diligent researchers attempting to expose sugar as a deadly white, for which he encountered many efforts to discount his findings. Yudkin's experiments with animals showed repeatedly that excessive sugar consumption was a greater risk-factor for cholesterol, triglyceride and atheroma deposits (the name of the plaque deposits that form and even define the condition, atherosclerosis) than either fats or other carbohydrates (from say potatoes or flour). Human subjects have also been used and these also showed raised triglyceride and cholesterol levels as well as weight increase from eating a sugar rich diet. These results were immediately refuted by the sugar industry as irrelevant because the level of sugar consumption was not realistic, when in fact the yearly average of 50kg a year is only that, an average and in fact many people consume 200kg and more every year and these levels far exceed the doses given by Yudkin and his contemporaries such as Professor MacDonald also from England, Dr Reiser from the USA, Prof Cohen from Israel and others.

The immune and nervous systems are also knocked for six with too much white sugar constantly in the system, with links to both bronchitis and sinus infections. Research has repeatedly shown that sugar consumption directly affects the ability of white blood cells to deal with bacteria in direct proportion to the amount consumed. Most colds and coughs and more serious diseases can gain access to the human organism when it is already compromised by the white blood cells trying to rid themselves of the excessive sugar. The correlation between excessive sugar consumption and illness is startling and disturbingly unregistered by the general population (I noticed a very similar coincidental illness of the respiratory system affecting many children where I live immediately after pesticides – intended to knock out the respiratory system of insects – are sprayed on the fields surrounding us, a coincidence that worryingly only became blatantly obvious when I pointed out the timings of the children's illnesses and the sprayings).

Sugar is also a direct irritant to the digestive system as it has high osmotic pressure, insomuch as it sucks water from membranes and tissues it comes into contact with in the digestive system, drawing the water away from the mucous membrane for instance, leaving it red, raw and inflamed, a condition that is made worse by this sugar intake being repetitive, as well as the other deadly whites compounding the problem (especially refined salt, which is even more osmotic). This constant irritation and cellular damage is a definite avenue that allows such conditions as irritable bowel syndrome or cancer to get an initial foothold.

Gastric and duodenal ulcers (also known as peptic ulcers) most likely find their root cause in sugar consumption, complying with the irritant example above. As these peptic ulcers are fairly common (as one would expect if sugar was at the heart of the aetiology) the pharmaceutical industry has conveniently come up with a whole range of drugs to help alleviate suffering. Of course, the simple advice of cutting out sugar from the diet would be a step too far for the doctors, who fail to uphold the advice of Hippocrates entirely, who clearly stated 'food is your medicine'. Instead of dealing with the root problem and actualizing a cure, by cutting refined sugar from our diets pharmaceutical giants offer us balms to ease our symptoms, such as Aluminium Hydroxide and Magnesium Hydroxide, Domperidone, Famotidine, Glycopyrrolate, Lafutidine, Menpenzolate, Misoprostol, Omeprazole, Oxyphenonium, Pantoprazole, Pirenzepine, Propantheline and Ranitidine, (all sold under numerous trade names, being either antacids, antimuscarinic agents, proton-pump inhibitors, prostaglandins or histamines). Clearly a winner for the pharmaceutical corporations, who definitely don't want the answer of cutting out sugar to be well known as this would reduce their client base considerably. The side-effects from the above peptic ulcer drugs would also be avoided, effects ranging from diarrhoea, constipation, dizziness, stomach aches, headaches, sore tongue, arrhythmia, vomiting, liver problems and many more, which if left untreated will lead to other diseases, often more serious than the initial ulcer.

Gallstones often display symptoms as indigestion and are usually present in people who are also suffering a couple of the following: diabetes, obesity, hiatus hernia or elevated blood levels of triglyceride and insulin. Research from New Zealand on patients with gallstones indicated they occurred far more readily in those who consumed the most sugar, which is no surprise as it is probably sugar causing the ailments in the first place. Italian and English research showed there was an association between those who consumed more sugar, and a greater propensity to become a Crohn's Disease patient (there is still no causal factor accepted for Crohn's Disease, although sugar and white flour are the prime candidates).

Damage to the teeth, perhaps the most accepted problem associated with sugar consumption, displayed as caries, where sticky acidic residue forms plaque that damage the teeth. The sugar industry vehemently denies any association and blames bacteria found within plaque, *Streptococcus mutans*, as being responsible. This *Streptococcus mutans* does indeed attack the dentine, producing caries and flourishes on a specific carbohydrate within the plaque, dextran, which is far more readily built up in the presence of sucrose, proving the sugar industry's denials to be ridiculous. Tooth decay is only seen as being wholly determined by the residue on the surface of the teeth because of all the toothpaste and toothbrush adverts, confusing our perception of reality. The acidification of the bodily system caused by sugar has just as much of an impact on the strength of teeth, as this acidification is alkalinized by calcium (and other minerals) being removed from the teeth and bones (hence sugar is also an aggravating risk factor in osteoarthritis). This means that sugar causes a double whammy on teeth, attacking them from both outside and inside. If sugar were to be eliminated from the diet, the positive affect on the health of teeth (and the entire organism) would be significantly greater than the questionable benefits ever achievable from brushing with sweetened, chemically laced toothpaste.

Acne and seborrhoeic dermatitis also appear to have a correlation with the intake of sugar, with the latter being more common amongst those who eat the most sugar. Acne is probably also caused to some extent by sugar (and the other deadly whites) as it interferes with hormone production at a critical stage of maturation, puberty, where hormone production is a defining feature.

How sugar impedes other aspects of hormonal production and effectiveness will be a source of new research, as so little appears to be understood about this at present. There are a few examples, and if these were to be extrapolated out to consider other hormones, sugar indeed appears a serious risk factor. Amongst the immeasurable interferences it causes, either known or as of yet unknown, the biological mechanisms for how sugar causes depression and tiredness are fairly well understood today. For good brain functionality the amino acid, glutamic acid plays a crucial role, the production of this amino acid is determined by B vitamins produced by bacteria in the gut and as the consumption of sugar encourages detrimental bacteria to be produced at the expense of the helpful bacteria, there is a knock-on effect on the production of the B vitamins and glutamic acid, leading to tiredness and a lack of cognitive performance. If this condition is allowed to continue, as it often is, drugs are prescribed for depression or sleep deprivation. The production of the hormones, melatonin and serotonin, is also interfered with by the consumption of sugar, adversely affecting mood as well as sleep patterns. If this situation is allowed to continue, far more serious cognitive neurological conditions can manifest such as Parkinson's, neuropathy, epilepsy, depression or schizophrenia. Sugar also adversely affects other delicate hormonal balances, notable amongst these are insulin, cortisol and oestrogen. It is well understood that negatively affecting these hormones also causes other dysfunctions within the body's chemistry, from other hormones being produced to heart disease and of course diabetes.

There has been little study done on the affect of a continual hormonal imbalance, although from the work done already on insulin, a hormone that is most definitely linked to sugar consumption, the artificial and constant excessive requirement of this hormone to balance out blood sugar levels causes more severe problems than simply blood sugar levels. This elevated and imbalanced blood sugar level is of course the basic foundation that identifies diabetes and with this disease alone there is still an awful lot that is still to be understood. In fact the truth about diabetes needs to be re-understood, as the knowledge of this disease was superior as long ago as the 1930s, although economic rationale has suppressed this information. It seems only logical that sugar should play a major role with diabetes, as it is excessive consumption of sugar that is a major factor in unbalancing the blood sugar levels. Prof Yudkin also showed there was striking evidence to implicate sugar with diabetes, as well as its association with diabetic nephropathy (kidney disease), which accounted for 15% of those with kidney disease in the UK, (25% in US), as long ago as the 1960s and 70s, when Yudkin was doing his work.

The list of other ailments sugar is implicated in, as a causal or aggravating factor, is fairly comprehensive: including the few from above, as well as hypoglycaemia, mood swings, Alzheimer's, learning difficulties, aggression, ADD/ ADHD, concentration difficulties, migraines, anxiety, mental disorders, epilepsy, Candida, eczema, varicose veins and haemorrhoids. Sugar also lowers the effectiveness of hormone, enzyme and gland production, as well as causing chromium, potassium and copper deficiencies (the deficiency of which is being frequently associated with Type 2 or age-onset diabetes). Chromium not only alleviates sugar cravings but also helps with attention deficit disorder (ADD). Sugar also adversely affects calcium and magnesium absorption, as well as preventing the release of linoleic acid (Omega-6) and the bio-assimilation of several other nutrients. Lowering vitamins B6, B12 and E levels, creating acidification within the body, as well as promoting inflammation. These all hamper proper brain and cardiac functioning and cell reproduction. Sugar has also been shown to weaken the retina, damage the pancreas and kidneys, whilst adversely affecting asthma and multiple sclerosis. It also causes premature aging and is addictive, with serious withdrawal symptoms. Not so sweet now, huh?

The tide is turning

The fact that sugar causes diabetes, especially Type 2, is beginning to be seen as irrefutable (as with the correlation between cigarettes and lung cancer, the message appears to take an unreasonable amount of time to filter through to the general public). What we fail to appreciate is that diabetes manifests itself as a wide range of symptomatic diseases, not just diabetes defined as irregular blood sugar, but also heart disease, cancers, kidney disease and of course obesity. These diseases either progress to a fatal conclusion or continue to lay the foundation for a never-ending string of medical complications, which themselves will become fatal. As the basic cause of the catalyst for illness, that of excessive sugar consumption, is never addressed, all manner of illnesses are allowed to prevail. It is this simple, although of course by the time the patient is aware of this (if at all), the continual sugar consumption has caused diseases that have become chronic (incurable), because in many instances the medical profession refuses to act in a forthright manner with regards diet. It is no good politely suggesting that a change of diet would help, when in fact it should be made clear to actualize a real cure at an early stage of many diseases, all that has to be done is to cut out sugar completely from the diet, (just as it would be wise to cut out all the other deadly whites) before the diseases reach a chronic condition. Sugar even interferes with the utilization of prescription drugs, making its consumption even more problematic and adding to the doctor's failure by not insisting that sugar intake is severely reduced. Even rats live for 30% longer if their diets are rich in starches as opposed to sugar.

Professor Yudkin demonstrated that not everyone was equally as susceptible to sugar 'poisoning'. It is a deadly white for everyone, although 30% are more sensitive to the adverse affects of sugar consumption and are therefore more susceptible to heart disease, diabetes, cancer, depression or any of the other diseases of civilization. Such a sensitivity would help to explain why only a proportion of smokers get lung cancer, if some are more susceptible than others to begin with and for those that are particularly sensitive, lung cancer could develop without even being a smoker.

Yudkin was perhaps the greatest contributor in attempting to sway the public away from the pernicious sugar industry, with his life's extensive scientific research and his book "Pure, White and Deadly', first published in 1972. As he was one of the foremost antagonists of the sugar industry (and those companies dependent on sugar), Yudkin experienced continual attempts to erase and discredit his efforts to bring to light the dangers of sugar. This was done by the food industry applying pressure on those who had him speak at conferences or printed in publications, a route taken constantly to mute out voices of opposition to these dealers of the deadly whites. Food companies sponsor many health talks, conferences, research, publications even education faculties, quite deliberately, out of economic sense not caring sense, as all they need ever do is threaten to withdraw finances (sponsorship) to silence opposition. A good example of this is The British Nutrition Foundation formed in 1967, financed initially and significantly by Tate & Lyle, Hovis and McDouggal, and from their lofty academic position The British Nutrition Foundation has been able to apply leverage in guaranteeing very little scientific research reaches the public domain if it could jeopardise its sponsor's finances.

Consumption rises unabated

In the late-1970s sugar accounted on average for about 17% of the calorific intake of the population, a figure that seemed ludicrous and dangerous to Yudkin at the time. There were of course those consuming more than this, and as demonstrated in the next couple of pages, most of the population, especially the children today, obtain much more than this in calories from sugar consumption, with 50% being more widespread than could seem possible, let alone reasonable or acceptable. The fact that today sugar accounts for as much as 50% of some people's calorific intake, whilst the diseases Yudkin stressed were associated with sugar consumption have continued to escalate in incidence, adds further weight to the notions that (a) the drugs don't work and that it is indeed (b) sugar that is a major risk factor in the establishment and or escalation of the diseases of civilization.

Today in Britain, we eat about 25 times the amount of processed sugar than we did 200 years ago. There has been a slight decrease in the past few decades of sugar consumption, more than compensated for by the increase in fructose and artificial sweeteners. The danger with sugar is that even to consume well below the average of 50kg a year, is for many, a dangerous amount, let alone that many consume up to fourfold this quantity. For the quarter to a third of the population who have elevated intolerance to sugar, to consume any is problematic, although as this is never medically recognised the continual harm caused by sugar consumption will only be recognised as a problem when it causes a diagnosable ailment such as heart disease or diabetes. It has been shown that the death rate from heart disease is 5 times higher for those eating the average of 50kg of refined white sugar a year, as opposed to 10kg. With 60kg consumed a year, the death rate is a whooping 10 times that of those eating just 10kg.

50kg annually is surprisingly easy to achieve, considering four cups of tea or coffee a day with two sugars is 15kg of sugar over the year; a can of coke or other sugar water every day is over 15kg a year. Even something as innocuous as the jam on two slices of toast a day can amount to about 8kg of refined sugar in a year. These three alone already account for about 40kg a year, before all those biscuits, cakes, ice-cream, chocolate and alcohol is counted. Sugar is incredibly difficult to avoid, even supermarket bread has sugar in it, as does over 90% of all items in the average supermarket, it's even added to cigarettes, emitting a sickly acidic smoke, which is also carcinogenic.

Some authorities are currently putting the average yearly consumption figure nearer to 75kg. Add to this at least 15kg of high fructose corn syrup (HFCS), a figure that is rising rapidly, as this cheaper sweetener is being more commonly substituted for and added alongside sugar in ingredients. Then there is approximately 5kg minimum of dextrose and all the artificial sweeteners, which churn up a whole new heap of troubles, being ingested to an astounding 10kg plus a year, of pure chemical poison. Figures vary enormously from source to source, although the levels of HFCS, dextrose and the artificial sweeteners combined puts the average sugar intake at over 100kg a year (or 400,000 calories).

WHO have recently stated that in order to curb public health problems, added sugar should not contribute any more than 5% of daily calories. Which is an admirable amount to aim for, although percentages aren't everyone's top subject, so if WHO say 5%, what are we eating and more importantly what are we feeding to our kids that will guarantee them a safe and healthy future?

Surely as a parent our only role is to nurture and raise healthy, happy children who have the best chance possible of achieving a fulfilled and contented adulthood. What are we giving to them? Prepare to be shocked, as the vast majority of the population have been deliberately kept in the dark about what we are giving our kids, so to shine the light on the crazy situation the food industry have been solely responsible for creating, let's look closer at some figures:

One level teaspoon of white sugar equals about five grams, which at four calories a gram gives 20 calories for every teaspoon of sugar. The following is the average from observing a few families at one of my children's schools and includes only the food given to a child aged from six to eleven (primary school).

Breakfast: Bowl of coco-pops (portion size - 50g) equals about 5g of added refined sugar (all cereals with added sugar have a similar amount), small glass of orange squash (200ml) has about 10g of added white sugar.

Packed Lunch: White bread cheese sandwich has about 1g in two slices (although white bread is also full of 'naturally' occurring sugar due to it being almost pure carbohydrate), cereal snack bar has about 10g (most cereal bars average this, regardless of how healthy the packaging makes the product appear), carton of blackcurrant squash (200ml) 10g, packet of crisps (with the problematic polyunsaturated fat, as well as usually a little sugar or sweetener added).

Tea: Pack of sweets (60g) 30g of added sugar (all sweets are a minimum of 50% sugar, usually nearer to 80%), squash (200ml) 10g of sugar.

Dinner: Fish fingers, chips and peas with tomato ketchup, 10g, Ice-cream (50g) 10g at least of added sugar, similar if vanilla or one with sickly bits in.

Evening snack: three choc chip biscuits, 11g, hot chocolate (packaged not cocoa) has up to 15g of added sugar in a 200ml mug.

This all totals for an average day's food, a staggering 122g (nearly 25 teaspoons) of added white sugar, or about 490 calories worth, which is more like 30% of all calories from daily (Monday to Friday) food ingestion, some way off WHO's 5%. For a weekend, this figure of 122g could easily be doubled, as it could for holidays and days out etc. Considering that non-school days account for nearly half of the year, this 122g average is raised by 50%, giving roughly 180g daily average intake of added sugar. Remember this is just an average, many children will be spending much of the day gorging themselves on sugar-laced treats and can easily consume an astonishing 250g and more of added sugar a day. This 180g daily average, equals just over 67kg of added sugar being eaten by a primary school child in a year, a figure that will be applicable to many five year olds as well as 50 year olds. To cap it all off, if one was to compare the weight of healthy nutrient-rich ingredients eaten in a day, just a few grams, compared to the 80% of carbohydrate-rich processed foods that comprise the average diet, hundreds of grams, an answer to the pervading illness of mankind is laid bare.

What makes this even more shameful, is that all this delete-rious dietary input is being supplied by the children's parents and guardians, as well as the stark fact that as a percentage of body weight, this ratio of detrimental food input, increases the problem substantially. For me to give my three-stone daughter a doughnut is the equivalent of me eating four doughnuts (as I weigh nearly 12 stone). It gets worse, because all that sugar is playing havoc with their development at a critical stage of growth, physically, mentally and hormonally, whilst constantly weakening the immune system. Often we give kids a sweet as a supposed treat, elevating the status of these sweets and increasing their desirability. Although what really pisses me off, is the fact that this proliferation of sugar (and other deadly whites) in the food chain could easily have been prevented. Ultimately it is not our fault, as the government has failed in its role of 'steering mankind' to a healthy future; all they have done is 'control our minds', unequally distribute the wealth, whilst the duplicity of economics has held sway.

Natural, no added, unsweetened, foods that sugar?!?!

The figures above are just for added refined sugar, the natural sugars have been deliberately excluded, not just because the added sugar is what is being looked at, but the natural sugars create a whole new ballpark of confusion, as we will see. If all sugars were included in the above example, the calorie count attributable to sugars would easily exceed 50%, probably nearer to 60%, which is frankly unbelievable, particularly if one considers that only a century ago sugars would have provided about 10% of total calories and added white sugar no more than 2 to 5%. Is there any real surprise that a diet consisting of sugars and processed foods leads to ill health?

My research has led me to work out some fairly complicated mathematics, although for this little exercise in trying to translate as simply as possible the amount of sugar in foods, I failed. This was because it was either near on impossible to separate or identify the added refined sugar content from the naturally occurring sugars. Some of these naturally occurring sugars have a greater concentration and calorific content than added sugar. In some fruits, for instance a banana weighing 140g, has 17g of sugars (obviously naturally occurring) and contains 125 calories, 68 of which come from the sugars. Which makes little sense (to you or I!) when trying to assess the nutritional and health impact of a banana; 125 calories (which would take 10 minutes to burn off by cycling or running at full pace) is the same as can be found in 45g of raisins or half a pack of Starburst (weighing 30g), of which the Starburst has 17g of sugars, the raisins have 30g that sugars, meaning the banana has the same 17g of sugars as the Starburst, while the raisins have double. I hope you can see where the confusion begins to creep in here, because it's blatantly obvious that a banana is a healthy item of food, whilst Starburst are only negative, although from the observation of the numbers alone this is not apparent.

Misdirections and ignorance

In Britain presently there is talk of taxing sugared foods, with the latest initiative trying to get people to consume no more than six teaspoons a day of sugar (120 calories, about the same as the WHO 5% recommendation), or about 30g a day which totals just over that 10kg a year figure mentioned earlier as a healthier average. Brilliant idea, but how will they achieve this with just words? As shown from the above average dietary regime, how will this apply to reality? Considering the new average for added sugar consumption is nearer to ten times this at 100kg a year, meaning the average resident is eating 275g a day. If sugar is not actively removed (and not just replaced with HFCS or sweeteners) how on earth is the average consumption going to drop to 10% of that of today? Surely the only answer is to remove all food with more than a teaspoon of sugar from the food chain, which I don't see happening soon.

This educational programme of six teaspoons a day is bound

to fail, regardless of the health sense it makes. It's the same as trying to educate the public about eating five-a-day portions of fruit and vegetables, a message that has only resulted in a shambles, with the food industry being allowed to deliberately muddy the logic. Not only do the majority of people fail to achieve five-a-day, with one-a-day a struggle for many, this whole five-a-day issue is mired in controversy, especially considering what is allowed to be labelled as providing one-a-day, whether that's on a fruit-winder sweet with over 60% sugar in it, or a glass of cheap concentrated juice, full of sugar or sweeteners, both are actually negative dietary inputs, definitely not the same as eating one of five portions of fresh vegetables a day (this whole five-a-day fiasco is looked at in a little more detail in the White Lies chapter). The level of consumer confusion about this message is on a par with the misunderstandings inherent in passing on a simple message about how much sugar is in a food item and whether that's in naturally occurring sugars (which just means carbohydrates or fructose in most instances), or is added white sugar.

If the government and health agencies in the UK want to limit sugar intake to just six teaspoons a day, it is an impossibly small amount to ingest if one's diet is dominated by processed and packaged foods. The message from the health agencies really should state that the aim is to wean the population off the processed foods and establish a dietary regime that incorporates predominately raw food ingredients being mixed together, very much as we did before the 1950s. Can you imagine the confusion and fuss that such a clearly stated message as that would cause? The food industry lobbyists would be in hyper-drive and the threats to the government about loss of earnings and jobs would be astronomical. However, it would be the solution, and after just a five-year period the health index of the entire nation would have gone through the roof, the National Health would have saved itself billions and the population would have repositioned itself onto a path that leads back to evolution, not the current cul-de-sac that is devolution.

There's a whole world of other sugar - here's Fructose

Moving onto other sugars that do not start out as a sugar cane or beet, it's worth beginning with fructose, as this is relatively new to Europe, gaining widespread use in only the last decade. In America it gained popularity about 30 years ago and from this earlier introduction it is noticeable, with no recourse to epidemi-ological or statistical analysis, as it is visually in full view that Americans have gotten bigger in line with the rise in consumption of fructose. If you assumed fructose was a generally safe sort of sugar obtained from fruits, it's definitely worth delving just a little deeper before we move onto the rest of the sugars and sweeteners.

Fructose is beginning to emerge as the number one sweetener. It is also proving to be even more harmful than refined sugar, although as of yet there have been none of the long-term reports; when these become available in a few years we will already have been suffering the consequences of its excessive consumption for too long. Fructose, as with sugar, needs to rob nutrients from other parts of the body in order for it to be metabolized, although worryingly with fructose, the burden falls primarily on the liver, which is already under severe strain from all the other negative dietary and environmental inputs. The liver deals with only about 20% of the glucose consumed, as every cell in the human body utilizes glucose as its energy source, but not fructose. It is left to the liver to utilize this fructose, which in cases of excessive consumption it cannot (excessive could be deemed as little as 20g a day) and the only solution the body has is to covert this fructose to fat. Hence why this recent surge in fructose consumption is a significant contributor to obesity and morbid fat deposits throughout the body.

As just mentioned, a common misconception is that fructose is from fruit, which of course it can be, but when found as an ingredient in a processed food item, it is not. More and more sugars are coming from corn, such as dextrose (which is basically pure glucose) and HFCS (high fructose corn syrup), with yearly production rising by at least 5% year-on-year. HFCS was first developed in the 1950s, and by the mid-1980s it had its foot well and truly in the sweet door. There is no similarity whatsoever between the bioavailability of the fructose when eaten as an apple, or that available from industrial sweet fructose, derived from corn starch after chemical and heat processes. HFCS is actually a product at the end of a highly toxic chemical procedure, even a waste product from the ethanol industry. Conveniently for the ethanol industry and very inconvenient for human health, this waste is also a type of sugar, which, with some inspired economic management and chemical tinkering, made it available to be used instead of and with the huge quantities of cane and beet-sugar already used in processed foods, drinks, medicines and confectionary (this is not the only method used to obtain HFCS). The Corn Refiner's Association has an advertising campaign and website called sweetsurprise.com in which it refutes all claims about any differences between sugar and HFCS, or any links with obesity and mercury; to read this biased site as the only source of information about HFCS would certainly lead to an erroneous truth. The site's section on nutrition and health clearly points out that a balanced diet is key to a healthy life, offering what a balanced meal looks like; interestingly, nowhere does it mention that HFCS forms a part of this healthy balance. Although, by even addressing what a balanced diet is, they can argue that the site covers all aspects of health, done for the benefit of the consumer, even offering FAQs, where they handily rebut every previous scientific article that may have pointed out the obvious detrimental health implications of repeated consumption of HFCS. Quite where the mercury came from in nine out of 20 samples found in common processed foods from a recent consumer report on HFCS is still a mystery (although mercury is used in the production chain of obtaining ethanol and HFCS), it would certainly be a sweetsurprise to find out.

HFCS, sometimes labelled as simply fructose, is far more processed than refined white sugar. HFCS is known to atrophy the pancreas of humans, thereby damaging insulin production and is seen as a direct cause for the recent rapid increase in obesity and diabetes. HFCS also damages the heart, liver and testes, as well as disrupting copper metabolism within the body. The results are clearly palpable; everyone's getting fat and the fat are getting fatter from this increase in fructose consumption, being the number one reason for the sudden rise in morbid obesity in the past 20 years. Especially true in America, where its excessive consumption is well advanced, since HFCS's intro-duction to Coke in 1984 (it was not used in European Coke, with American coke lovers not happy with the change in taste, going to the lengths of importing Mexican coke, as this contained no HFCS). Total negligence by the FDA and all the other health authorities, whose responsibility is allegedly to look after the public; to highlight this calamity of fructose use, the European Food Safety Authority has just agreed that because fructose has a slightly lower GI (Glycaemic Index, a lower GI requires less insulin) than sucrose, if food manufacturers replace 30% of sucrose with fructose (which will be HFCS) they can label their products as healthier! The only result will be a surge in morbid obesity in Europe paralleling that of the USA, as consumers are deceitfully hoodwinked into believing that their purchases are healthier. Only the bank balances of the fructose and food producers will become healthier, not the public (Tate & Lyle are by far the biggest HFCS producers in Europe, so any loss in incomes from sugar becoming demonized will be more than made up for by increased revenues from HFCS and other sweet-eners they control, such as stevia). It is a remarkable coincidence that after stretching the waists of the American public for nearly 30 years, the food industry is slowly replacing fructose with normal sugar in America, and other sugars, such as those derived and patented from stevia. Instead of learning from the American mistake, we are blindly following their lead.

The blame for this rise in HFCS and indeed for all the corn derivatives found throughout the food chain can be traced back to President Nixon. In 1971, seeking re-election and desperately trying to distance himself from the calamitous situation in Vietnam, it was decided that the only way to win public favour would be to halt the rising food prices, initiating a drive of mass production of corn, wheat and soy (these sectors of the food industry in the US contributed significantly to financing Nixon's re-election campaign). Monsanto leapt at the chance to provide GM crops to actualize this programme of mono-cultural agriculture, which did indeed provide a surge in these crops, to such an extent that there was a significant surplus. This surplus was the trigger for ethanol and HFCS being produced from corn, further helped along by the increase in taxation and reduction on quotas of imported sugar (no doubt as a result of lobbying from The Corn Refiner's Association).

There is strong epidemiological evidence suggesting that since this introduction of HFCS into Coke from 1984 (with other soft drink manufacturers following soon after) there has been a surge in obesity. A surge that fructose has to be responsible for, by not only damaging the pancreas, its consumption raises triglyceride levels in the blood and as a consequence of this the hormone responsible for triggering the satiated mechanism called leptin (when the stomach tells the brain it has eaten enough), is interfered with (refined white sugar as we have seen also has a detrimental effect on hormonal production), making it possible for overeating to occur, helped along its way by the brain's pleasure senses being stimulated by this constant sweet input. This of course makes HFCS (and sugar) a dangerous addictive substance, particularly in relation to obesity, although the president of the Corn Refiners Association unsurprisingly insists that HFCS is indistinguishable from sucrose once absorbed by the body.

HFCS has become common in the UK food chain over the past few years and exactly as with the case in the US a couple of decades ago, obesity levels are soaring, with many people now weighing in at an astounding 50 stone, some even bursting the scales at 80 stone (no household scales go beyond 30 or 35 stone, most only to 20). To put this into perspective, Britain's first obese man, Daniel Lambert, weighed in at what was considered an unbelievable 53st in 1806, charging a shilling to view his naked bulk he made a fortune (Lambert almost certainly had a very rare genetic predisposition to obesity, today's obese are just fat from eating too much HFCS, sugar and the other deadly whites, whose only genetic excuse is the damage done to leptin production). The average weight today is on average 3 stone more than the average from the late 1960s and it has been proven that much of this gain is due to diet not physical inactivity, rates of which may have increased, but nothing like as dramatically as the rise in processed foods consumed.

HFCS has even been replacing the sucrose that the bee-keeping industry feeds its bees, which could have something to do with the subsequent colony collapse problem affecting bees currently (a pesticide used to control mites in hives has also been implicated, as has the class of pesticides known as neonicotinoids, also the fact that the pollen of agricultural plants is bereft of nutrients once common and natural; all four of these variables are injurious, new and probably the reason for this colony collapse). There is no doubt that HFCS and any fructose added to processed foods should be avoided, as should all processed foods, if you have any concerns about your health.

Some are more 'natural' than others

Continuing with the other alternatives to white refined sugar, aside from cane and beet sugar and HFCS, firstly, what can very loosely be called the natural sweeteners, although don't assume natural in this instance means safe or healthy. All of the following natural sweeteners still have to appropriate nutrients from the body in order to be metabolized (for the body to break them down to become bio-assimilated). Firstly the Sugar Alcohols (a misnomer as they are neither sugar nor an alcohol), such as Xylitol, which is made from corncobs (without the corn kernels, the commonest form of xylitol), or utilizing what is left from the sugar cane stalk after sugar is refined from it or it can be derived from birch wood waste. Glycerol, a waste from soap manufacture is also conveniently sweet, so a profit can be made out of this waste product, often finding its way into medicines aimed at children. Sorbitol, Maltitol and Mannitol are all processed from corn starch using toxic chemicals. The last of the most commonly met sugar alcohols is Erythritol, which for some variety, is fermented corn starch. All of these carry fewer calories than white refined sugar, being their only advantage, they are all the end products of exceedingly unnatural processing, involving extremely dangerous chemicals and high temperatures. Organic birch xylitol is probably the best of this bunch of sugar alcohols, if one had to choose. The sugar alcohols are digested in the main by the small intestine, although if any more than 30g are consumed a day (20g for mannitol), there are problems with bloating, flatulence and diarrhoea. There is even advisory information on some products about the importance of establishing a digestive tolerance (what I'd call a diarrhoea threshold), asking you to eat enough so that you literally shit yourself, then use this as your individual digestive tolerance level, remaining at just below this level and with continuous ingestion, the body will adapt within a fortnight. Do we really need the sweet stuff this bad?

Juice Concentrates, most often from dates, grapes, apples and pears, are usually the closest to a natural product and if they are from a good source and not heavily refined, can make an excellent and beneficial addition to food, although of course only when eaten in moderation, as there has been a tendency to over-emphasise the natural fruit sweetening from usually apple, although this still demands an unnecessary burden on the liver to deal with the elevated fructose content. China has recently been producing enormous quantities of apple juice concentrate to add as a sweetener to anything from baby foods to jams and a whole array of processed foodstuffs.

Other types of natural sugars include, Maltodextrin, derived from corn, potato or rice, with Maltose and Malts being fermented grains, traditionally barley. Fructooligo-saccharide is made from the inulin found in Jerusalem artichokes, onions, wheat and bananas. Inulin doesn't require insulin to be converted to energy, making it a good thing for diabetics, but when taken in even a seemingly insignificant quantity, just a few grams, there are many adverse reactions.

Tagatose is made from lactose and therefore brings with it many of the health worries about dairy consumption, especially a product that is entirely made from the problematic milk sugar, lactose.

Trehalose is naturally occurring and can be found in foodstuffs as diverse as mushrooms, honey, shrimps and lobster. Although unsurprisingly, it is derived from corn starch when produced commercially, as well as being heavily refined.

Honey is also heavily refined and therefore depleted of most beneficial nutrients, with the natural sugar, levulose, getting converted into glucose. There is some confusion over levulose, which could be argued as being the only real 'sugar' and certainly the only one mankind should be consuming. There is an extensive body of evidence stretching back beyond Hippocrates (who had a particular interest in honey and its curative abilities) associating honey with well-be(e)ing. Honey and Maple Syrup are unquestionably preferable to every other type of sweetener when unrefined, being sweet and beneficial, so long as consumption is in moderation.

Agave syrup is often highly refined, being 80% fructose. For health benefits only buy unrefined, otherwise avoid, as the refined supermarket product (even most of the ones in the health stores) are also known as Hydrolyzed High Fructose Inulin Syrup (HFIS), with its very high fructose content making it as detrimental, if not worse than HFCS. Be very wary of this new product pretending to be natural and used for 1,000s of years, which admittedly, the Aztecs made alcohol from, but they drank it unrefined, not by the ton made from massive steel containers, heated to extremely high temperatures and mixed with dangerous chemicals and acids.

Coconut Palm Sugar is produced from the nectar, the sap of cut flower buds of the coconut palm, meaning the coconut crop is sacrificed (another can be grown as with all crops, although the alternating from flower nectar back to coconuts impinges the coconut productivity by as much as 50%). It is low in carbohydrates as well as having a reputed lower glycaemic index rating than refined white sugar. It does have a desirable treacle-like flavour and depending on the quality and unrefined status, it can provide a good compliment of minerals and vitamins. As with agave, when that was being championed, the truth has been somewhat veiled by those pushing it, solid research will undoubtedly verify the true GI and fructose position of coconut palm sugar.

Stevia is a very sweet herb, native to Paraguay, having been used by the Indians there for millennia. Many hail it as the best alternative to sugar and indeed it appears to be so, but only when consumed as a dried unprocessed whole leaf, which has a slight liquorice aftertaste; sadly this is actually illegal in the EU. The recent fuss that has been made over stevia by the FDA and food producers only underlines its true potential. The sugar-pushers have been clambering over themselves to most efficiently (i.e. economically /cheaply) extract the sweet stuff, whilst the ensuing battle continues with Cargill (Coca-Cola) having patented methods of extracting the steviol glycosides known as Reb-A (Rebaudioside from the Latin name for the plant *Stevia rebaudiana*), being pushed as Truvia. PepsiCo have Reb-D, with others coming thick and fast, such as Reb-X, and Monsanto with their Purevia. Commonly mixed with dextrose and erythritol and sold under various names, all weighing heavy with semantic psychology, stressing the naturalness of the product in an attempt to sway the consumer that it is healthy and pure, when in reality it is just another heavily processed denatured chemical that the body will have serious problems adjusting to, and in the long term will cause a whole new heap of problems. It's all very sinister, particularly when one considers that the natural product of stevia leaf was banned by the FDA, who didn't consider the pure leaf form of stevia to be safe for human consumption (irrespective of its longevity of traditional use, with no health issues attached). Now that patents have been awarded and signif-icant investment and taxes are looming, suddenly a heavily processed and certainly not a natural product has miraculously been awarded the green light from the FDA, as stevia had been banned from being sold not only as a sweetener but as a herb!

It has been suggested that the FDAs initial reluctance to award stevia a GRAS (Generally Recognized As Safe) status was because of pressure from Monsanto in attempting to maintain its market share with their diabolical aspartame and neotame sweeteners, whilst giving them time to extract and patent the steviol glyco-sides. Currently stevia, regardless of how processed it is, is being marketed as natural, when clearly it is not, although the consumer has absolutely no chance of seeing through the confusion. I also make herbal food supplements (from the knowledge I obtained from the extensive research for this book) and recently fell foul of the law as stevia is considered a novel food item and as such is not classed as fit for human consumption in the EU. The rationale for this stems from a 1999 report that suggested more scientific evidence was required to establish stevia's safety, although this report strongly suggested it was the steviol component that had already caused lesions and cancers in laboratory rats, not the whole leaf. So what happens? After patents are awarded for this flagged ingredient, this miraculously becomes safe whilst the rest of the plant in its green natural state becomes legislated against. The upshot for my Culinary Caveman powders is that I have to remove stevia from the Green Gaia Goodness and the Purple Purifier, although I could replace this with the denatured and industrially produced stevioside and steviol!! I trust you see the obvious face of big business heavily influencing legislation irrespective of logic and health. I've also got a bit of a bee-in-my-bonnet about stevia, as I need to reformulate and re-label my products (although I notice many other green powder producers do use raw stevia, I'm not going to snitch on them as I know that being a tiny independent I will be the one getting squashed and made an example of).

The simple answer is to avoid all of these sweeteners unless they still bear some resemblance to what it looks like when it has grown from the earth, not processed via laboratories. Stevia only has health benefits if consumed in moderation and unrefined; once refined and processed any health benefits are negated, although industry will quote the unrefined benefits, even if no longer applicable once processed.

Getting dark and dirty with the artificial sweeteners

Moving onto the artificial sweeteners, these are not carbohydrate rich, some are classified as proteins and are calorie-light, if not calorie-free. It's the protein bit that needs to be remembered, as it is these proteins that are another one of the definite variables in this search for the causes of the present manifestation of the diseases of civilization. Starting with the oldest, Saccharin, being over 125 years old, this ranges from 200 times to 700 times sweeter than white sugar and has always been known to be a carcinogen, although it is permitted to be added to thousands of foodstuffs. Next time you see that little packet of sweetener at the table, next to the packet of white or brown sugar in a restaurant, cafe or hotel, instead of thinking that this is for those who may be diabetic or health conscious, think Benzoic sulphimide. The result of chemical reactions involving toluene (used in explosives), anthranilic acid, nitrous acid, sodium nitrate, hydrochloric acid, sulphur dioxide, chlorine and finally ammonia, which yields saccharin. Oh the wonders of science. What a fatal coincidence it is that after all these deadly poisons are reacted together, the result is sweet tasting and calorie-free. President Roosevelt championed Saccharin in 1907 and it has been controversial ever since, always managing to squeeze out of trouble. This said, saccharin is slowly being phased out, only to be replaced by some far worse alternatives, such as:

Aspartame, which is 200 times to 600 times sweeter than sucrose, originally invented as an ulcer drug, unfortunately it was accidentally found to be also very sweet. Before it quietly slips out of use, it is so bad that it warrants its own chapter in Book 2 in this series, as this is a variable into the aetiology of the diseases of civilization all by itself. Aspartame is particularly destructive, as demonstrated by the correlated rise in certain neurological diseases since its introduction to the food chain in 1982. Deserving its own dedicated book (there are many, such as 'Sweet Poison' by J. Starr), this one is particularly pernicious.

Which brings us nicely onto what is essentially an aspartame remix, brought to us, as with aspartame, by those good people at Monsanto, introducing Neotame. This can only be considered as the nuclear bomb of the sweetener world, being an astounding 13,000 times sweeter than sucrose! Neotame fallout is surely going to screw us all right up, especially as it already has FDA approval and has gone global (E961) and to cap it all, Monsanto have wrangled it so that it doesn't even have to be listed in the ingredients, even finding itself in some organic and natural products. So for your benefit here's what's in it: Aspartame, which is made from 50% Phenylalanine, has caused seizures in lab animals; 40% Aspartic Acid which caused holes in the brains of lab animals; 10% Methanol, well known to cause blindness, liver damage and death. These are then added to 3-di-methyl-butyl, which is on the EPA's (Environmental Protection Agency) list of most hazardous chemicals. The end result will ultimately be cell death or more personally, your death.

Sucralose, is 600 times sweeter than white refined sugar (confusingly named so as to mimic sucrose) and is commonly known as the brand Splenda (which also contains dextrose and maltodextrin), owned by Tate & Lyle. If you believe a word from their website, which makes out that Splenda is a life-saver, where they are proud of their heritage (slave trade?) and holistic and healthier approach. Healthier than what? Cyanide? It may be calorie-free but research shows that its consumption causes insulin spikes, which with continual use will lead the consumer straight down Diabetes Drive. Unsurprising, considering that it takes these far from inert chemicals to make it: trityl chloride, acetic anhydride, hydrogen chlorine, thionyl chloride and methanol in the presence of dimethylformamide, 4-methylmor-pholine, toluene, methyl isobutyl ketone, acetic acid, benzyltri-ethylammonium chloride and sodium methoxide. Industry argues that only a fraction of sucralose is absorbed and all is flushed out in the urine and faeces; science says that up to 6% remains, accumulating in the liver and kidneys, and you can be sure once there it's not inert. It also shrinks the thymus gland (an immune system regulator) and harms beneficial intestinal bacteria. The Centre for Science in the Public's Interest (CSPI) an Italian non-profit organization, places saccharin, aspartame and acesulfame K in the avoid category, soon to be joined by sucralose, which they found caused leukaemia in mice, making it a carcinogen along with the rest of its artificial cousins.

Acesulfame K, the K is for potassium and very similar to saccharin. It is 200 times sweeter than sugar (sucrose). In laboratory rodents, acesulfame K has produced lung, breast and rare organ tumours, various forms of leukaemia, and chronic respiratory diseases. Surely there is no need to go on, and there is definitely no reason to consume it, unless you again take the word of industry who swears its safe whilst independent scientists swear its harmful.

Sugar, sugar, everywhere

We didn't need any of these natural or artificial sweeteners to evolve. The caveman had no use of them and neither should we. All the sweeteners should be avoided as all they are doing is contributing to our ruin. They are heavily chlorinated, highly artificial with absolutely no health benefits whatsoever. These sweeteners and HFCS have been added to the food chain with little health consideration, the only consideration has been that they are cheaper than sugar, keeping food costs down and profits up.

The annual global production of white refined sugar is about 160 million tons, increasing more than 2% year-on-year. So prevalent and in demand is the sweet stuff, that sugar cane and beet can neither keep up with demand, or keep up with the changing times and cheapness of chemical alternatives. Sugar itself has been superseded by a sweeter and cheaper sweetener, that being HFCS. As well as of course, the worrying omnipotence of the cancer causing, heart stopping, MS inducing, attention deficit and diverting, artificial sweeteners, notably aspartame and saccharin. Even without the sweeteners, we would still be in dire straits, sadly with the sweeteners it looks like we could be in even more serious trouble.

In the early 2000s a WHO report advised that sugar should

never exceed 10% of daily calorific intake, a very liberal amount considering how much is actually consumed. It cited several reports that suggested that consumption below these levels was an effective preventative for many of the diseases of civilization. The sugar industry in the US went ballistic at this proposition (notably the US Sugar Association and World Sugar Research Organization) lobbying the US Congress to abandon its $406m funding of the WHO, threatening to bring the WHO to its knees if the report was publicized. With considerable success it would appear, as the limit in the US was finally set at a staggering 25% of daily calories to come from sugar, set by the US's FNB (Food and Nutrition Board), a board funded unsurprisingly by M&M, Mars and a consortium of well known soft drinks manufacturers. WHO have finally seen sense and recently stated that added refined sugar should not exceed 5% of calorific intake, let's hope this message gets worldwide exposure.

Current press coverage and the scheme of taxing sugared products is all an orchestrated cloak and dagger exercise. Sugar is blamed for making people fat, allowing sweeteners, stevia and HFCS to become market leaders, all still owned by the same conglomerations as the refined white sugar. In the meantime the food industry is hedging its bets on the hope that the pharmaceutical world will be able to cope with the rise in obesity. Sugar is slated as being the ultimate bad boy in the war on obesity, when in reality it is just the tip of the iceberg and only the first of the deadly whites, there are still six others to come. Sugar might raise your blood sugar level, but then so does a slice of white bread in exactly the same way. We are entering into extremely dangerous industry-led propaganda years, and that is the point of this book, to remove the polish sprayed on by industry and reveal the true grain.

Laying the foundations of ill health

I trust this chapter has demonstrated how the increased presence of sugar in ones diet can lead to multifarious considerations as to how diseases can manifest, be that as a consequence of sugars ability to interfere with hormonal production and levels, or create acidification and inflammatory conditions, or just make you fat from all the calories. Almost single-handedly this first chapter has implicated sugar as being a major risk factor, and that is of course the rationale for starting this book with sugar. However, as the following chapters unfold, they themselves will follow a similar route of blame and accusation. Sugar has been undeniably an insidious addition to the diet and one that is totally removed from what would have been eaten by our caveman ancestors.

Today, sugar has managed to slip into all kinds of food from baby formulas, to ready meals, and of course the huge range of sweets and cakes. What I would argue sugar does is that it lays down the initial damaged foundation blocks that once the following other deadly whites are added, builds an ever increasingly damaged organism that becomes progressively more difficult to actualize where the tangible problem or blame lies for the rise in the diseases of civilization, let alone where to find a cure.

Phew! So ends the first deadly white. If you thought any of it to be controversial or just too depressing to be told the truth (as ignorance is truly bliss), it might be advisable to stop reading now, or perhaps just skip to the appendix. If you want to know more, bless you for your inquisitiveness and solid faith, because I'm afraid it only gets worse from here on in.

The Second Deadly White

Milk

"Watch out, Watch out, there's a Humphrey about" "Full of
Natural Goodness" "Milk's Gotta Lotta Bottle"
(Milk Marketing Board advertising slogans)

The benefits of milk in regards to our health are emblazoned
everywhere.

How on earth can it be bad for us?

Milk has always been there. It was even given away free at school
(and still is to many under-11s); it's so healthy, providing us with
all the calcium required for strong bones and growth. Everyone
knows that milk is good for us.

The reason everyone knows this is not because it is the truth,
it's because the advertising, propaganda and indoctrination has
been so successful in getting a particular point of view across,
that this is the only view seen. A view, I hasten to add, the Milk
Marketing Board (MMB) and the Dairy Council have paid
handsomely for in Britain. The Dairy Council, run by the dairy
industry, has a business objective to "proactively promote the
nutritional benefits of dairy and protect it from inaccurate and
unfair publicity" (as quoted from their website), even if the
"inaccurate and unfair publicity" often happens to inconve-
niently be the truth, as it is the Dairy Council who themselves are
being inaccurate. Irrespective of the truth, they will protect it and
promote it, with a lot of funds to do so. In the United States, the
dairy industry spends over a third of a billion dollars a year to
maintain its market position, paying off dieticians and doctors,
whilst also funding researchers, taste-makers and celebrities to
push and plug the white stuff.

Nixon got a milk-tache

As long ago as 1971, dairy representatives handed President Nixon a three million dollar cash-gift (invoiced as a contribution to his re-election campaign). Nixon, as we saw in the last chapter, is not only the man responsible for the surplus in corn that instigated the addition of HFCS to the food chain, he also had a seriously maladjusted sense of morality and justice, particularly with his involvement in the Vietnam War. It was with his approval that Laos and Cambodia, both barely involved in the dispute, were blanket bombed (as well as Vietnam) with napalm and Agent Orange (for which he was no doubt paid handsomely by Monsanto and Dow, who made these catastrophic, hell-inducing, chemical weapons). He may not have been President at the onset of the war, but his staunch anti-communist agenda justified the slaughter in his mind when he was President from 1969-74 (his predecessor, Johnson, desperately wanted the war to end). Nixon is the only President ever to have been impeached, due to his involvement in burglaries, phone tapping, spying of opponents, bribery and financial wrongdoings (known as the Watergate scandal). His hatred of communism (and socialism) extended to assisting in the coup by the murderous Pinochet in Chile, toppling the popular Marxist, Allende.

Back to the three million dollar cash-gift from the dairy industry: what on earth would any business be doing this for? Unless it was to broker for unwarranted favours, which is exactly what happened, as within two days Nixon agreed to raise the price of milk, earning the dairy industry a cool $3.24 billion in extra yearly revenue, making that cash-gift a very sound investment. Hearing of one unethical transaction is the same as seeing a single rat; if there's one, there's a dozen.

What's it all worth?

I digressed, sorry. If you go to any of the dairy websites around the world, the message is always the same, promoting milk as a vital component of a healthy diet, guaranteeing healthy bones and teeth. This pretty much amounts to the backbone of the entire industry's argument, and as we will see, it is a spineless statement, because no independent scientific research substantiates these decades old claims.

What it all boils down to, in this up-to-the-minute, short-term profit, economic world, is how much is it all worth? This is why the mouths have been so loud in favour of dairy, with those not in favour quickly quietened. Milk (dairy) contributes a massively loud 14%, or £117 billion a year of total EU agricultural output. For the UK this figure is about £3.3 billion, which is a third of the value of the entire harvest of fresh fruit and vegetables. That's why the dairy industry has such a loud voice, although in terms of volume it should be pointed out that agricultural produce only accounts for 0.7% of GDP (gross domestic product, how much a country produces in total worth of all goods and services), industry accounts for significantly more at 21.1% and the service sector (banking, insurance, hedge funds etc.) an astounding 78.2%, which accounts for why bankers appear to be running the country's finances and money today defines what the public considers to be economy.

Whilst looking at a few figures, it's worth noting that the EU still subsidises dairy farmers to the tune of £11 billion a year, which works out to about £1.40 per day per cow (allowing for 21.5 million cows on state benefits in Europe). This means that European cows have an income higher than over half the world's human population, who survive on less than £1.30 per day.

Marketing and promotional expenditure of $350 million every year by the US dairy industry keeps the public there consuming an average of over 100kg each and every year, with 250kg being fairly common (a kg is roughly a litre of milk, although of course cheese and other dairy derivatives come by weight not fluid measure). I have seen estimates that put dairy consumption as early as 1992, at 750g per day, which amounts to

275kg in a year. Consumption and general availability of all manner of processed foods utilising dairy has definitely increased since then, so a 100kg average is very conservative. Also in the US, the Dairy Management Incorporated spends over $170 million in marketing, with an emphasis on targeting sales to young children (attempting to make them lifelong addicts) and mothers, in very close partnership with amongst many others, Kraft and McDonalds. Which is not a problem if milk was as healthy as they say it is, anyone can be in partnership with whomever they like, but suspicion has to be alerted when deleterious packaged food producers and fast food giants collude. How can there not be a whiff of conspiracy?

A Victorian country idyll and sporting prowess

Much of our traditional, timeless, countryside imaginings of cheese have been seeded and paid for by the Dairy Council. Even the Ploughman's lunch was a figment of an advertising companies imagination, thought up as a way to invoke a sense of history and rural idyll for cheddar, coming up with the Ploughman's lunch in the 1960s. They also sponsored the Milk Cup football trophy and the Milk Race cycling event for many years. This twinning of a product with a sporting event, participated in by supreme athletes, gives a great association and an illusion of health and unrivalled sporting prowess achievable by consumption of the sponsors' product. The Milk Cup is now the Carling Cup (lager producer), which is stretching credibility a bit far, as is Coca-Cola and McDonalds sponsoring the Olympics. Usain Bolt certainly does not run the 100m in 9.6 seconds fuelled by Coke and Big-Macs! There is no doubt that the Milk Marketing Board and the Dairy Council fulfilled their brief, doing a fantastic job in marketing milk and dairy produce. Now we need to unlearn the propaganda and learn the truth about modern milk.

What doesn't seem to concern anybody is that all this free milk and dairy consumption has had the opposite effect on the very things it was clearly argued by the industry that dairy facilitated, namely strong teeth and bones, as today we are plagued with teeth cavities and osteoporosis, affecting an ever younger demographic. The dairy industry obviously refutes any accusations there could be any harmful affects of milk, even presenting it in such a threatening manner, that if this food group were to be excluded from the diet, serious illness could result from the nutrients it exclusively offers not being consumed, which is pure scaremongery and bullying. In the real world of biology and nutrition, there is nothing exclusive about milk's nutrients, and there is far more independent, scientific evidence suggesting it is the exclusion of dairy that leads to better health, such as the largest demographic study ever made, Dr Campbell's seminal 'China Study' (published in 2006), which clearly points to this and the many adverse affects of dairy consumption (more on this amazing study later). It amounts to a similar state of affairs as seen in the last chapter, where the sugar industry completely dominates and suppresses all negative research and knowledge.

Did you hear the one about milk being good for bones?

First off, let's get to the bottom of this myth, that milk with its rich calcium content, benefits bone growth. As Britain is one of the largest dairy consumers (actually eighth in the world, after Finland, Sweden, Ireland, Holland, Norway, Spain and Switzerland), it would follow that Britain is benefiting from all this milk and cheese in the diet. A good indicator of this would be our exemplary teeth and lack of osteoporosis and weakened bones, where a comparison of our incidence of osteoporosis against a nation that consumes little dairy, would show the palpable health benefits of all this dairy consumption.

Well I hope you are sitting down, because the actual truth is that the nations that consume the most dairy have by far the highest incidence of osteoporosis, whilst those consuming the least dairy have the least incidence of osteoporosis. An illogical outcome if milk were so good for bones. The Bantu of Africa for example, who eat a sparse, mainly vegetarian diet with no dairy, consume just over half the RDA at 400mg of calcium (RDA set at 700mg), only show signs of osteoporosis when they become acculturated (move to the cities and change diet and lifestyle). The Taiwanese also have a particularly low calcium intake, averaging only 130mg, although teeth and bone problems are very rare there. The inhabitants of Pitcairn Island in the Pacific also eat no dairy and they have long been extolled as being some of the healthiest people in the world. So there is nothing illogical, it is just because we assume dairy is good for the bones and this is only because the dairy industry has misled us for generations.

This implies that there is very little connection between calcium intake and osteoporosis or dental problems, which is very confusing, although there are other factors involved, as we will shortly see. One of which includes the Inuit, who average the highest calcium intake of almost triple the RDA at 2,000mg, although they suffer from some of the highest rates of osteoporosis, with up to 15% less bone density than Europeans. The blame here however lies in their high meat intake of 350g per day and not their milk intake, as a high meat protein intake (not vegetable protein) significantly raises the blood acid levels and consequently this leads to calcium loss from bones to alkalinize the bodily system. This acidification caused by animal proteins (including the protein from milk) is often neglected, with sugar taking the brunt of the blame for this acidification, when meat and milk proteins are just as liable.

All of this came as a bit of a shock to me. Go and check for yourself, do an internet search for 'dangers of milk' and read someone else's opinion, there are plenty of doctors and professors voicing themselves and none of them appear to be very positive about milk. Conversely, search for the 'benefits of milk' and read the opinions, almost exclusively from the dairy industry, as there is no independent optimism, apart from those advocating raw, organic, grass fed cow's milk, which is immensely hard to find, being illegal to sell in most shops.

And that's just the start of it

Ready for a real shocker? Research actually shows that dairy consumption can deplete the body of calcium . . . What? This is because there are certain nutrients that promote the retention of calcium within the bones and teeth and there are those nutrients that promote the excretion of calcium. Amongst those nutrients that retain it, magnesium, potassium and vitamin D are crucial and it is these three that we are often deficient in, in the industrialized world. Particularly important is magnesium (abundant in fresh greens and all but missing in modern milk), which has to be present and eaten in balance with calcium to help with assimilating dietary calcium, controlled by the parathyroid gland, which is already struggling due to our deficiency of dietary iodine and selenium. The nutrients that promote calcium excretion are protein from animals, phosphorus and sodium, all of which the modern diet has a vast excess in. For the body to successfully assimilate calcium it requires not just magnesium, it also needs phosphorus to be consumed in equal proportions. We have a daily excess of phosphorus (phosphates are also added to many foods as an acidity regulator) as well as cow's milk having six times the phosphorus found in breast milk, inhibiting the assimilation of calcium further. Further exasperated by the fact that the protein content of cow's milk is at least three times that of breast milk (I mention breast milk here because *Homo sapiens* have evolved on this). This excess of phosphorus and protein in cow's milk, therefore does not encourage calcium retention, it only encourages its excretion. Also, even with ideal human health and a perfectly balanced diet, only about 20% of the calcium from milk could ever be bio-assimilated. With green leafy vegetables and nuts it is possible to bio-assimilate nearer to 40%, with the best source for calcium being stinging nettles, peppermint and seeds, all more readily utilised and bio-assimilated due to their excellent and balanced magnesium content.

Basically, our diets repetitively have too much of the stuff that removes calcium and not enough of the stuff that stops this thievery, with the widespread deficiency of magnesium preventing bio-assimilation. Calcium is constantly being depleted within the body, removed from the bones and teeth, which of course results in weak bones and teeth, as this imbalance to the homeostasis is never rectified. Calcium's prime role within our diet today is as an alkalinizing agent for our overly acidic diet, for which milk can't be solely blamed, it is all the Deadly Whites together causing this increased and sustained acidification.

A curious aside, taken from the world of cheese-making, is that if pasteurized milk is used to make the cheese, calcium chloride has to be added as the heating of the milk makes the calcium unavailable (destroying the enzymes that make the bio-utilisation happen), clearly demonstrating calcium is already deficient and is never going to be found or utilized by the human organism from pasteurized milk.

This in a nutshell underlines one of the major problems with modern dairy products, insomuch as heating negates any benefits it could have had. Emphasis should fall on the word *modern*, as consumption of dairy is not new, just as many of the diseases of civilization are not new. What is new is the rise in incidence of a few particularly devastating diseases, such as cancer and heart disease.

Are there any changes in the use and production of dairy that could account for the more recent changes in the type of diseases afflicting us over the past century?

There have been plenty.

It's not like it was in the old days

Hopefully a very brief overview on the history of dairy and the changes in dairy production may identify any causative agents for the changes in the diseases of civilization. The oldest documented evidence of processing milk (not just from cows, also from sheep and goats) to cheese comes from those wonderfully illustrative Ancient Egyptians, from about 2,500BC. As animal stomachs have been used for storage and transport, since long before the caveman, the coincidence of a stomach having rennet in the lining and the mammalian milk curdling in them, would have led to such cheeses as feta having a considerable antiquity. When rennet is added to milk, the whey and curds separate with the curds setting to a wobbly gel, whilst the whey is the liquid part. Little Miss Muffet can attest to both of these forming at least a part of the diet in the past. Cheese and butter would have constituted the major uses of milk in the past, as milk could only have been consumed near to the farms, although refrigerated transportation soon changed all this.

Today, we consume more low-fat liquid milk, less whole-fat milk and less butter and more cheese than at the turn of the twentieth century, as well as all the new processed foods containing various extracted bits of milk (which makes it harder for those with lactose intolerances to ascertain what has milk derivatives; words, prefixes and chemical names containing casein, lacto and whey will all be milk based). Cheese was the main part of dairy consumed in the past, which has far less lactose than milk, cheddar having about 5% of that of milk, with hard aged cheeses such as Parmesan, having none or very little. The word, cheese, comes from the Latin, *caseus*, which is also where the word casein is derived from, the main constituent of cheese. Dairy produced in the past was all from unpasteurized milk, producing strong regional variations in cheese, as is still the case throughout France today. Today in England we have little knowledge beyond cheddar (developed in about 1720), with nearly all supermarket cheese being pasteurized. This means that most dairy no longer provides the benefits it may have done in the past with regards its changed and depleted nutrient content.

Walking milk factories

The biggest change of the last 100 years or so has to be that in the past, all cows grazed outside on grass and herbs, with the milk being unpasteurized; whereas today, cows eat pellets and the milk is pasteurized. 100 years ago (and long before) a farmer would have had 10 to 20 cows, all hand milked and fed on lush, diverse meadows of grasses, herbs and flowers, with the manure being used as fertilizer, allowing a range of fecund organic vegetables to be grown. This sustainable and proven method lost out to huge herds and hugely expensive milking parlours, now even computer controlled, administering varying ratios of feed and drugs to individual cows. Even though large herds have become the norm, the total number of cows has actually fallen in the past 100 years, although the amount of milk these produce has risen by up to 600% per cow. Production was in the region of 1,360 litres per cow per year in 1900, rising to 2,400 litres in 1950, continuing on a steep slope until the turn of the twenty first century, with production topping an astounding 7,700 litres per cow per year. The current world record stands at 32,000 litres in one year by MyEverGreenView-1326 in 2009/10, an American Holstein (a breed developed from Friesian Dutch imports to the US in the early seventeenth century), a particularly ironic name for a cow predominately living with only a view of a concrete shed! In Britain cow numbers fell from 3.2 million in 1980 to 1.8 million in 2010, whilst average herd size grew from 80 to 113 over the same period with each cow seeing an increase in production from 5,400 litres in 1995 up to 7,315 litres in 2010.

There has also been an associated gradual depletion of the nutritional profile of milk over the past hundred years, because as milk production increases per cow, the nutrients put into this milk by the cow have to be increasingly diluted. To boost production to these modern extremes, the cows could never graze enough (if they were lucky in the first place to ever graze), so the feed became forever higher in protein and nutrient derivatives, from corn, soy and worryingly other animals, even cows. Enforced cannibalism doesn't sound very natural, ethical or safe, which is why BSE spread and vCJD came into being from stray prion proteins found in cows and chickens. Cows are of course vegetarian, their whole physiology and digestive system is geared towards chewing grass and herbs all day, every day. In so doing, they can be nurtured to provide between 1,500 to 2,500 litres of beautiful fresh milk in a year, as was common before WWII. There is little comparison between this traditional meadow fed milk and modern supermarket milk, apart from them both being called milk. Making the comparative life of modern cows even worse is that dairy cows today only manage around three lactations, with the cow slaughtered at no more than 4 years of age, becoming too ill and unproductive by this early age, whereas each cow would have been productive for ten to fifteen years a century ago, living to 20.

The powerful force of economies-of-scale has made increased herd sizes a necessity, if the expensive machinery for milking and pharmaceutical programmes is to be implemented (which is exactly the same trick/business model used on the agricultural sector, enslaving farmers into debt for machinery, decreasing diversity and increasing reliance on pesticides and seeds). In the 1990s many cows were changed to the Holstein breed (a process known as Holsteinization) as these were proving to be reliable milk factories on legs, naturally having more growth hormones within them, taken full advantage of by coaxing them with a cocktail of other growth hormones and antibiotics to produce up to 80 pints of insipid, chemically laced, nutrient weak, white water, every day. That's before its pasteurized, where it loses most of the remaining nutrients, whilst retaining a proportion of the chemicals and bacteria. The nutrient profile of milk has been further changed recently as potassium has been limited in the feed to curtail 'milk fever', exasperating the common human deficiency and further unbalancing the crucial ratio of sodium and potassium, as sodium (found in salt) is already excessive in the modern diet. Magnesium is also a co-worker with these minerals, which is also deficient from the modern diet. Unsurprisingly, the best sources of magnesium and potassium are to be found in the green leaf vegetables such as parsley, sorrel, chickweed, comfrey, nettles and dandelions, all of which were extensively eaten in the past (by both humans and cows), all absent or excluded today.

The goodness of milk begins with a healthy natural range of nutrients made available from grazing, not just grass, but all the herbs and flowers growing in the meadows; it most certainly does not mean pellets of grain and refined oils, enriched with industrially produced nutrients. There is such a huge difference in the quality of milk from different pastures, that grass-fed alone is not a guarantee for top quality, nourishing milk. If the grass used for grazing is a commercial rye grass, grown on depleted soils using dangerous agro-chemicals, the milk will be less nutritious with dangerous chemicals compared to traditional grazing on diverse organic meadows. There has been up to a hundred-fold increase in the use of fertilizers on grazing lands, with corresponding decreases in the species diversity of these grazing lands as a result of the aggressive pushing of agro-chemicals by the pharmaceutical corporations, with considerable coercion from government agencies. The best solution would have been to maintain the species diversity of grazing lands, as the meat or dairy from cows grazing on these industrial grasses is always significantly inferior to the meat or dairy produced from traditional farming, where a meadow (or a ley) full of clover, deep-rooting burnet, vetch, chicory and cocksfoot and many other grasses are used for grazing. The manure from cows grazing lush pastures is subsequently richer, this fertilizes the soil, making future crops more nutritious. Everyone's a winner in this small-scale economy, fulfilling the true definition of 'good household management'. When the ante is upped and everything has to fall in line with the modern version of economic viability, there begins to be losers, with the first loser being health; the health of the cow, the land and the consumer.

It's not like that on the telly

A common image of milk production probably comes from television, no doubt a children's program or a period drama, with a small farm and a dozen or so cows milked one at a time, in traditional tiled barns, roaming chickens and ducks, with green fields, red tractors and smiling farmers. The reality couldn't be further from this vision, which is full of concrete prisons, shit everywhere, with the cows lucky if they even see the sunshine, let alone a blade of grass. Most organic dairy comes from cows, who the imagination likes to assume are grazing happily in the sunshine, (often corroborated by a picture on the packaging of cows contentedly grazing), when actually they live in the same concrete compounds, only they are fed on organic feed (the same is true for most organic chickens); unless you have seen where it comes from yourself, never assume the best, always the worst, as that will inevitably be nearer the truth. This lack of sunshine means the milk has very limited vitamin D, just as it is deficient in magnesium, selenium, iodine and many other essential nutrients, many of which require vitamin D to help them be synthesized and bio-assimilated, as indeed does calcium, as a lack of vitamin D inhibits the production of the hormone calcitriol, a calcium regulator working in conjunction with the parathyroid gland, which itself is weakened due to the lack of dietary iodine. Milk products are also often fortified with vitamin D3, usually sourced from dehydrocholesterol, which is most commonly extracted from pig's skin, brains, raw fish liver or sheep's skin. Certainly not vegetarian or even close to being kosher, not to mention an easy route for cross species contamination of pathogens.

There was a time not so long ago (still the case in parts of rural France and Switzerland) that the first milk and cheese of the year, after the cows had been put out to graze in the meadows, after spending the winter inside, were a cause for celebration. At this time of year, the milk, butter and cheese are richer in nutrients and flavour with a deeper yellow colour. This is why Swiss chocolate is so prized today, because some chocolatiers in the past only procured their milk from particular breeds and regions renowned for their rich, lush, spring meadows full of flowers. These produce the finest milk and ultimately the richest, smoothest chocolate. Sadly this is a secondary consideration (if at all) in today's world of economic viability. Guernsey and Jersey cows are also renowned for their golden creamy milk, although less productive they are making a come back today as the tide slowly turns against the Holsteins and the present model of milk production.

That meddling Pasteur fellow

Most of the goodness that is present in fresh raw milk is lost when it is pasteurized, regardless what the dairy industry may want you to believe. Further degradation occurs with the time passage from farm to supermarket and from fridge to use. The residue from any toxic chemicals, such as pesticides the cow munches on, often remain unchanged after pasteurization, as do many of the bacteria that were supposed to have been eradicated by the brief heating, such as certain *listeria* and tuberculosis strains. As many of these endocrine disrupting and carcinogenic agricultural chemicals are fat soluble, these toxins can be found in the fat, with butter having 21 times the fat concentration of milk (which equates to 21 times the harmful chemicals and growth hormones), hard cheeses have 10 times (it also takes about 10 litres of milk to make a kilo of cheese) and ice-cream has 12 times the fat content of milk. Toxins have also been shown to atrophy, with a test on a Ben & Jerry's vanilla ice-cream finding 200 times the safety levels of dioxin present. What about all those products that haven't yet and probably never will be tested?

Raw milk contains enzymes and all the goodness from the grazed grass and herbs, two of these enzymes are *phosphatase*, assisting with the absorption of calcium and *lipase*, helping to hydrolyse and absorb fats. As the enzymes are destroyed with pasteurization, milk is harder to digest and could well be the main cause of dairy intolerances. Raw milk also has a high quantity of Omega-3 and a low amount of Omega-6 in an extremely healthy ratio, lost when pasteurized, as is the butterfat, which is homogenized or removed in pasteurized milk. This butterfat has been shown to help the body utilize and absorb minerals and nutrients in the water fraction of the milk, as well as being an anti-carcinogen. Research from the 1930s and 40s showed drinking raw milk could solve certain gastro-intestinal problems and predating this, in 1911, Dr Charles Porter, after completing 27 years of intensive research and analysis, published 'Milk Diet as a Remedy for Chronic Disease', advocating only unpasteurized milk. The same applies for the work carried out by Dr Crewe of the Mayo Clinic, who success-fully treated a whole range of illnesses with raw milk from cancers to tuberculosis and many more. The fatty acids found in raw milk, such as butyric acid have been shown to be anti-carcinogenic, whilst the lauric acid is an antiviral, antifungal and antibacterial agent, the caprylic acid has similar antiviral capabilities, whilst the palmitic and stearic acids are useful to lower cholesterol levels. All these fatty acids are pretty much destroyed by pasteurization and are completely absent from skimmed milk, although of course they can still be found in unpasteurized milk. There are also plenty of healthy bacteria in raw milk, which help to proliferate beneficial bacteria in the intestines, which in turn feeds the whole immune system.

With the mechanization of the dairy industry after WWII, the traditional methods no longer remained economically viable, unpasteurized milk soon became near impossible to find. The dairy industry has since focused on the economics, whilst the health aspect was neglected. It can't be true that all dairy is bad for humans, particularly as its use has a considerable history. It is only *modern* milk from *modern* cows that is bad for humans. Which is why the Maasai of Africa and the yak herders of Tibet still thrive on dairy today, just as Europeans appeared to have done so in the past.

The FDA tell us raw milk will be the death of us

A bit of pseudoscience and the creating of a 'scare 'n' smear' campaign about the pathogens in raw milk by the dairy industry soon put most people off it. With the marketing propaganda proclaiming pasteurized milk is the same as raw milk, without the nasty bacteria, such as *salmonella* and *campylobacter*. Which is possible, although the incidence is extremely remote from well cared for, grass fed cows, using careful sanitary milk collection techniques. When was the last time someone was infected with TB from raw milk? Whereas BSE, foot-and-mouth and the more recent bovine tuberculosis and *E-coli* scares, all predominately originate amongst modern dairy cows.

The FDA's website is very clear about the serious health implications from drinking unpasteurized milk and eating unpasteurized milk products, stating there were 1,500 reported incidences of illness from 1993 to 2006. It doesn't state what these illnesses were, beyond just sickness, certainly no deaths, and a quick calculation shows that the figure of reported adverse affects is only 107 people a year from a population in the USA exceeding 320 million. From the number of pages devoted to this issue on the FDA site and the accompanying videos, the assumption is unpasteurized milk is the bane of public health, preying on pregnant women, the young, sick and elderly, when the truth is only a paltry 107 people reported becoming sick from its consumption each year (that's a miniscule 1 in 3 million chance across the whole population). Hundreds of thousands report illness related to aspartame, millions are adversely affected by legal prescriptions (with a minimum of 120,000 dying), unrecorded millions have problems with pasteurized milk but no, according to the FDA *unpasteurized* milk is the danger to American citizens. I trust you see the obvious influence of the dairy council in this scaremongering. The French eat unpasteurized cheeses all the time and there is no evidence to suggest they are falling like flies to this clear and present danger. Any isolated problems appear to stem from unsanitary production not the unpasteurized milk *per se*. So, don't believe the headlines, just like the subheading for this section.

Raw milk is such a niche market today, unless you live in the country, it is unlikely you would even come into contact with unpasteurized milk from traditionally grass fed cows, particularly as it is illegal for supermarkets to sell unpasteurized milk. What a strategic manoeuvre this was by the dairy industry, on a par with giving out free milk at schools, totally confusing us from an early age about the rightful place of this modern milk in our diets. How much did it cost to achieve this? And how difficult was it for the lobbyists from the dairy industry to convince the non-scientific politicians to pass legislation banning sales of raw milk due to health concerns raised by their own questionable research?

The implications run much deeper than the above

All of the above only implicates dairy consumption as not being as healthy as we might have once thought it was. Thoughts that we have seen have been moulded by continuous and expensive marketing campaigns. Such misinforming of the public of any real truths about calcium content and our bones worryingly only wipes the top off a frothy frappi-latte, especially when you see independent research indicating dairy as being a significant causal factor in:

Certain types of cancer, notably of the breast and prostrate, as further expanded upon later in this chapter. Rheumatoid arthritis, a serious form of osteoporosis, caused by the diet stripping calcium from the bones, becoming increasingly common amongst juveniles. Also childhood and adult diabetes, both of which sugar, meat and white flour intake are as much to blame for. There is also Insulin Dependent Diabetes (IDD), which has an incidence that runs in tandem with those countries with the highest milk consumption, headed by Finland. It is increasingly being shown from research that Bovine Serum Albumin (BSA, Bovine means it's from cows) is a prime cause of IDD, especially amongst children, particularly those who were introduced to cow's milk before four months of age. Then there are various gastro-intestinal and respiratory disorders, such as gastroesophagal reflux, constipation, nasal congestion and asthma. There has also been shown to be links between dairy and iron deficiency anaemia, where the intolerance to lactose and or casein results in intestinal bleeding, which over an extended period of time results in iron stores becoming depleted. *Listeria* has been shown in studies to survive pasteurization, as does *salmonella*. Milk is also implicated with teeth cavities, irritable bowel syndrome and Crohn's Disease, where all patients tested with Crohn's, also had *Mycobacterium paratuberculosis* RNA within them, which solely originates from milk surviving the pasteurization process. Multiple sclerosis (MS) is also beginning to be linked with whey, which is indiscriminately used in many processed foods; MS is absent from all non-dairy consuming cultures, surely not just a coincidence.

In the natural world, when an infant reaches about two years of age, it is weaned and breast milk is no longer offered. In line with this weaning is the human's reduction of the production of the enzymes rennin and lactase that break down the casein and lactose, ceasing completely for 75% of the world's population upon weaning, because from the age of three the gut biota should be able to assimilate most food. Without these enzymes (lactase and renin), the vast concentration of casein in cow's milk clogs up our intestines, preventing the digestive system from absorbing nutrients. With regular consumption, milk leaves an increasingly hardening, virtually impermeable coating on the inside of the intestinal membrane, severely restricting absorption of nutrients, as well as filling us up with mucous, detrimentally affecting the respiratory system. It is very often this lack of the enzymes, renin and lactase that causes the casein and lactose intolerances, manifesting as one of the illnesses just mentioned.

Amazingly, the medical profession very rarely, if ever, considers dairy as being even a minor causal factor for any of these illnesses. Even if cow's milk is still full of pus, hormones and glue, as well as loads of other things that Mother Nature didn't put there when she was working out a dietary plan for calves. Cows with Johne's Disease have heavy diarrhoea and these cultures get into the milk and when consumed the results are argued by some as resulting in Irritable Bowel Syndrome (IBS) and Crohn's Disease. They are commonly tainted with disease-causing bacteria, such as *salmonella, staphylococci, listeria,* deadly *E. coli* and *Mycobacterium paratuberculosis* (possibly another of the agents causing Crohn's disease; a form of life-threatening chronic colitis), as well as a virus' known to cause lymphoma and leukaemia-like diseases and immune deficiency in cattle. Dairy cattle are infected with bovine immunodeficiency viruses (BIV = cow AIDS) and bovine leukaemia viruses (BLV) worldwide. Cows, in a sentence, are extremely unhealthy, full to the brim with viruses, bacterium, antibiotics and growth factors, living to only 20% of their natural lifespan; there should be no surprise their milk is unfit for human consumption. In fact, the only surprise is that we drink and eat it at all.

Cow's milk also has significantly less of the essential thyroid hormones, such as thyroxine, which could account for the recent surge in dyslexic, autistic and ADD syndromes, at least as a significant contributory factor. It is the thyroid gland that is over and above all the other glands, crucial for proper human development. The thyroid is essential before birth in early development, making sure the DNA blueprint is copied and assembled correctly, hence why iodine is so important, as this is essential for the thyroid and for hormone production.

And there's more . . . There are also definite links with dairy consumption and childhood ear infections, pneumonia and a whole batch of baby and childhood allergies, intolerances and complications from sudden infant death to rashes, colic, wheezes, disturbed sleeping, tight stomachs, severe constipation, aggressiveness, tantrums and more. Then there is the increased risk of heart attacks, strokes and atherosclerosis, as the fat content of milk and cheese is directly attributable to the clogging of the arteries, the world's biggest killer. All a little more serious than a jovial white moustache, or is that a pustache!

A few million pus cells in your tea madam?

It is old news now that pus, hormones and glue can be found in milk and dairy products. Old news it may be, but still next to nothing has changed. There is still at least a gram or two of pus in every litre of milk, with up to 400 million cells per litre being permissible (around 2 million cells per teaspoon). Bearing in mind that bacteria/pus cells can double every 20 minutes at room temperature, or double in two days in a fridge, it's best to start with none. This is the case whether it is organic, or not. Much of this pus is as a result of the over-worked and severely stressed cows, which are quite literally on the brink of collapse, the majority suffering from mastitis and serious teat stress from where this pus originates, with the ever present faeces also a major risk factor. There is still pus in organic milk, but at least it will have some of the hormones and antibiotics missing, although there is still plenty to choose from, be it pituitary hormones, steroid hormones, hypothalamic hormones, thyroid and parathyroid hormones or gastrointestinal peptides and over fifty other growth hormones. Often dairy cows are slaughtered after only three or four years of abject slavery, when they could easily live to beyond 20 (producing milk for at least 12 years), having had all their organs and glands relevant to milk production saturated in growth hormones and antibiotics. Slaughtered dairy cows rather surprisingly make up 20% of the beef on the market, ending up as cheap mince, sold onto fast food chains and as value meats for supermarkets, where these chemicals and pharmaceuticals have accumulated within the fatty tissue. The overuse of antibiotics is making more pathogens resistant, drastically increasing the possibility of a catastrophic cross species disease, resistant to our present pharmaceutical armoury.

With regards the glue comment, this would be from the protein casein, of which there is up to 300 times more in cow's milk than in human breast milk. This casein has been used for a very long time as furniture glue, as well as the glue to stick labels onto bottles and more recently as a polymer in plastics. This glue manufacture constituted a major use of cow's milk, particularly in the 1950s, when dairy use was declining, which is when the Milk Marketing Board (with a big budget), stepped in to convince us of the benefits of modern milk.

Growth hormones and Monsanto

Returning to growth hormones, as these in particular need to be singled out as a major and significant worry. Scratching a little deeper here, it is hardly surprising that the name Monsanto quickly comes to the surface. Monsanto have sunk half a billion dollars into developing their own growth hormones, as the economic implications of quicker growing cows that also grew larger glands such as the mammary to accommodate more milk production are clear. What wasn't made clear by Monsanto was the association with tumour growth, as these growth hormones act like fuel cells for cancer. This association of breast cancer and dairy containing growth hormones is becoming unquestionable as more independent research replaces the erroneous, pseudoscientific research that Monsanto has continually been allowed to carry out themselves, especially in these times of self-regulation. Some of Monsanto's research even correlated growth hormones with tumour growth, but still the FDA allowed dairy with added growth hormones to enter into the food chain. A decision influenced by Monsanto, who stated that these growth hormones, also known as IGFs (Insulin Growth Factors) were safe, based on their in-house research showing the IGFs were destroyed in the human gut. If this was the case, then the whole purpose of IGFs and indeed breast milk (and all mammalian milks) would be redundant if it were destroyed before carrying out its duty. Of course they are not broken down before they can be put in the bloodstream, this is precisely the reason nature put them there in the first place. Subsequent independent research (not paid for by the dairy industry) has shown that these IGFs are of course not broken down; protected from the gastric juices by the protein, casein, only being broken down at the end of the digestive system, where it should be, so as to enter the bloodstream, allowing all these miniscule growth switches (which is what IGFs essentially are) to course around the body wanting to attach to anything and complete their mission of activating growth. Casein is used to encase pills, protecting the pill from digestion until it reaches the intestines, where it is broken down and the drugs are released to complete their assignment. This clearly reveals that it is well understood by the pharmaceutical and medical world that IGFs (as for all drugs) are not destroyed, as it is the job of casein to protect the IGFs and all other hormones from early digestive degradation. These IGFs are a major risk factor for the initial growth of cancer cells, particularly in areas where growth constantly occurs in the adult body, such as the areas associated with reproduction (there is of course cellular re-growth constantly taking place in the whole body, from the skin to the organs). However, of all the growth hormones, IGF-1 is unique. This is because IGF-1 is the only identical hormone (of the thousands of hormones) that is shared by humans and all the other 4,700 mammalian species. Human IGF-1 blood levels can rise 10% after consuming a glass of milk, so how far a step is it to postulate that these growth hormones are encouraging and switching on the growth of cancers?

Monsanto entered the market with rBGH, going by the trade name Posilac in 1994. The 'r' stands for recombinant, where they have sliced together these bovine growth hormones (BGH) with engineered *E.coli* bacteria. Monsanto's involvement in *E.coli* is made all the more sinister by the fact that the most deadly form *Escherichia coli* 0157, suddenly appeared 'as if by magic', or, far more likely from a laboratory, found almost exclusively in association with dairy farms. As the Holstein breed of cow has more naturally occurring BGH, this was the breed selected and pushed beyond the limits of all other breeds for milk production. With Posilac, its main purpose was to increase the number of these IGFs, in the hope that more milk is produced, which it did, with about 15% more milk being produced as a result. Also, from Monsanto's own data, Posilac increases mastitis by 79%, with a 19% increase in somatic cell counts (pus and bacteria), as well as increased incidence of enlargements and calluses around the foot and knee region, with a 55% risk of lameness and a 40% reduction in fertility. Thankfully, most of this rBGH milk stays in the US, being banned in Canada and the EU. Which brings to mind a theory from the 1990s in the US, where the sudden spike in breast cancer rates was being blamed as being psychosomatic, being caused by all the television and press attention this cancer was attracting from its sudden escalation. What an incredible coincidence, that a substance known to encourage tumour growth (rBGH) and once allowed to join the food chain, sees a correlated rise in tumour growth of the organs it was supposed to encourage the growth of, notably the breast (and prostrate) in another species with exactly the same growth factors. The psychosomatic theory has the sordid, sour smell of a diversionary tactic, using some in-house scientific research, in an attempt to draw the public's suspicion and gaze away from themselves, as Monsanto knew full well of the definite danger they had put consumers in. Every scientific report confirms that this rBGH increases the amount of IGF-1 in milk, so milk from cows hooked up on rBGH can and does create serious GBH!

Considering that the American government was already buying up a billion dollars worth of surplus milk every year; why on earth would they want more? Particularly more of a product that had definite risks attached to it and very limited exportability, as no other country wanted anything to do with it. It only profits Monsanto, which further demonstrates that when Monsanto say 'Jump!' the FDA answer: 'When, where and how high?'

As just mentioned, there is IGF-1 in the milk of all mammals, with more being present in sheep, goat and cow's milk than in human milk. This is to be expected, considering the rapid growth these mammals undertake. A cow doubles in size from its original birth weight in 47 days (growing from a 15kg calf into a 250kg cow in a little over a year); for a goat this birth weight doubling is achieved in only 19 days; and for a human, birth weight doubling occurs in a comparatively slow 180 days. As this IGF-1 is the same chemical whatever mammal it is found in, a human should most definitely not have any extra dietary IGF-1, the body creates its own when required, so any excess when not required is unquestionably going to be undesirable. Insulin growth hormone circulating around a body already awash with other chemicals (both natural and industrial), whilst being deficient in protective minerals such as iodine, selenium and zinc, logically can only lead to problems. As the human body may not be signalling for any particular growth, these IGFs aren't directed anywhere specific, instead they just circulate in the blood until utilised by whatever it comes into contact with. Any stray cancer cells (these are made every day naturally) or established cancer cells (all those other carcinogens we are exposed to daily from agricultural, industrial and domestic pollutants encouraging cancer growth), absolutely love it, as has been repeatedly proven in laboratories. Growth factors from cow's milk are so good at doing what 'they-say-on-the-label' about encouraging growth, milk is fed to cancer cells for them to do what they do in the body, grow, when culturing cancer cells in a laboratory. The very substance that works so well for cancer growth in laboratories, where they also use the hormone, prolactin, again from milk, is the very substance that many of us are munching and gulping through a quarter of a ton of every year!

That last paragraph is worth reading again, especially if the full impact did not hit home on the first reading. It underlines a very significant danger associated with cow's milk and any possible correlation with cancer, notably breast cancer. Although to confuse the public even more, a book by the British Medical Association (BMA), in association with the cancer societies on breast cancer makes absolutely no mention that there is any correlation between dairy and breast cancer, only mentioning that there is no scientific evidence to link them, which there definitely is, stating only soy as being problematic, whilst clearly stating it would be ill advised to not consume dairy and its beneficial nutrients. Prof Plant in her book 'Your Life in Your Hands' and Dr Campbell's huge epidemiological investigation 'China Study' most certainly refute this dangerous stance of the BMA, with hard scientific evidence. A simple epidemiological comparison of countries that do not consume any, or a limited amount of (non-human) mammalian milk with those consuming a lot, such as Europe, clearly underlines this clear and present danger posed by modern milk.

A new market highlights the dangers

Asian people of the Far East are renowned for their lack of consumption of dairy, the fact that the majority of them are lactose intolerant obviously plays a part in this decision (25% of Caucasian people are also lactose intolerant). Here fascinating cultural, demographic and epidemiological comparisons are available to study. Which is exactly what Dr Campbell in his seminal 'The China Study' undertook, with a huge comprehensive study of the Chinese population, being by some distance the largest study ever undertaken looking at the association of nutrition and health. The study produced over 8,000 statistically significant associations between various dietary factors and disease. The single food substance that created the most correlations with cancer growth was repeatedly dairy, notably casein, which makes up nearly 90% of cow's milk protein. Campbell showed conclusively that casein was a significant factor in the promotion stage of cancer, where any one of a multitude of carcinogens modern humans come into daily contact with actually begins to grow as a cancerous tumour. In his studies he found that the effects of dietary animal protein were so powerful that cancer growth could be effectively switched on and off, depending on the levels of protein consumed. The book blew me away and I was delighted to find that it only gave further corroboration that the Culinary

Caveman theory was on firm footings.

Amongst the populations of these Far Eastern countries, such as China and Thailand, the incidence of, for instance breast cancer, is much greater in the largest cities, where the diet has become more westernized, incorporating dairy by-products in processed foods, burgers etc. Whereas, the rural dwellers, still eating a traditional, predominately dairy-free, low meat diet, suffer far less from breast cancer and all of the diseases of civilization. The reasoning for the Chinese to traditionally avoid dairy extends as far back as the time of Emperor Shen Nung, from approximately 2,737BC, who ordered a thorough understanding of culinary knowledge, with a scientific study of the beneficial aspect of foods, this scientific observation of the nutritional aspect of food had continued virtually unbroken for nearly 5,000 years. The Chinese are only falling sick with these diseases of civilization when they reject their own cultural food and take up western food, in the same way they have taken up western consumables and western agricultural practices.

The Japanese, who only until this generation have also avoided dairy, (an old Japanese friend used to say that the English smelt to her like sour milk), have in every other aspect lived in parallel with any resident of any modern European city. They have been exposed to the same industrial pollutants, urban pollutants, domestic pollutants, wear the same clothes, work in essentially the same offices and factories as anyone else, be they in Nagasaki, Tokyo, Los Angeles, London or Copenhagen. The only real difference was dietary. Until recently the Japanese had much lower incidences of cancer and heart disease, with the rise of westernized fast food and an associated decrease in iodine from less traditional food (seaweed), there has been a rise in the diseases of civilization. If everything else is identical, then surely the change in diet has to be at least a candidate for the change in incidence of the diseases of civilization in recent Japanese history.

The Japanese have conducted interviews since 1946 amongst tens of thousands of residents in relation to their diet, lifestyle and illness every year, initially done so as to observe any adverse affects from the nuclear fallout from the bombs dropped by the Americans. From analysing these figures, it can be seen that in 1950 the average dairy consumption was 2kg per year per person, by 1975 this had risen to 50kg. The height of the average 12 year old girl over the same period had increased from 4' 6" to just over 5', whilst her menstrual cycle began after 15 years 3 months in 1950, by 1975 it had dropped to 12 years and 3 months. Quite what those 59 bioactive hormones (all of which are species trans-ferable) found in milk have to do with these changes is only a matter of opinion.

What is the chance that growth hormones cause growth, and that oestrogen and progesterone affect ovulations?

Which wraps up growth hormones and their dangers, bringing us onto another modern change that milk has undergone, one that has been significantly covered up by the food industry, although its adverse affects could be even more dramatic to human health.

Lab coat Vs Mammary

Introducing formula milk, the dried milk for babies, which as we will see is only a formula for disaster and is barely worthy of the name 'milk'. At least the other deadly whites are a pale shadow of their former healthy self, formula milk is two steps further away, as it is a pale shadow of its former cow's milk self, and it obviously isn't even processed human breast milk. Cow's milk, without wishing to sound dumb, comes from a cow, a totally different species and one that diverged approximately 80 million years ago from a shared common ancestor of humans.

The impression given from the marketing and advertisements for these formulated drinks, is that they are the culmination of years of intense scientific enquiry by teams of white-coated scientists in laboratories, full of glass beakers and Bunsen burners, incessantly experimenting with different concoctions to get as close as possible to guarantee perfect future development both physically and mentally of our babies, formulating a milk even better than nature herself! As if . . .

The ingredients are truly horrendous, the bulk is dried milk, whey powder, milk fat and lactose, sweetened with galacto-oligosaccharides and fructose, with loads of industrially and chemically derived minerals and vitamins added to form what looks like an impressive and substantial list of nutrients; although if all the individual nutrients from coconut milk were listed it would be just as long with the added bonus of it being naturally balanced and real as opposed to artificial and made up.

Mother's breast-milk is a truly extraordinary liquid. It is a complex delivery system for a whole array of nutrients and hormone messengers to coordinate growth, exclusively designed for our species. Our old friend Hippocrates was very weary of cow's milk and was more than suspicious that it was the root of many ailments, from respiratory complaints to diarrhoea and childhood allergies. Much more recently, America's second biggest selling book, after the Bible, 'Baby and Child Care' by Dr Benjamin Spock, clearly mentions cow's milk as a health hazard, recommending, unsurprisingly, only human milk for human babies. Have the Americans actually been reading this book? Or has it just sat on the shelf, next to the unread 'Brief History of Time' by Hawkins, as a meaningless egotistical symbol of alleged intelligence.

The marketing disinformation and pseudoscience of these formulated drink sellers, has over generations become ingrained as what can only be described as 'cultural brainwashing', all carefully engineered and manipulated by the food industry. This also extends to how milk, human milk, this initial building block in life is viewed, as it has been all but eradicated by residents of urban agglomerations and replaced with formula milk. Most mothers now supplement their own milk with a powdered variety from a tub, more often than not, switching to bottles within a few months, often weeks, if not days after giving birth. This switch away from natural breast milk is done in the firm belief that the science behind the formula milk is more advanced and in tune with the needs of our precious babies than dirty, pathogen-ridden nature could ever be.

Culturally, breast-feeding has become side-lined, seen as being a nuisance and a bit impolite, with a certain yucky element to it, extolled by and adhered to only by militant mums. Which is clearly madness, this is the start to life that nature has deemed best after millions of years of harmonious evolution, not the product of some male executives of a corporation seeking only monetary gain and short-term profits. The only goal of the formula milk producers has been to ensnare as many mothers as possible into their web of deceit, helping them to grab as large a share as possible of the global market for their white powder. A market that is today worth in excess of $11.5 billion, growing at an extraordinary 9% per annum, making up an astronomical 40% of the baby food market. Asia is the fastest growing market, with over 50% of the global share, which is all the more extraordinary considering the fact that 75% of Asians are lactose intolerant! Which can only mean a particularly painful extended period these Asian babies endure, until some form of natural tolerance can be ascertained. Mother's are very quick to blame the baby for the crying, tight stomachs and sleepless nights, instead of blaming the real culprit, the formula milk. Perhaps this would be a little too close to blaming the mother's decision to use it in the first place.

Historically, if for whatever reason a mother could not breastfeed prior to the twentieth century, various grains, such as oats soaked in water, made a suitable breast milk substitute, with regional variations in recipe applicable, with coconut milk making a fantastic option for tropical climes. For those with greater finances in the past, a wet nurse would have been employed, essentially a surrogate breast. The earliest formula milks appeared in the early twentieth century, although they were generally unpopular (amongst babies and parents), with evaporated milk being the preferred substitute until the 1950s, when formula milk finally toppled this dominance. The 1950s is of course the decade that sees the introduction of so many consumables, in tandem with the rise of the advertising agencies and the diseases of civilization. From here on in the truth gets lost in the murky world of economics and advertising. Such as the fact that breast milk has 10,000 living cells in every teaspoon, formula milk has none, neither does it have the same enzymes or hormones. It most certainly should never have been allowed to get to the position where today, with new mothers believing that there is little difference between breast milk and formula milk. It's not as if there is the option to buy breast milk. There are underground networks and some hospitals do a donation system, where they freeze excess breast milk to give to babies in need in the hospital, although it certainly is not freely (or even moderately expensively) available.

There has been considerable concern from doctors and mothers about the rise to prominence of formula milk. WHO and UNICEF, along with all health agencies around the world, have long agreed that it is indisputable that the best course of good mothering and disease prevention is breastfeeding, with very strong recommendations to do so for at least the first 6 months, if not a year. As long ago as the 1978 boycott of Nestle, people have been attempting to draw the public's attention to the fact that formula milk is the worst option for the present and future health of your baby. The boycott of 1978 was prompted by Nestle's presence in Africa and their aggressive method of promotion and advertising of what was proving to be a dangerous substitute for breast milk (it is still ongoing, for more on the boycott go to www.babymilkaction.org). There was plenty of evidence from many regions of the world correlating the lack of clean water and unsanitary conditions when preparing the formula milk at home, that it was leading to the direct poisoning and malnutrition of many babies. Such deaths and diseases that could easily have been avoided had the false ideology and aggressive profiteering of the processed food producers been left in Europe and America. Well over a quarter of a century later and nothing has changed, the same aggressive marketing is still being instigated, although focused on Asia now, repeating the false claims and associations of enhanced intellect, health, sleep and growth from consuming formula milks.

Samples of formula milk are given out free at hospitals and clinics throughout the world, with doctors and nurses offered incentives to promote these products. Vouchers are given to those on state benefits in England for free formula milk, hardly enforcing the message that breast milk should exclusively be given and encouraged for the first six months, as mandated by the WHO. If the public repetitively sees these products in maternity units and at the doctors, supposed havens of medical knowledge, it looks as if such havens are endorsing the formula milks (many of which do, if there is a bit of cash involved). If used from birth, or at any time thereafter, the quantity and quality of breast milk is adversely affected. It is also lactation that can act as a powerful contraceptive, so to stop this or interfere with this, increases the chance of population growth, especially in those countries with little education (by education I mean freely available information about the benefits of breast-feeding) and other forms of effective and easily available birth control.

UNICEF state that a formula-fed child is up to 25 times more likely to die from diarrhoeal disease than a breast fed one and four times more likely to die from pneumonia. At least 100,000 under fives die in China every year from formula milk causing diarrhoeal and respiratory conditions. In some developing countries, even though exceedingly poor, they still have incredible rates on consumption, with up to 65% of children on formula milk, money which would be far better spent on a selection of vegetables for the mother to eat to help produce healthy milk. In Laos, a sweetened coffee creamer made by Nestle gives the visual look that it is some form of infant milk, with a mother bear cradling a cub; there have been numerous incidences of mothers exclusively feeding their babies on this, with predictably malnutrition and death of the babies and infants being the result.

It's not fair to just blame Nestle, Danone is no better. With their Cow & Gate brand, with laughing cows offering babies protection from infection. Danone also sits on the governing body of the Global Fund for Improved Nutrition, without declaring its conflict of interest as being the second biggest baby food and milk producer. Danone advises governments about nutritional needs, whilst of course promoting their own wares as being at least as good as nature. It's all duplicitous and sickening, if not criminal and deadly.

Conveniently left out of the adverts for formula milk

The following is a very brief synopsis of the results from hundreds of scientific studies, looking at the correlation between incidence of illness and use of formula milk, with each disease having had several independent investigations from different parts of the world. This research shows the incidence of all the following were far more frequent amongst bottle-fed babies (under 12 months), being in some instances completely absent from those who had been exclusively breast-fed; very often the incidence rises in relation to how early breast-feeding was ceased:

Gastroenteritis, giardia, haemophilus influenza, meningitis, necrotizing enetrocolitis, otitis media (ear infection), pneumococcal disease, respiratory infections, bronchitis, urinary tract infections, anaemia and iron deficiency, thyroid diseases, constipation and anal fissures, esophageal and gastric lesions, reflux, Sudden Infant Death Syndrome (SIDS), general infant illness, wheezing, allergies, eczema, neurological, psychomotor and social development disorders, poor thymus development and visual acuity and lactose malabsorption. Breast fed babies had a much lower incidence of diarrhoea (one of the biggest killers in the developing world, killing as many as 20% of babies in some regions), with the oligosaccharides in human milk preventing many pathogens, from *salmonella*, *E.coli* and enteroviruses taking hold. With *E.coli* (as with most pathogens), the artificial feed given to cows significantly increases the acidity of the cows digestive system, with up to 40% of cattle now containing *E.coli* bacteria within their newly acidified guts, these pathogens already being acclimatised to the cow's guts acidity are less likely to be killed by the acids in the human stomach when and if they are transferred from cow to human, via meat and milk consumption (various studies have demonstrated that pasteurization does not kill all these pathogens).

Long-term studies, beyond the first 12 months of life, have correlated all of the following with a formula milk regime as opposed to a breast milk one:

Undescended testicles, bedwetting, autism (with a higher incidence amongst those not breast fed, or weaned off the breast within a week or two after birth), appendicitis, lower bone density, childhood and adult cancer, Hodgkin's Disease, leukaemia, testicular cancer, CVD (Cardio-Vascular Disease), atherosclerosis, coeliac disease, Diabetes Types 1 and 2, *Helicobacter pylori* infection (commonest cause of stomach ulcers), IBS, Crohn's, ulcerative colitis, juvenile rheumatoid arthritis, mental health dysfunctions, MS, obesity, lowered protection from toxins, stress resilience, tonsillitis, vaccine response and speech and language development disorders. Finally, bottle fed children have a lower IQ compared to breast fed children, although part of the problem here could be the plasticizers such as biphenyl-A

(BPA has been shown to be detrimental to development and is extensively used for nipples and bottles, slowly being phased out), although the lack of thyroxine in cows milk must also be worthy of a portion of the blame.

To expand briefly on this link with formula milk and diabetes, when incompletely digested protein fragments enter the bloodstream, the body recognizes them as foreign invaders that have to be eliminated. Sadly some of these protein cells are almost identical to the beta cells that make insulin, which are also destroyed and as this process continues, Type 1 diabetes is an almost certain outcome. Statistical epidemiological analysis shows that genetically susceptible children, who were weaned from the breast too early, have a greater chance of getting Type 1 diabetes than a smoker does of developing lung cancer. Genetics is being exaggerated as a causal factor in diabetes because this removes responsibility from industry, and as is repeatedly being shown, industrial scientific research often has at its core purpose a rebuttal of real scientific evidence. For instance, as a simple example, with identical twins, this genetic link doesn't hold true, because if one twin gets diabetes there is only a 13 to 33% chance of the other twin getting diabetes, which surely would be nearer to 100% if diabetes was genetically determined.

Breast-feeding has also been shown to have beneficial affects for the mother, such as lowering the incidence of, amongst other cancers, breast, thyroid and uterine, as well as protecting against osteoporosis, rheumatoid arthritis, stress and improving sleep. Babies breast-fed sleep on average up to 45 minutes more, the opinion that babies drink more from a bottle and so sleep it off for longer is an advertising 'fact', not one based on reality. There is also a stronger parent-child relationship amongst those breast-fed for longer, with up to five times less child abuse and neglect amongst breast-fed children. Breast-feeding has also been shown to help with the proper development of the jaws, palette and as a consequence also the dental arch, as well as the airways, nose, ears and eyes. Bottle-feeding is a factor in improper jaw development, narrowing the dental arch and causing tooth crowding (as elaborated upon by Dr Page in his books 'Your Jaws: Your Life' 1 & 2, recommended reading, covering health issues very often neglected, even by the dental profession, apart from his refusal to see mercury as a serious problem, which it most definitely is).

If baby formula milk wasn't contentious enough, let's have a quick look at its systemic contamination with melamine, most commonly found as a kitchen, work surface top. Melamine contamination of formula milk in China in 2008 left 54,000 babies hospitalized, four died, although the true figure could have been much more, with many developing kidney stones (this was uncounted), with the contamination spreading as far as Taiwan and South Korea. What had been happening was that Chinese dairy farmers had been adding a melamine-formaldehyde-cyanuric acid mix to their dried milk, which when tested gave a false higher protein content, allowing them to pass off their substandard dried milk for a higher price, which is very scary. Nestle guaranteed that their stringent safety procedures meant that such contamination would be impossible in their brand. Well surprise surprise, tests in South Africa showed melamine in Nestle baby formula products from locally produced milk. Nestle allegedly tracked this to contaminated cow feed, and if Nestle are to be trusted (which is most definitely open to debate), the melamine was not directly added to the dried milk, as in China. Which is actually more worrying than direct contamination, as it means that an unnecessary chemical can pass from feed to milk to humans relatively easily. Melamine by itself is not particularly toxic, often resulting in no more than the formation of kidney stones, although regardless of the toxicity, it underlines that this distressing practise of artificially inflating the perceived protein content is global. What about all the other undiscovered practices of adulterating the nutrient content of raw foods, done so with absolutely no concern for safety? Not that it mitigates this shocking behaviour, which would probably not occur in a smaller fair-trade, personal business world, as farmers worldwide are forced to sell to the multinationals at the lowest possible price. These corporations have no care for the livelihood of the farmers, who in turn have no respect for the corporations and cannot really be blamed for trying to scrape a few more pence out of unfair deals from each ton of their incredibly hard-worked for produce.

All of the above paints a very bleak picture of modern dairy farming and the milk that comes from it. There has always been a risk that the consumption of dairy can lead to cardiovascular difficulties and that the insulin growth factors could contribute to cancer growth. As cancer is an extremely old disease, this could well have always been a variable for the manifestation of this particular disease. There are of course fundamental differences between the dairy of today and of the past. Notable amongst these is the preponderance of cows not fed on grass and that pasteurized liquid milk is extensively drunk and processed further into a panoply of processed foods. It is hard to emphasize clearly enough that there truly is no comparison between the light yellow, nutrient-rich, dairy produce from the past, or the Deadly White milk we have today. It's the same scenario as with sugar and the upcoming Deadly Whites, where traditional = healthy, and modern = deadly. Compounding all of these problems is that dried whey by way of formula milk, most definitely is not the start to life nature had meticulously planned for.

A convenient link from this deadly white to the next is the fact that the word 'dairy', has the same root in Old English as dough, implying a 'bread-kneader'. This either demonstrates the antiquity and eminence of bread, and or, that the churning chores of butter and cheese making were seen in the same light as kneading. From Middle English, the word dairy implies a room for a *deye*, who would be a milk woman or farm servant who would have done both the churning and the kneading. At a later time the occupations became split, with the baker being responsible for the bread kneading made from the next chapter's ingredient.

The Third Deadly White

Flour

"Give us this day our daily bread."

This is not a slogan that has seeped into our consciousness via an advertising campaign by Hovis or another baker. This is an extremely ancient truism, adopted by the Christian church, no doubt as an attempt to make their theology more palatable and recognisable to the general public, who most definitely enjoyed a loaf long before Jesus turned a few barley loaves and a couple of fish into a meal for 5,000. Bread is as old as dairy if not significantly older; exactly like dairy, it was also a previously healthy staple that has been processed today in its raising and manufacture and become unhealthy.

How old is bread?

How long bread has been made for is impossible to say with any certainty. Dates get pushed back each year, with current evidence putting the harvesting of wild barley at about 23,000BC in the Near East, probably also accompanied by the harvesting of wild wheat. This is 14,000 years before the definite domestication of these grains by 9,600BC in Jordan and 9,000BC in SE Turkey. It is the propensity of grains to be made into flours and then bread that no doubt influenced why these grains were domesticated in the first place. It is unlikely grains were first domesticated and then discovered that they could be made into flour and conveniently into bread. It is only a recent assumption in the West that a loaf of bread has to be made exclusively from wheat flour, taking the shape of a loaf, bought from the bakery department of a supermarket. When thinking about bread from the past, it's best to think more along the lines of unleavened flat bread, such as a pita, tortilla, chapatti or a small roll, being made from any number of flours. There is no need to be restricted to exclusively grass grains either, there are also hazelnuts, acorns, chickpeas, other legumes, hemp seeds or the seeds of the chenopods such as Fat Hen and quinoa and many more, all utilised for their potential in making flour.

The earliest evidence for the harvesting of wild grains is still not proof bread was being made from these harvested wild grains, it's only a probability, even if a very likely one. The first documented proof for bread making comes from the ancient Egyptians, who cultivated emmer wheat for their bread, as illustrated in some wonderful wall paintings from the third millennium BC. Also from the same period, the Sumerians (Mesopotamians) already had hundreds of recipes for bread, pastries and rolls, with laws protecting the quality of flour and bread made from it. Bread was a staple throughout the classical period of Greece and Rome as well, with loaves being preserved from Pompeii (with a somewhat crispy crust), baked in 79AD. Barley was also used as a currency amongst the Sumerians, indicating the pre-eminence of this grain. Money today is still referred to in English as bread or dough, a reference to the fact it also fulfilled the role of a currency and a very important barter item in the past.

Up until 1815 (beginning in 1266), both ales and bread were controlled and policed by the local Assizes (regional courts) in England and Wales. It was effectively self-regulating, as business was predominately conducted locally, with those selling underweight or adulterated goods easily ostracized from the community by being fined, excluded from trading, put in stocks or imprisoned. From 1815 with the onset of the Industrial Revolution, free trade reigned and suddenly there were 50,000 bakers in Great Britain, all competing with one another. So much so, that many bakers actually began the practice of underselling due to the massive competition. Underselling is when an item is sold for less than the production costs in the hope of attracting custom and making more profit from other items sold. Adulteration with cheaper ingredients, such as adding sawdust, plaster, crushed chaff, chalk, alum and clay was a common method employed to keep costs down. This food adulteration was often carried out along the lines of organized crime, whose underhand ethics, secrecy and lack of morals seamlessly blended into the workings of modern industry, corporations and the global conglomerates of today.

In the past, this adulteration was far easier to mask amongst whole grain flours and far more difficult with white refined flours. These initial white flours also required considerably more milling, having to separate the husk and the bran from the endosperm, as well as the extra drying and grinding to make it 'soft'. As a consequence, only the rich could afford the refined white flours. This paradoxical fashion is of course now fully turned on its head, with the rich eating 'artisan' whole-grain loaves, with the poor subsisting on the chemically adulterated white-sliced filth.

Milling

Throughout history, each stage of technological innovation has only marginally degraded the nutrient content of the flour, although with modern white flour, this degradation has leapt off the scale. The original hand grinding with a pestle and mortar caused minimal degradation, with the resulting flour being consumed very soon after, preserving a very high proportion of all the available nutrients. This method of grinding grain and seeds has an unknown length of continuance, possibly extending as far back as the beginnings of our own species, *Homo sapien sapiens*, to any time from 120,000 to 45,000 years ago. There are countless natural depressions in rocks that could have been utilised for this purpose, although being exposed to rain and other erosional factors, the evidence of crushed seeds and grains has long since disappeared.

There is a vast array of novel regional inventions for how best to grind the grain and seeds, using all manner of giant pestle and mortars, predominately rotated by humans or animals. This very manual method was sufficient until around the Byzantium period in Turkey and the Hellenistic era of classical Greece and Rome in the third century BC with the invention of the watermill. It appears that the Chinese came up with similar water and windmills contemporaneously, with there being some inference that the Babylonians may have come up with a similar device as early as 1,500BC, although evidence for this has yet to be found. Large millstones have a tendency to survive in the archaeological record and from current evidence this only extends as far back as a couple of centuries before the time of Christ. The slow yet persistent pressure of the traditional wind and water mills, as well as those using animals steadily turning millstones, resulted in a coarse flour with an excellent range of the nutrient content left intact, which would have degraded only slightly with good storage if successfully kept free from rodents, weevils, damp and water.

In the late nineteenth century, with the increasing industrialization of milling, flour became much easier to mass-produce if the germ was removed. This was because the germ, containing most of the goodness, oxidises relatively quickly and can easily create rancidity throughout the flour. The germ contains the Omega oils and other fats, with a small amount in the bran, with B Vitamins found in both, although only a miniscule amount of this nutritious content is found in the endosperm. Without the germ and the bran, the remaining starchy endosperm produces flour that could last as long as it took the rodents or weevils to eat it, which became less likely, as even weevils cannot survive on white flour alone, which surely shouts out the fact that neither can humans. The germ makes up about 14% of the total weight of a grain of wheat, the bran only 3%, with the starchy endosperm being the remaining 83%. To the early flour producers, this loss of 17% weight was more than compensated for by the advanced longevity that the flour remained sellable, storable and useable. These early industrial millers, one would hope, had no comprehension that their actions were to significantly contribute to future malnutrition and the diseases of civilization.

The white flour made from just the endosperm still had a small proportion of nutrition remaining at the end of the nineteenth century. However, throughout the twentieth century milling became completely mechanized, with the grain getting roller milled with metal rollers at forever increasing speeds. So fast in fact, that since the middle of the last century the velocity of the metal rollers creates temperatures that are high enough to damage the nutrients, reaching temperatures as high as 400 degrees Fahrenheit, robbing what little was left in the endosperm. This is a much higher temperature than when bread is baked, where it only reaches about 170 degrees Fahrenheit. Such modern milling reaches temperatures so high that wholegrain flour is also partially denatured. There is a recognised correlation between these steel rollers and the incidence of duodenal ulcers, caused by the refined flour feeding the Heliobacter pylori bacteria, which today has found an unsuspecting host amongst 50% of humans, this bacteria is being seen as a risk factor for other diseasesd such as stomach cancer.

Neither modern wholegrain, whole wheat or white flours are even closely comparable to the original flours and their full compliment of nutrients available from the traditional methods, for as long as time cares to remember, before the nineteenth century.

Far from being the best thing since sliced bread

None of the health problems that follow appear to have been prevalent when wholegrains were used for bread production. It seems obvious, that if there were such significant associated adverse health problems as there are today with heavily processed flour, the continuity of bread and the growing of grains would not have perpetuated. There is, just as with sugar and dairy, something with modern flour and bread production and its use across so many processed foods that is detrimental, not necessarily the raw ingredients of the flour itself. The start of this problem must have something to do with the amount of nutritious content that is lost with the production of modern white flour, compared with traditionally stone ground whole-grain flour, as a quick look at those nutrients lost clearly indicates.

Amongst the minerals, 89% of the cobalt and strontium, 86% of the manganese, 85% of the magnesium, 78% of the sodium, zinc and potassium, 76% of the iron, 71% of the phosphorus, 68% of the copper, 60% of the calcium, 50% of the molybdenum and chromium and 16% minimum of the selenium (if there is any to begin with) is lost; amongst the vitamins 80% of thiamine (vitamin B1), 75% of the niacin (B3), 72% of the pyridoxine (B6), 67% of the folic acid (B9), 65% of the riboflavin (B2) and 50% of the pantothenic acid (B5) is lost, as well as at least 50% of the vitamin E, if not much more; 95% of the Omega oils and fibre is also lost as is about 35% of the protein (many of these losses are on the conservative end, some studies suggest even greater losses). In total, about 30 nutrients are removed by the refining process, a predicament that early dieticians and nutritionists identified as being a serious health problem for the consumers of these denatured breads, especially as bread (flour) is a staple.

As a consequence, in an attempt to put some of the nutrients back into flour and bread, from the 1930s iron and vitamins B1, B2 and B3 were added. This is known as fortification or enrichment, the addition of what are heavily processed and industrially produced nutrients in an attempt to put a portion of the goodness back that has been removed and or destroyed by processing. There is very little actual biological or scientific evidence suggesting this fortification makes much difference, as the human body has trouble in bio-assimilating these isolated nutrients when they are taken from their original complex web of nutrients. Nature's intricate balance is ripped apart and the picture put back by industrial man is an unrecognizable, pale imitation. In fact iron is very often found in toxic levels in elderly people, a risk factor in encouraging heart attacks, strokes, arthritis, cancer and other age-related illnesses, quite possibly as a result of this unnatural fortification of white flour. From the 1990s, vitamin B9 (Folic acid) has been recognised as a very important nutrient, essential for cell reproduction and is deficient from the average diet, with noticeable health suspicions. Folic acid was therefore the fifth nutrient to be added to this fortification or enrichment, which itself is laughable terminology; if you were robbed of £30 and given a fiver back, would you feel enriched? Instead of educating the public to seek out whole foods that have a natural richness of these essential nutrients, the modern food industry (backed by the modern health industry and the government) assume it is being responsible and caring by harking on about their scientific approach to improving the consumer's health. That's what the advertising might give the impression of what is going on, the biological truth speaks a very different story.

This extends to leading consumers astray and deliberately causing confusion when it comes to relaying the nutritional information in relation to wheat (and other grains) on packaging, or in literature. This is because the nutrient figures given are very often for wheat and other grains in their unrefined, uncooked state, which is totally unrealistic, painting a very false picture, because wheat and most of the other grains are inedible until processed and/or cooked, which results in a sizeable proportion of the goodness being lost. This is when the nutrient content should be ascertained, after production or cooking, as this is the state they are eaten in, not before cooking and processing (the same as the dairy industry using nutrient figures for milk that were determined from grass-fed cows before WWII).

What you are also getting from eating modern bread, which is most definitely not of any nutritious consideration, is the agricultural chemicals (agro-chemicals). In tests, over two-thirds of bread had residues from these agro-chemicals within them, with chlormequat, glyphosate, malathion and primphos-methyl being the most common. These four, as well as most agro-chemicals, if not all of them, are linked to headaches, nausea, heart palpitations, genetic and DNA mutations, as well as being carcinogens. A loaf with a millionth of a gram of these toxins in it will not kill you straight away, although science has never confirmed that these known toxin's bio-accumulation is safe; all science has ever done is confirm their danger, even when consumed in infinitesimal amounts. These agro-chemicals have in fact been blamed as causing a very specific type of intolerance to flour, with the other intolerance to flour coming by way of the proteins and as we are seeing, it is proteins that appear to be causing all manner of problems for the human organism. This brings to mind a quote from Sir Peter Medawar: "The human mind treats a new idea the same way the body treats a strange protein; it rejects it." The meat industry has completely indoctrinated the public about where protein comes from, it certainly is not exclusively from meat; bee stings and snake venom are even types of protein.

Grains provide a good level of protein content, essential for humans, but the modern species, being monopolized by wheat, along with the removal of the nutrients, means that often the only nutrient left is this protein, either gliadin or glutenin and we all know that 'too much of a good thing becomes a bad thing'. This problem with the proteins is looked at after we break the drudgery of bad news with some positivity offered by the healthy substitutes below.

Alternatives to white wheat flour

The reality and health problems of our daily bread being almost exclusively made from refined wheat flour is, as we have just seen, a new one. Flour is merely a powdered state obtained from grinding or milling any of a number of cereals, nuts, grains and seeds. Flour sounds like flower because it is derived from the French, *fleur*, meaning blossom, as well as a reference to fineness and beauty. Flours, producing various textures and versatility can, were and still are made from any of the following:

Amongst the nuts, acorns have an ancient use and no doubt this is connected with the veneration that the oak tree has amongst the earliest mythologies worldwide. Acorn flour was used until well into the Middle Ages in Europe and after, often being the saviour of entire communities when crops failed, its use as a flour is well documented by the Native Americans and is today still used by Koreans. Today we all assume acorns to be poisonous, which is not true, they merely need to be boiled or roasted first (or the crushed nuts soaked in moving water overnight), as with some beans and pulses, while a White oak tree produces acorns that can be eaten raw. Almonds make an extremely nutritious flour, whose flavour and versatility is considerable. Chestnut flour is still popular around the Mediterranean, especially Corsica, where it is made into bread that stays fresh for more than a fortnight, it is also the original ingredient for polenta, as well as several varieties of cakes and pasta. The Romans are responsible for taking chestnut trees with them wherever they colonized, helping spread this highly desirable nut tree across much of Europe (there is some debate about this, as it could also be a natural spreading). Coconut flour, made from the meat of the coconut has fantastic fibre content, excellent healthy saturated fats and a low carbohydrate content, making it a superb and healthy diet choice. Peanuts (which are of course a legume but included here with the nuts as their name causes much confusion) make an excellent protein rich flour with a broad range of amino acids. Always seek out organic peanuts, as often peanuts are used in crop rotation with cotton, the growth of which is responsible for about 30% of total agricultural pesticide usage worldwide, saturating the soil in poisons, to be sucked up later by the peanut bushes (no doubt the cause of the recent rise in peanut allergy, it's not the peanut it's the pesticides causing the problem but the huge agro-chemical corporations swerve the blame with their own highly questionable research refuting any responsibility; a mould found on peanuts has also been blamed for this allergy but this could easily be a part of the cloak and danger techniques employed by the pharma and food corporations). Nut flours were the original flour used in cakes, known as tortes, originating from across Central Europe.

There is a broad range of grains that can be made into flour, including amaranth, a common feature of South and Central American cuisine, with an ancestry as old as the human inhabitants of the continent. Championed by the Aztecs, it is becoming more popular in health stores today across Europe and North America, as is quinoa another early domesticate from the same region, both being rich in protein and other nutrients (quinoa is not actually a grain it is from the *Chenopodium* family, which also includes the beets, chard, spinach and Fat Hen, whose abundant seeds found throughout Neolithic archaeological sites suggest this was an ancient staple. Quinoa has become so popular recently that its price has trebled, worryingly causing shortages and price increases for the locals who depend upon it). Buckwheat (not related to wheat) has a fantastic range of all the essential amino acids and was once, along with barley, one of the most popular flours (being the flour of choice for Christ and his loaves). The demise of buckwheat has been to the detriment of human health. Buckwheat is still used in crepes and pancake recipes, making the popular soba noodle in Japan and the Russian small pancake, blinis, as well as being the only food allowed on many Hindu fasting days across India. Corn, another

South and Central American domesticate was another staple of the old Meso-American cultures, as well as holding special godlike reverence. Rice has been used for both pastries, breads and noodles for centuries in Asia, with an excellent range of nutrients, which sadly today is just another of the Deadly Whites discussed in its own chapter later. Rye has a mixed history, being highly nutritious, with its historical use being predominately from more northern latitudes, where other grains cannot be grown as successfully. Its use in whiskey production spread it across the world, especially to America, although it would appear its initial curse/infamy, was that it was susceptible to fungal infection from *Claviceps purpurea*, known as ergot, from which the hallucinogen LSD was synthesised in the early twentieth century. Literature is heavily biased against this ergot poisoning, it certainly didn't appear to initiate a summer of love as LSD did in 1967, as its effect was seen as the work of the devil in the Middle Ages. Personally, I take all reports of this poison with a pinch of salt, just as the alleged deadly qualities of certain psychedelic mushrooms, whose main danger appears to be showing the truth of heaven and hell and the true dominions of god and Mother Earth, an obvious threat to the Christian pantheon and dominance. Millet has a fantastic although mainly lost history, being native to north Africa and was reputedly used as a staple in China before rice, being very high in nutrients as well as an anti-fungal and one of the least allergenic grains – its use is well overdue a resurgence. Sorghum and Teff, both native to Africa, have long been used there for flours and flatbreads, sharing a similar high nutrient and low allergenic profile as millet. Wheat flour from various wheat species takes many forms, such as durum, emmer, kamut and spelt, all having been used for flour for millennium without the health problems associated with modern wheat flour.

Seeds have also been utilised to make flour, amongst these hemp must be the most important, with its superlative ratio of essential oils and other nutrients, its use diminished undoubtedly because of its association with cannabis and marijuana utilising the flowers, for what is also one of the plant kingdoms best pharmaceuticals, whose criminalisation has been one of the worst 'economic' decisions of the twentieth century. Flax seed shares many unbeatable health qualities along with hemp seeds, as well as many non-food uses, from paper to cloth manufacture, which as with hemp was seen as a threat to the cotton and paper industries (and indeed the health industry) in the early twentieth century. Ancient Indian scriptures state that to obtain nirvana, flax seed has to be eaten daily and that's just on its nutritional capabilities, hemp obviously has more levels of nirvana associated with it. Other seeds such as pumpkin and sesame, can also be made into flour as they contain excellent quantities of nutrients and extremely low allergenic rates.

Legumes have many species that can be dried and made into flour, such as chickpeas, whose main use in European cuisine is as hummus, whose modern supermarket version mixes it with huge amounts of poor vegetable oils rendering it unhealthy and inflammatory. Chickpea flour, known as gram flour, is traditionally used to make several Indian flatbreads such as chapattis, and in Italy it is used for Ligurian farinata (a flat bread very similar in shape to a pizza). Beans such as aduki, broad, various members of the kidney bean family (*Phaseolus vulgaris*), peas and soy all can be dried and made into flour, with various culinary uses around the world.

Even some roots have the capability to yield flour, notable amongst these is Cassava, the source of tapioca, which is essentially dried starch, the same method commonly used to produce potato flour, although the whole potato can be dried and made into flour.

A major problem today is that food is rarely cooked from scratch i.e. from raw ingredients. Flour is hardly ever used and if you wanted to make your own bread it would cost more than a supermarket loaf, so with the passing of the generations since it was common to make your own bread, it is now a novelty to do so, as it would be to make rolls, pasta and pastry from scratch using any of the plethora of flour types above. There would have to be an incredible shift in not just diet but also food production to allow for the flour types above to once again become more commonly used. However, consumer power could champion this, but only if it became economically viable for the food industry to make products from 'alternative' flour, which could within a generation become the norm. Education has to shift in line with diet and this is never going to happen if there is not a shift in the various mechanisms controlling society. The mere fact that most of us associate only wheat with flour, and that talk of any other flour is seen as extreme culinary alternativeness, is most worrying. As these 'alternative' flour varieties are obviously healthy, it has taken considerable expense in marketing to allow the rise of sliced white filth to rule. Such a affective campaign of cultural brainwashing has been undertaken, that those who advocate the real healthy flour types have been ostracized, sidelined as an anarchist, lefty, hippy and dope smoker (even a caveman).

Clearly none of the above varieties of flour warrant any mention in a book entitled The 7 Deadly Whites, although these had to be included as their incredible health and dietary capabilities have been totally neglected in favour of just two grains, wheat and corn, whose modern variants and production leaves us with essentially little less than a poison. The culinary and health injustice is phenomenal and I hope you can see that from the very brief synopsis of alternative flour types above (they also add a pleasant positive aside from the general negative tone so far encountered).

Today, the heavily processed flour from wheat and corn provides in many instances well over half of the diet by weight and calorific content for the majority. The adoption of wheat and corn and its processing has not been done for the health benefit of humans, they have been allowed to dominate only because of the profits that can be made (before mentioning any 'conspiratorial' theories about deliberately dumbing-down the populace, which of course has been one of the convenient consequences of this bias toward processed wheat and corn). Most of the above varieties of flour also have no gluten content, or very little, and thus avoid one of the major food intolerances of today. Even wheat, well known for its gluten content, if consumed in its organic, whole-wheat status, has significantly lower levels of problems for those who suffer from intolerances, as its historical continuance signifies.

Wheat camouflaged

Of course bread is only one of the many uses of wheat flour today. Wheat can also be found as hydrolyzed vegetable protein, dextrins, emulsifiers, modified food starch, vegetable gum, starch or protein, gelatinized starch, natural flavouring and any number of combinations and derivations of these names (although not exclusively from wheat as it could be derived from corn as the more substantive list of corn derivatives indicates in a few pages, which very annoyingly, labelled ingredients do not need to specify the origin of such strange chemical sounding names on the ingredients list).

More obvious food items made with wheat include different kinds of bread (even health store ones with rye and other flour usually have wheat in them as well), crumpets, muffins, pastries, doughnuts, cakes, biscuits, pies, tortillas, pizzas, beer, bouillon and stock cubes, bran, many cereals, condiments such as most dressings, crackers, couscous, semolina, as well as processed meats having a varying percentage of wheat as a filler in them such as sausages, falafel, breaded and deep-fried foods, gravies, ice-cream, pasta, pies, puddings, soups, baking powder, soy sauce, as well as many sweets and chocolates. Non-food sources of wheat include a plethora of cosmetics, bath and hair-care products, medications and vitamin pills, pet food, glue, wallpaper paste and many more.

Means of distribution

As of 2012, global corn production topped the agricultural commodity charts with 916 million tons (mt); wheat weighed in with 675mt, with rice coming in third with 480mt. These three alone give a world harvest of just over 2 billion tons, and when other cereals such as oats, barley, rye, millet, keff and quinoa are included, this world harvest rises to at least 2.5 billion tons. If this were to be divided by the world population of seven billion, there would be an amount of 360kg per person per year, or a kilogram per person every day. As it is estimated that currently only 20% of this grain production makes it to a human plate or dish, this still provides for 200g of grains for every person on the planet every day. This is sufficient (particularly as children eat substantially less), especially if it is wholegrain (and this doesn't include all the vegetables and other foodstuffs that the more wealthy residents can indulge themselves in). I appreciate this is a gross over-simplification, although a good simple example shows that seven billion human beings could easily be sustained from just a few grains (three predominately). Not that the population would have remained at seven billion for any more than half a second, with a global net increase in population of about 80 million per year, or 200,000 a day, or 2.3 every second.

Since the late 1960s the world's grain harvest has in fact trebled, whilst the human population has a little more than doubled, although this excess has more than been used up for in other uses, namely bio-fuels (20%) and an increasing amount of animal feed (35% to 40%), meaning there is less for human consumption than two generations ago. That 35% animal feed equates to about 760 million tons of grain, enough to feed in the region of 2.5 billion people. Cows to put it simply, are not designed to be eating grains, they have very complex digestive systems devoted to grass and herb grazing, and as we have already seen, by feeding them grains the stomachs of cows are as much as a hundred-fold as acidic as they would be if fed grass and herbs. So less cows with better crop rotation incorporating grazing lands equals better fertilised land (from the grazing cows directly fertilizing the fields they graze), as well as better crops and better meat and milk, with far less chemicals being required, so everyone is a winner – a bit of a no-brainer really.

So what made wheat *numero uno*?

The answer has been heavily influenced by the aggressive marketing of the American exported model of bought seeds, fertilizer, pesticides, mono-culture and heavy machinery. In Europe, America and parts of Asia this has not only ruined the natural diversity of the countryside, turning once fertile soils into drug dependent sick soils, this agricultural model has also emptied the villages from what was just after WWII a multitude of small-holdings and resident farmers, all diversifying and contributing to the local community of each and every village. Land that formerly housed several families and fed many more, is more often than not just one giant wheat farm today, employing no staff, only temporary contractors for the planting, fertilizing, combine harvesting and regular pesticide sprayings. The internal infrastructure of the countryside has been pulled away and the people devoted to its sustainability and health have been forced out. As mentioned above with cows and grazing rotation, household management economics is much better off with traditional techniques, where the land and people win, the new form of economics only favours a few global corporations with the land and people being the losers.

Weighty consumption

Returning to the health problems related to the explosion in the consumption of the Deadly Whites. If the average teenager and adult of the industrialized world is consuming over 60kg of the sweet stuff in a year as well as at least 100kg of dairy, refined flour must be topping the scales with a bulging 125kg, if not considerably more every year. These three total a third of a ton of unnecessary food that is eaten every year. These figures represent the lowest estimate for the average adult (as well as being true for most kids), which ignores the fact that many are consuming 225kg of dairy, 150kg of sugar and 275kg of refined white flour, or two-thirds of a ton in a year! If all of that were laid out on a (huge) table it would certainly be a visual shock (as long as the table didn't collapse), especially if it was stood next to the diminutive pile of fresh fruit and vegetables that had been consumed in the same year.

Compounding this dietary excess is the double-edged sword that for many, as their weight increases, their exercise levels drop in an inverse relationship. If exercise levels were to increase in tandem with the consumption of processed foods over-heavy in 'energy' potential, then a large percentage of obesity would never manifest, as the fat stores would be readily converted to energy as exercise regimes increased. Diabetes levels would of course still be rising due to all the phenomenal quantities of insulin required to break down all the processed sugar, dairy, flour and the increase in HFCS. As we know, the buck stops at the exercise regime, with the majority of the public doing less, which is a real shame as exercise level could and would be a contributing factor to the solution as to how to prevent many of the health problems currently occurring.

Some of the problems with white flour

White flour isn't naturally as white as that found in packets, there has been some form of bleaching taking place to achieve this colour. Bleached with a variety of agents such as chlorine, chloride, nitrolysl or benzoyl peroxide (with other chemical salts added), the same bleaches used to whiten paper or clothing, some of which remains as residue, even after the flour has been further heat-treated. These chlorines, especially chloride oxide, combine with whatever proteins are left after refining to produce alloxan. Chlorine, peroxides and bromates are all now banned in the EU, a good thing too, because alloxan is used in laboratories to induce diabetes in animals as it destroys the insulin producing cells in the pancreas. So there was already a well-established scientific link between white flour and diabetes, which the food manufacturers conveniently forgot to tell anyone about. For some reason, the US food safety agencies continue to refuse to ban this chloride oxide.

A few years after the Second World War ended, the Danish government noticed a correlation between the marked decrease in the incidence of cancer, heart disease, high blood pressure, diabetes and kidney ailments amongst those that had been eating only unrefined flour during the war, when all refining had been banned. More recently the Canadian government banned the fortification of wheat flours with artificial supplements and encourages the production of only wholegrain varieties of bread and pasta. The Swiss government recognising the adverse health problems associated with white bread increased the tax on white breads, using this as a subsidy to make wholegrain bread cheaper to produce and buy (a programme which some commentators say has failed to prompt increased sales in wholegrain bread sadly).

This refinement of flour from just the starchy endosperm means the flour is consumed and bio-assimilated (broken down into glucose), causing a sudden rise in blood glucose levels, exactly the same as sugar, thus linking white flour once again with diabetes. It was erroneously assumed for a very long time that only sugar raised blood glucose levels. The mere fact that white refined flour is so similar biologically to sugar, significantly adds to the constant strain the pancreas is under. Refined white flour definitely has causative effects with obesity and heart disease, as well as contributing to the whole list of diseases of civilization, notable amongst these:

White flour raises the level of bad cholesterol (LDL) in the bloodstream, leading to a narrowing of the arteries, resulting in strokes, thrombosis and other cardiovascular diseases, such as atherosclerosis. Refined flour leads to an increase of fat storage and sluggishness, making it even less likely that the fat will be burnt off with exercise. Also the lack of dietary fibre found in white bread can lead to Crohn's, irritable bowel syndrome (IBS) and even cancer of the colon.

Compounding the detrimental health effects of white bread, is the fact that it is made with both sugar and salt, added before the baking process, when milk powder is also very often added. Further complications arise as the bread is frequently eaten with more dairy, in the form of butter and cheese, or heart clogging margarines, with the deadly white of sugar again featuring in the guise of jams and spreads with packaged, processed dairy products almost guaranteed to contain five of the deadly whites. If it has a long shelf life, which invariably processed foods do, they are certain to be chock-full of preservatives and additives, many coming from the earlier processing stages of the grain, as the earlier list of wheat derivatives and the forthcoming list of derivatives of corn indicates.

I can remember making glue at school with just flour and water and when I experimented at home my mum went ballistic at me for blocking the sink and ruining a rug, part of the carpet and a towel after it had dried and set hard as concrete. Well today, these are the ingredients that make pasta, bread, cereals and so much more, and unsurprisingly it still does the same thing, turns to glue in the intestines, with little to no fibre content helping transit, as it clogs the digestive system, hinders digestion and creates a slothful metabolism. Hardly surprising that this creates constipation and painful to pass, hard stools.

The world of gluten intolerance

Many people suffer from gluten intolerances, which is the protein found within wheat, of which those with the highest protein content have been cultivated for bread manufacture, creating the soft and high rising (elastic) loaves preferred today. 75% of this particular type of protein within modern strains of wheat is called gliadin, it is this, more often than not, causing the gluten intolerance when it enters the intestines. This intolerance can manifest as any number of the inflammatory conditions associated with the bowels and digestive system, from Crohn's to irritable bowel syndrome.

About 45% of people in the UK suffer from food intolerance, with wheat topping this list of intolerances. Wheat intolerance differs from coeliac disease, which is a life long allergy to the gliadin protein (gluten) found in wheat (and some other grains), affecting about 1% of the UK population, where even a tiny amount of gluten can cause damage to the small intestine, and continual consumption can allow very serious symptoms to prevail. Coeliac disease can be inherited, and by abstaining from all gluten there will be no symptoms associated with this disease, with a blood test successfully diagnosing the disease. Some symptoms of coeliac disease include bloating, diarrhoea, fatigue, mouth ulcers, vomiting and weight loss.

Other symptoms for gluten allergy (whether it be called IBS or coeliac) include asthma, chronic indigestion, depression, dyslexia, hyperactivity and aggression, infertility, memory loss, muscle cramps and pains (even sarcomas, cancer of the muscles) and schizophrenia. A gluten allergy can begin in the early stages of life during weaning and be a life long condition, the only remission from which is to avoid all gluten.

Another type of allergy to gluten is one caused by the pesticide residue found in wheat. This is an allergy that is becoming far more common due to the widespread use of chemical pesticides and fertilizers and their slow bio-accumulation in body fats throughout the human organism. The human body links this poison from the agro-chemicals as being associated with the protein (gluten), and to protect itself antibodies are created to reject varying segments of the gluten molecules, with each individual person creating antibodies to varying segments in the gluten molecule. This creates difficulty in establishing whether the individual has a gluten allergy, further complicated by the expense of testing for different antibodies, and further compounded by the fact that each grain has its own type of gluten (essentially very similar to the increase in peanut allergy, its not the peanut *per se* causing the allergic response, the peanut is just a carrier for the poison from the pesticide attached to the peanut).

Remediation of this allergy can be achieved by switching to organic grains, although a period of elimination would be required because the body would still reject the protein for a period of time, as it cannot be expected to know the difference between a poisoned protein or a beneficial one, particularly as a previously healthy one was causing the problem in the first place. This gluten allergy and intolerance is just as applicable to all grains containing gluten, and as discussed later there is even more controversy with this as some authorities erroneously label some foods gluten free when in fact they are not, notably corn, which most supposed experts contest doesn't contain gluten. Talk about confusing, it's a veritable minefield of proteins and grains. With regards to the allergic response to glutens caused by pesticides and chemical fertilizers it has to be recognized that for those that eat organic grains, this allergy has a much lower incidence, exactly as would be the case in the past when no chemicals were applied to farming and the associated allergic response was exceptionally low – this is not a coincidence.

Other symptoms associated with gluten intolerance include a form of migratory arthritis, which travels from joint to joint, never staying in one place as is the case with normal arthritis, and can flare up and then disappear periodically. Gluten intolerance can also take the form of peripheral neuropathy, symptoms of which are a loss of sensitivity, a tingling or pain experienced in the arms, hands, legs and feet. Gluten has also been symptomatic of ataxia, a neurological disorder affecting the control of muscular coordination in varying forms of severity. These conditions and ailments are diagnosed by doctors as any number of different diseases, all of which have dispensed varying drugs and creams for, when very often the only real cure is to adhere to a gluten free diet (or at the very least a diet that is free from processed white flour goods).

For those with wheat intolerance, this intolerance could be associated with the whole grain not just the gluten part. There are no hard and fast rules, only individual observation about which other grains, such as rye, barley and oats also cause intolerance. After eliminating certain grains, these may well be successfully reintroduced to the diet with no adverse symptoms, as is the case with many food intolerances. Symptoms of wheat intolerance can range from bloating, constipation, diarrhoea, eczema, fatigue, flatulence, headaches, mood swings and upset stomach. This range of symptoms makes wheat's intolerance very difficult to diagnose correctly, often being confused with any number of other ailments such as coeliac or IBS (as they share a number of symptoms), which itself could be caused by wheat intolerance. Regarding the figures of 1% suffering from an allergy to wheat or its constituent gluten, this alone accounts for roughly 600,000 people in the UK, and it is generally agreed that there is probably a similar amount who have the allergy but have not been diagnosed. This brings the figure up to 1.2 million, but it doesn't end there, because a brief look through the symptoms reveals that these are actually affecting even more people, but only temporarily, which means realistically as many as 2 to 3 million in the UK alone could be suffering various severities of allergies to wheat, a figure that is forever rising, especially for those being adversely affected by the bodily accumulations of pesticide residues. This represents a vast client base for drug companies, a client base that would be diminished considerably if the simple advice of eliminating white flour from the diet was given and adhered to. I just wanted to put that thought out there.

Pitfalls of the Paleo-diet

Many diets today, for instance the Palaeolithic Diet (also known as the Caveman Diet), call for the exclusion of all grains from the diet as the caveman apparently wasn't eating these before agriculture, a fact I would dispute. Being the Culinary Caveman it may be assumed that I would advocate such a diet, but I am also an archaeologist, anthropologist and nutritionist and have many reservations about what is being claimed that our ancestors ate by way of the Paleo-diet (as claimed by nutri-tionists with little to no understanding of prehistoric habitats and diet). I believe the adherents to these diets are merely highlighting such food intolerance or allergies that affects a significant minority, claiming it to be an unnatural foodstuff for humans, which somehow misses the point. Humans have eaten grains for a considerable period and certainly for much longer than agriculture has been around. If we weren't eating them before agriculture appeared they would never have been selected for domestication in the first place, and as mentioned at the beginning of the chapter, we have harvested wild grains of barley for at least 25,000 years (probably much longer), which is over 15,000 years longer than agriculture has been around, which surely indicates that such grains have always been a part of our diet. Today, for those with coeliac and a genuine predisposition to an allergy to the protein found within grains, obviously the grains should be avoided, for the rest of the population, if they were to solely eat organic, wholegrain, unprocessed flours the argument put forward by Paleo-diet adherents would be flawed both archaeologically and biologically.

117

Vegetarian Mahayana Chinese Buddhists, from an unknown antiquity, developed ways of utilising the protein content from wheat for their benefit, making a similar item to tofu from gluten, as their diets may well have been deficient in protein. This isolated protein from wheat is known as mock-duck or seitan today, and is made by washing dough in water until all the starch dissolves leaving the gluten, it can then be fried or cooked any number of ways and can be very hard to differentiate from meat in a dish (being a vegetarian, at times in Asia I have had to question that the meal served in a restaurant really didn't have chicken in it, only to be shown the seitan). There is no evidence that this pure gluten causes, or caused detrimental health problems for the Chinese, nor for that matter did soy, which today receives much bad press about intolerance toward it and associations with breast cancer, which seemingly didn't affect the Chinese. What needs to be understood and emphasised is that it is *modern* denatured flour from wheat that is the danger, and its danger is much worse than merely gluten intolerance. Obviously gluten intolerance by way of pesticide residue is a relatively recent problem, as is diabetes caused by white flour. The facts that white flour clogs digestion, is a factor in atherosclerosis and heart attacks, as well as causing obesity and diabetes are all considerably more worrying than gluten intolerance. I would argue that all white flours should be avoided, whilst people suffering from such intolerances should be better educated about where this stems from. To blame all grains and even legumes, as is the case with Paleo-Diet adherents, is actually erroneous and sends the wrong message about what food we should be eating. If you have no intolerance to gluten, why would it be advisable to not eat organic, stone ground rye bread or peas?

It must be remembered that the vast majority of people who initiate such fad diets are themselves intolerant to certain foodstuffs, hence their evangelist approach in marketing their diets and their rationale in initiating them. For the majority of the population the only thing missing is better education and information regarding the best and safest foods to eat. In this light, no one from any dietary background could reasonably argue that avoidance of all the Deadly Whites is not a practical and safe approach to diet, nutrition, longevity and health.

Corn Walking

All the above is predominately pertinent to only wheat, the flour of which is mentioned in detail for the main of this chapter because in Europe this is the number one flour used. Europeans in the past where predominately wheat eaters, with rye, barley and oats also making important contributions to the diet. This is not the case in the US and South America, where as the Aztecs called themselves 'corn walking', corn is often a major component of the diet. As briefly mentioned in the introduction, derivatives of corn are used in every industry and carry names in ingredients lists that give little or no indication that it may have originally originated from corn, as this slightly more comprehensive list, although still only fractional demonstrates: Acetic acid, alcohol, alpha tocopherol, artificial flavourings, artificial sweeteners, ascorbates, ascorbic acid, aspartame, astaxanthin, baking powder, calcium citrate, calcium fumarate, calcium gluconate, calcium lactate, calcium magnesium acetate, calcium stearate, calcium stearoyl lactylate, caramel colour, carbon methylcellulose sodium, cellulose microcrystalline and methyl, cetearyl glucoside, choline chloride, citric acid, cocoglycerides, crosscarmellose, crystalline dextrose, cyclodextrin, decyl glucoside, dextrin, dextrose, d-gluconic acid, erythorbic acid, erythritol, ethanol, ethylene, ethyl acetate, ethyl alcohol, ethyl maltol, fibersol-2, food starch, fructose, fumaric acid, gluconate, gluconic acid, gluco delta-lactone, glucosamine, glucose, glutamate, gluten, glycerides, glycerin, glycerol, HFCS, hydrolyzed vegetable protein, hydroxypropyl methylcellulose pthalate, inositol, invert syrup, iodized salt, lactate, lactic acid, lauryl glucoside, lecithin, linoleic acid, lysine, magnesium citrate, magnesium fumarate, magnesium stearate, malic acid, malonic acid, malt extract, maltitol, maltodextrin, maltol, maltose, mannitol, methyl gluceth, methyl glucose, methyl glucoside, methylcellulose, modified cellulose gum, modified food starch, mono and di-glycerides, monosodium glutamate, olestra, polydextrose, polylactic acid, polysorbates, polyvinyl acetate, potassium citrate, potassium fumarate, pregelatinized starch, propionic acid, saccharin, simethicone, sodium carboxymethyl-cellulose, sodium citrate, sodium erthorbate, sodium fumarate, sodium lactate, sodium stearoyl fumarate, sorbate, sorbic acid, sorbitol, stearic acid, stearoyls, threonine, tocopherol, triethyl citrate, unmodified starch, vanilla flavouring, vanillin, vinegar, vinyl acetate, vitamins, xanthan gum, xylitol and zein.

What a boring paragraph. Although I trust you get the picture, that just as with wheat, corn is omnipresent and for those with intolerance or an allergy to either corn or wheat, it is nigh on impossible to avoid them without prior knowledge and information about where they might be found. It staggers believe just how so many different ingredients can be made from a cob of corn; you can be sure that the list of deadly acids and chemicals used to obtain the list above is just as long if not more so than the resultant derivatives. It is this modern processing again that is the danger, taking a previously healthy raw ingredient and making it into any number of unhealthy chemicalized ingredients. Incredible as it may seem, irrespective of the exhaustive derivatives, there is one derivative that stands head and shoulders above all the others in its association with risk factors in relation to the diseases of civilization, and that is corn oil, which is dealt with in the next chapter on fats and oils as this chapter is about flour, which may be troublesome enough, but as will be seen, corn oil (and the other vegetable oils) takes the whole problem a very large step further down our devolutionary journey.

This is what links wheat, corn and flour to so many grains and underlines the dangers of them all, as processed foods that have found themselves ubiquitous across the whole food industry. Names on ingredients lists rarely look as if they could be derived from corn or wheat, they can even say gluten free when it's not. It all just makes so much more sense to stick to a whole food diet: a potato is always going to be a potato, just as a leaf of kale and other fresh produce are. Even if poisoned with agro-chemicals, at least it is a good imitation of what a fresh, raw ingredient should look like, and the further a food source can be traced to the grower and the soil it was grown in, the safer the consumer will be. As the consumer is also the general public, this makes good household management on a national level, and when it comes to processed foods it's a lottery, or a dangerous game of Russian health roulette.

All knowledge and information these days is freely available, the only obstacle is separating the truth from the bullshit, and there is an awful lot of bullshit out there, as well as there being an incredible amount of caring people whose only *raison d'etre* is to get the truth to as many people as possible, often not even for any financial gain. You might have bought this book, putting a few pence in my bank account but I genuinely don't care if you borrowed the book or stole it, if it has helped you then my objective has been accomplished.

Wheat does not monopolize gluten

A serious bone of current contention is that unbeknownst to most GPs, dieticians, nutritionists, etc., is that corn also contains gluten, It's not identical to wheat gluten but still its various proteins can cause the same adverse response as wheat gluten. Corn gluten feed was one of the first products industrially made from corn as early as 1882, so the presence of gluten in corn has always been known, the confusion arises because it's not chemically identical to wheat gluten, with its very high proportion of gliadin. This gluten content of corn causes many who eliminate wheat from their diet but not corn to feel despair, as their symptoms have remained exactly the same, and it is all to easy for this to lead to the erroneous assumption that it was never gluten being the root of the reactions. They assume they have cut gluten from their diet, when of course they haven't, if corn has been substituted for wheat, or is still continued to be consumed. Often packaging incorrectly states that corn is gluten free, when all corn products, even those heavily processed such as HFCS, can cause the same symptoms for those allergic to gluten. It is important to point-out that this is not strictly true for everyone, and the elimination of wheat will remedy the gluten intolerance for some, even if corn is still consumed, whilst for others it makes no difference and the suffering continues unabated as long as corn is still consumed. Recent research has shown that corn prolamins (zeins) contain amino acid sequences that resemble wheat gluten immunodominant peptides, these can readily cause the same problems as wheat gluten. Compounding this is the stratospheric rise of genetically modified corn and the use of agro-chemicals on corn crops, and of course the use of corn oil to cook wheat products with. Even something as innocuous as a tin of tomatoes could set off a reaction in someone with a corn (gluten) intolerance, as amazingly the citric acid used in it as an acidity regulator more than likely came from corn, which could lead to the consumer who suffers an adverse reaction to this product assuming it is the tomatoes they are allergic to. It's all so confusing, but it's not impossible to clear the fog, although it's going to be a mammoth task.

With corn and the flour made from it – from all available nutritional profile analysis – it appears that there is nothing like the degradation of nutrients that occurs with wheat flour when milled and processed. In fact, a traditional method of making flour from corn to make tortillas and the like in Mesoamerica, is a process known as nixtamalization, where the corn is soaked in lime (calcium hydroxide not the citrus fruit) or ash (potassium hydroxide), which actually improves the bioavailability of some nutrients, notably protein absorption and niacin (B3), a deficiency of which has been known to cause pellagra that can cause diarrhoea, dermatitis (the disease gets its name from *pella* – skin and *agra* – sour), dementia and death. I cannot refute these results of the minimal degradation of corn flour, although undoubtedly modern methods are far more degrading than ancient traditional ones, especially as nitxamalization is not done on an industrial scale, only the village level. That said, there is no question that corn's gluten content, as well as its pesticide residue, which is still bio-susceptible when in an oil form, will be causing a significant amount of adverse reactions, and it is these that need to be considered when judging what role processing has on extending the probability of falling victim to a disease of civilization. For these, processed corn and its multitude of derivatives is most definitely a factor, not necessarily just the flour from corn.

A common misconception, especially with coeliac disease and gluten intolerances, is that it is not just wheat that is the danger, as just shown with corn, it can also be other grains, such as barley, rye, soy and even quinoa. For all matters gluten, without me going on at length about it, if you feel it affects you please go to www.glutenfreesociety.org and read numerous case studies about this issue, as I could go on and on and still many readers would be tutting and thinking, 'well that isn't what I read' (from ill-informed literature); go and read the truth from those who have been affected by gluten for years and the stories of many doctors, scientists and nutritionists. All I need to do is outline the problems, this book cannot offer detailed evidence and solutions for all diseases and intolerances but it can definitely put you on the right path if required.

It has to be appreciated that one of the major problems with health is often the health professionals themselves. What they have been taught is simply wrong in many instances. This isn't a personal dig against health experts or even scientists, but what needs to be understood is that for every decade that passes, at least 25% of what was considered the truth at the beginning of a decade is by the beginning of the next decade proven to be wrong. This means that a whole quarter of what people thought was true in 2001, turned out to be wrong by 2011, whether it was about sub-atomic physics, archaeology or issues of health and causes of death, all are included in this 25%. This is very important to bear in mind, especially as very often the actual truth doesn't come from those ingrained in a paradigm sect, repetitively taught the same things every year, but from those who are free to roam in all fields of knowledge, as was the role of philosophers in days of *olde*.

Always remember it is personal, we all suffer differently and under no circumstance is there a rule of thumb; if there were it would be this: 'we are all individuals'. Listen to your body and what it tells you when you eat certain food. If you really are at a loss never take the opinion of just your GP, these days you are just another customer to many of them, as is the case with many nutritionists and dieticians, who often work by common denominators, not individuality, i.e. this food elimination or this drug works for 80%, so chances are it will work for you. Triangulate all information from all professionals, if all are saying the same thing then the chance of them being right is increased, but still it's never conclusive, especially as most don't even realise such fundamentals as what food contains gluten and in what food and other non-food items gluten can be found, from toothpastes to sweeteners and even stamps! Only you know yourself as you know yourself, have more confidence and learn how to listen to yourself and have more faith in yourself, as ultimately you will be the winner. To most people you are simply a proportion of an income, and sadly in most instances where money is concerned the truth can so easily be corrupted.

The age of the degenerative disease

It is surely worth considering, that just maybe this huge consumption of processed white flour (and the other deadly whites) is doing exactly as had been predicted, since before the 1930s. That is, damage to the human organism by degenerative diseases. This formative period of twenty or so years, so often quoted as some form of answer to the degenerative diseases, is in many cases just a result of eating processed foods for twenty years. Twenty years of imbalance must be the average length of time it takes before the sub-clinical condition, treated with drugs, with no attempt to halt the real cause, manifests as a disease of civilization, with more drugs available to not cure it. If the drugs were working and were truly the answer, we wouldn't be getting sicker.

So, if most of your diet consists of the above three deadly whites (sugar, dairy and flour), it can be seen that there is very little, if any, nutrition available. The excessive consumption also hinders the bio-assimilation of any nutritious food that may also be consumed, as well as being a very clear, major risk-factor in the diseases of civilization. It is worth mentioning that if the amount of fully healthy, unprocessed bread and unpasteurized dairy (to the tune of a quarter of a ton a year) was consumed, there would be less incidence of the diseases of civilization, just as there was 100 years ago, before most of the detrimental processing took place. If sugar was then eliminated from the general public's diet, how many would still fall sick from a disease of civilization? It's worth giving it some thought surely. Today we have the absolute luxury of having food from across the entire world at our disposal, although in the main our dietary choice is wrong for the simple reason that the above three deadly whites with their negative health associations form the vast bulk of our diet.

Continuing with this consumption of processed food items and the modern day corruption of previously beneficial ingredients becoming nothing short of poisons, we move onto fats and oils and their slippery and hidden role in the escalation of the diseases of civilization. Treading new ground for many from here on in, as most of us with some nutritional savvy know of the inherent problems associated with over consumption of processed sugar, dairy and flour, as these have been long documented, not so the dangers inherent in refined fats and oils. Prepare to be shocked (and I trust informed) as we move onto them.

The Fourth Deadly White

Fats/Oils

"Wherever flax seed becomes a regular food item among the people, there will be better health"
(Mahatma Gandhi 1869-1948, lawyer, activist, pacifist, vegetarian, leader)

If the chapter on sugar was a little confusing in establishing the fact that there are different types of sugar, some being essential for cellular and hormone messaging, whilst others, notably refined white sugar, removes nutrients from the body as well as detrimentally interfering with hormone production (as well as all the other adverse affects), and that energy has little to do with it, this chapter has similar ingrained erroneous cultural 'facts' that need to be erased.

With fats and oils there is a similar duality (some good, others bad), as well as negative consequences from not only the refining but the utilization of incorrect and damaging oils, in addition to the fact that the word 'fat' has predominately negative connotations associated with it, when in reality these natural fats are often essential in establishing and maintaining health. Indeed, this chapter veritably holds the key to opening the door to true health, a door that should be left ajar by its end. However, the opening premise is straight-forward enough, as it is applicable to all the deadly whites so far encountered, that being, take a healthy nutritious raw ingredient eaten for millennia and process it into a modern unhealthy and detrimental food item; although in this instance, even more pernicious is this deadly white, as its use spreads itself through most of the food chain with little thought or understanding of its inclusion and consequences.

There has been a steady succession of the food chain

becoming more processed and contaminated with chemically altered food derivatives, playing havoc with the human organism. The last three chapters may well have made you think twice about eating too much sugar, dairy or white wheat products, which can only be a good thing as their consumption is beyond excessive, needing to be kept to a minimum. These deadly whites adversely affect everyone, with a little bit of the immune system and general health being chipped away with each mouthful. The detrimental attributes of the first three deadly whites are of course well known publicly; the following chapter on oils unveils a web of public ignorance that has been once again instigated by the food industry. Whilst not wanting to scaremonger, here is where the shit truly hits the fan.

Artery clogging, heart stopping

The colour white might not automatically spring to mind when one considers vegetable oil, as the sunflower oil or olive oil used at home is a golden liquid, or at least a mild yellow. What one has to imagine is vast amounts of white margarine, or, rather prosaically, the white scum that clogs piping from the washing up and dishwasher, without even knowingly putting any more than a few drops from the frying pan down the sink, the accumulation on the pipes is considerable after only a year or two. An image that can be easily transposed to the human, with all that fat being produced from surplus glucose production by excessive carbohydrate input, not necessarily from consumption of fat *per se*, although this is also excessively consumed, as we are about to find out. These fats are all being deposited within the arteries, blocking them up like those domestic pipes, as well as being laid down on the thighs, buttocks and bellies, even around the heart and brain. This type of adipose fat, found around the belly and elsewhere, is certainly whitish.

Industrially, fat is not just literally white in colour, it is white as in the other deadly whites, in so much as it is a heavily refined product from a once relatively nutrient rich source, left severely depleted after refining. There is a vast nutritional and health difference between unrefined red palm oil, olive or sunflower oil and the varieties on the shelf of the supermarket, or the cheapest oils made from these to fry say, crisps. The pricier versions found on the supermarket shelf may be less refined, although often the extra price is merely a reflection of advertising, marketing and design costs, not necessarily the quality and health benefits of the contents. A common misconception is that oils are from vegetables and fats from animals, when in fact the only difference is temperature. At room temperature (roughly 60 degrees Fahrenheit) a fat is solid, be it from a coconut or cow, whilst oil is liquid. Although this is not a hard-and-fast rule, it's a handy guideline, because as we will see, often a fat contains oils and oils contain fats, which is only the start of the semantic confusion that swells from this particular topic.

A brief history of oil

A curious thing about vegetable oil is the lack of evidence of this oil until processing takes place. If you crush a walnut in your hand it feels a little greasy but that's about the extent of it. If you crushed seeds, there is little indication that oil is a component. Freshly crushed hemp seeds have a wet consistency but there is no oil as such, the same is true for every other seed, even nuts, crushing these gives the same wet paste.

From the archaeological record, olives appear to be the first vegetable used for oil production found in sites in Israel dated to around 17,000BC, where pits and associated pressing equipment have been found. These were probably wild olives, although as grafting is required to grow a new tree, the ancestry of olive tree cultivation could easily extend this far back. Earlier evidence found at a submerged site located on the south-west shore of the Sea of Galilee (Lake Kinneret), the site of Ohalo, is dated to about 21,000BC, with seeds, grains and nuts from over a 100 different species (from 100,000 seeds found) all adaptable by humans from emmer wheat, barley, olives, grapes and legumes, including flowers and twine being used. Any oil produced was primarily used for oil lamps, and evidence is inconclusive to suggest it was used as cooking oil, although it probably wasn't as we use it today due to the lack of metal pans. Older sites such as Dolni Vestonice in the Czech Republic could have had all plant evidence destroyed from earlier excavations, as is the case with many sites dug in the past, especially before 1980, as pollen evidence was rarely, if ever, the goal, with bones and stone tools being more visible rewards. Pollen analysis here could have shown how advanced the people at sites such as Dolni were 30,000 years ago, where already there is clear evidence for clothing, nets and artistic representation of 'Venus' figurines. It makes perfect sense to assume they were relatively well advanced in food preparation and knowledge in their early civilized life. Fortunately, new forensic and archaeological investigations are meticulously excavated and the evidence will soon surface that our utilization of plants for food, medicine and oils is considerably older than presently understood.

Olive oil was definitely being produced in Southern Europe from domesticated olives on a small-scale by 3,000BC, with the Chinese and Japanese almost certainly producing oil from soybeans by at least 2,000BC. There are no dates currently available for when the Native Americans of Central and South America began to make oil from peanuts and sunflower seeds, although this was almost certainly being done long before Christ. The commonest method to extract the oil from plants would have been to pummel them and boil them in water, skimming off the hot oil as it separates. Olives, coconut, sesame and sunflower seeds are unique, in that to produce oil from them pressing is sufficient, therefore retaining full nutritious content from what is called a 'cold-press'.

A quick note on what can be found on labels claiming to be

'cold-pressed' today, as unsurprisingly the food industry has managed to stretch and distort this term to produce a product that might very well not be as it first seems. A proper cold-pressed oil is the only real 'healthy' stage, as performed before the Industrial Revolution, when the method was to use a weighted press to squeeze out the oil. Today, seeds could be cold pressed and then have all manner of deodorizing and solvents added, although because the first process of crushing the seeds was done with no added temperature, the label can state it was cold pressed, with no indication that everything thereafter was detrimental and far from 'cold'. Even a press produces heat, although traditionally no more than 122 degrees Fahrenheit, whilst modern presses can exceed a damaging and denaturing 212 degrees Fahrenheit.

The residue from the squeezed seeds after the oil is removed is known as the seed cake and is often used as animal feed. Traditionally this would have been an excellent addition to the diet of domesticated animals such as cows and pigs, especially because in the past traditional pressing of the seeds to obtain oil only extracted as little as 10% of the oil from the seeds, meaning 90% was still available to be enjoyed by the animals it was fed to. Today there is little thought or care given to the build up of highly toxic chemicals from the chemical extraction method, which leaves as little as only 1% of the oil in the seed cake to be enjoyed by the animals, coupled with the fact that the dangerous chemicals used in the extraction process readily migrate from the feed to the milk and meat of the animals the seed cake is fed to, with only a miniscule fraction of the oils being available in the meat or milk when ate by humans.

The contraptions of extraction and refining

There was little refinement to this basic extraction process, either cold-pressed or crushed, boiled and skimmed off for millennia, until the 'stamper-press' was invented in the 1600s in Holland.

This was superseded by the early English Industrial Revolution machinations, with the engineer John Smeaton's roll mill being one of the first (a truly industrious fellow, as he also developed bridges, lighthouses, canals and harbours), used to crush vegetable matter more efficiently, used up until this was outmoded by Joseph Bramah's hydraulic press, improved upon in 1876 by V.D.Anderson's 'Expeller', a cage press that used screws and slots to increase efficiency a little further. Up until this time, the resulting oil was virtually unrefined, retaining most of the nutrients. Oil extraction took a turn for the worse in 1856, when the first patent for solvent extraction was given to Deiss of England, with benzene pumped over the presses, draining out of the bottom. This addition of benzene increased the amount of oil that could be extracted, although a known carcinogen, at this early stage of chemical production the resultant oil was not considered fit for human consumption, being used as an industrial lubricant or hydraulic fluid, or to make soaps, cosmetic and skin products, perfumes, paints and wood treatments (linseed and dammar resin are still used for hulls of wooden boats today). Benz's first engine was designed to run on peanut oil and Henry Ford built a car almost totally from soybean plastics and soy synthetic wool, which is where this and the other uses of these oils should have remained. If only . . .

In 1910 corn oil was first processed into cooking oil, with Mazola being available the following year. A year later in 1911 cottonseed oil was first developed, cotton producers were more than happy to turn their waste into oil, sold under the trade name Crisco and was one of, if not the most popular cooking oil until WWII, when soybean oil rose to prominence, itself toppled by Canola in the 1980s. Cottonseed oil has since been shown to seriously interfere with sperm production and the fact that over 30% of all the world's pesticide usage is devoted to cotton growing, flags this oil as potentially, if not severely hazardous. With the development of these oils, any notion of health is dropped and the world of chemistry takes over. Unlike the virgin cold-pressed oils of olive and coconut, the cold-pressed oils from corn, soy, cottonseed and many others are not desirable to taste, and most certainly not desirable to economical viability. So with oils from this juncture all undergoing several stages of processing to obtain what we buy in the supermarket, often being sold by the name 'pure' or even 'natural', this they most certainly are not. Firstly, impurities have to be removed from the oils or destroyed; this term 'impurities' gives the impression these non-pure entities are nutritionally undesirable, which is complete nonsense, as these impurities are often the nutritious elements that have the inconvenient tendency to limit shelf life and go rancid. So out they go, because economics always beats *oikonomia*.

The first stage of refining involves heating the crushed vegetable matter to around 230 degrees Fahrenheit and mixing it with toxic hydroxides and solvents (the four commonest types are a naptha, those being pentane, heptane, hexane and octane, all known lung irritants and nerve depressants), with this the fatty acids form soap, removed by being centrifuged and shipped to the paint, industrial chemicals and detergent manufacturers. Next comes the stage of degumming, where the lecithin is removed, as is the chlorophyll, calcium, magnesium, iron and copper by using phosphoric acid and water at 140 degrees Fahrenheit. Next it is further refined with caustic soda, better known as drain cleaner, to remove any remaining nutrients, usually just proteins by this stage. Next it is neutralized by filtering through what is called 'fuller's earth' (a natural product of clays and earth) – and still there's more, as by this stage it tastes, as one would expect, disgusting, so it is deodorized at 500 degrees Fahrenheit. This turns any remaining unsaturated fats into mutagenic ones, with the trans-fats being produced. All nutrients are now gone, as are most of the pesticides and hydroxides (which means there is some still there, as tests have conclusively demonstrated). As all nutrients are now gone, including those essential antioxidants, some are added to prevent the oil from going off, obviously not the natural antioxidants that were there to begin with, such as vitamins A, B3, C or E or the zinc and selenium, no, of course not, it's easier to just bung some more chemicals in to do this antioxidant business, such as butylated hydroxytoluene (BHT) or butylated hydroxyanisole (BHA).

All this refining produces the standard vegetable oil on sale in the supermarket, sold and marketed as pure, healthy, natural, low or high in this-and-that, just perfect to soak your fresh food in and cook. If that wasn't bad enough, there is still one more refining stage this oil is put through if the desired end product is margarine or other hydrogenated or partially hydrogenated oil (also known as trans-fats). The oil is heated up to 410 degrees Fahrenheit with hydrogen gas passed through it with a metal catalyst, usually a mix of aluminium and nickel, to obtain varying degrees of saturation. This is the sort of saturated fat that gives the natural ones such as coconut and butter a really bad name; there is no comparison biologically or chemically to the above refining process or the pressing of some coconut meat or skimming off the cream from milk and shaking it to make butter.

Trans-fats, pesticides, cells and bells; they need to be ringing

So there we have it, denatured cooking oil, which is usually obtained from fields drenched in pesticides using increasingly genetically modified crops, with traces of the pesticides and BHT or BHA still in them (all proven to be genetic mutagens and carcinogens, linked to kidney and liver damage, immune problems, infertility and behavioural problems in children). The margarines and other partially or fully hydrogenated fats, with their traces of pesticides, BHA or BHT and aluminium, are free to perform not only cheap cooking potentiality, they can also interfere with biological processes, almost guaranteed to in fact, as we are eating on average over 35kg of these every year (with many eating 75kg and more). Crucially, on a biological level and on the fundamental cellular level, these cheap processed fats have real trouble being broken down and change the permeability of cell membranes, damaging the protective barrier of the cell, allowing molecules that shouldn't be allowed into a cell to enter (such as the aluminium, pesticides or BHT) and allowing what's in the cell to leach out. Trans-fats also interfere with the energy and electron exchange reactions, often preventing the electric charge to give life to a cell, hampering a healthy flow of energy. All commercial oils are to some degree a trans-fat, as the molecular structure has been transformed (always for the worse, never better) in its manufacture due to the heat used; the extreme for a trans-fat is when it is fully hydrogenated.

After all the fuss made about them a decade or two ago, you would have assumed hydrogenated fats no longer exist. NO, industry has just changed the wording to mask them, increase consumer confusion, whilst doing sweet f-a about the detrimental ingredients. The words hydrogenated, partially hydrogenated and trans-fats rarely appear on labelling today, as consumers are rightfully weary of these, although words such as vegetable fat, mono, di-, or triglycerides have slipped in and reveal the very likely presence of hydrogenated/ trans-fats. There is no doubt that trans-fats increase natural cholesterol production, raise low-density lipoproteins (LDLs), with the new bad one going by the name of apo(a) or LP(a), and therefore are directly linked to coronary heart disease (CHD), raising serious reservations that the advertisers are clearly and falsely proclaiming their products to be healthy. Even if they have added a little olive oil or Omega-3, it is still nothing short of a dietary poison, as the refining process turns all fats into varying degrees of trans-fats.

The last two paragraphs I hope were clear, as it is within these that the real danger of these new cooking oils and margarines lurk, and it has only been since the 1950s that these have been marketed so strongly, all because of an erroneous and misinterpreted scientific report, which we'll be looking at after a brief summary of the history of margarine. I will be returning to the content of these last two paragraphs, as the fundamentals of health originate from the cellular level; if the cell is not healthy then neither is the sack of skin and bones comprised of billions of these cells, otherwise known as a human or any living thing.

Merci for the marge Messieurs Mouries et Bonaparte

Margarine, in its format as an alternative to butter, was first initiated by Napoleon III, setting a competition for a cheap source of fat that could outlast butter, won by Professor Hippolyte Mege-Mouries in 1869 with a mix of beef fat and skimmed milk. Reputedly tasting foul, which is not hard to believe, the future for this alternative to butter thus begun its journey, which today has different ingredients but still leaves a foul taste in the mouth and mind, even more disagreeable than its original. I shan't be using information from the Unilever site for this brief summary, a company that has been instrumental in the production and promotion of margarine since its Dutch founder bought the patent in 1871, but I shall give a couple of nuggets from their website: "Today's margarine is a nutritious food, part of a healthy balanced diet . . . its true nutritional power comes from the fact that it is a vegetable" and "Margarine consists of three ingredients: the best plant oils nature can provide . . . blended to contain essential fats... and water." So I must be wrong then and all the above chemical refining is just made up, as the professionals clearly state they only have your health as their focus. It just goes to show how easy it is to bury the truth within a semantic broth.

You've been an abhorrent scientific tease, Ancel Keys

Since Mege-Mouries' concoction, margarine has changed drastically, with the lard component gradually being phased out in favour of vegetable ingredients, usually sunflower or olive, done so with a big fuss being made by the producers, highlighting the polyunsaturated fats included, if only to a few percent, whilst moving away from saturated fat. This kerfuffle involving saturated fats was instigated by several scientific statements published in the mid-1950s by Ancel Keys, based around a growing suspicion at the time of a direct link between serum (blood) cholesterol levels and the incidence of coronary heart disease (CHD), stating it was all fats, with no distinction between animal or vegetable, which both raised this serum cholesterol level. Keys also stated saturated fats raised serum cholesterol levels and polyunsaturated fats lowered the level, whilst also specifying that it was hydrogenated vegetable margarine, shortening and animal fats that were the villains, with this last bit of Keys' statement being ignored by the makers of margarine, who pinned their marketing around Keys' alleged fact that saturated fats increased cholesterol, whilst polyunsaturated ones decreased it. Here was a clear corridor of corrupted scientific hyperbole that could be utilized to increase sales, whilst at the same time demonize the competition from the saturated fats of butter, animal and coconut. His research, the only one to make the correlation, was picked up by the food and health industries to prove the links between fats and cholesterol and heart-health; the fact his research has been disproved repeatedly and his methodology was completely unscientific seems to make little difference, as for some incredible reason the myth continues to perpetuate as an alleged biological and scientific fact, underlining the power of money and marketing.

Consider the diet of the Inuit, their fat consumption is astronomical although they have little heart disease; how can this be so? Are the Inuit somehow different to the rest of the human race? Of course not, that would be an absurd statement, the only adverse association they have is with higher rates of osteoarthritis. When Ancel Keys conducted his research in the 1950s, he simply threw away any evidence that contradicted his flawed lipid theory. He should have been arrested and put in stocks and publicly humiliated, instead of being lauded and put on the cover of Time magazine, paraded as a top scientist and allowed to revel in his fame. It is well overdue that this theory is thrown away, just as the ones involving sugar and energy, calcium and milk and meat and protein should be also. Ultimately, Keys and the skewered reportage of his results are responsible for millions of deaths from heart disease.

Using Keys' flawed science as an endorsement, the margarine manufacturers incessantly lobbied the US government emphasizing it was imperative for the nation's health that saturated fats were eliminated and their hydrogenated products, with some polyunsaturated fats thrown in, were put forward as the best and healthiest alternative to alleviate the problem of heart disease, a disease that had indeed began to see dramatic rises in incidence (although as we have already discovered, this rise can be more readily attributed to the surge of all the processed deadly whites that occurred after WWII, heavy in glucose production, whilst the consumption of saturated fats had remained fairly constant throughout the twentieth century). Several extensive scientific research results have shown that saturated fats are not to blame, as reported in the 1990s from the American Journal of Public Health and results from the massive Framingham experiment in Massachusetts in which the exact opposite was clearly demonstrated: for those who ate the most saturated fats the lower the serum cholesterol levels were. Evidence that merely corroborated a symposium of cancer specialists in Rome as long ago as 1956, when extreme caution was called for in allowing modern vegetable oils to enter the human body, as the association with cancers was already well established, let alone the associations with heart disease.

PUFAs

Some of the problems inherent with polyunsaturated fats (PUFAs) start at the most basic biological level, the cellular one, especially as the body needs fats for building and rebuilding cells and hormone production. When the body is presented with the wrong fats, by way of polyunsaturated ones instead of saturated ones (and monounsaturated ones to a lesser extent) it has absolutely no choice but to make do with these. The problem with using these undesirable polyunsaturated fats to make the lipid membrane of each and every cell is that they are highly unstable, and if they haven't already begun to oxidize and mutate whilst sitting on the shop or cupboard shelf or when used for cooking, they can easily do so when they have been intricately combined within cells, causing inflammation and mutation, allowing free-radicals to enter the cell and cause all manner of mayhem. In arterial cells these mutations can cause inflammation, clogging arteries, and when incorporated into skin cells, if they become mutated, skin cancer can be a possible result (the sun may cause skin cancer in some instances, the fact we think it is the only cause is because of the marketing and indoctrination from the sun-screen makers). Rats fed saturated fats did not develop skin cancers until their diet was switched to PUFAs. When these cells, made up with PUFAs are incorporated into the reproductive tissue, cancers and endometriosis can manifest here in the same way. Especially prone are these areas, as it is here that cell reproduction and division is far more common, as well as of course adversely affecting the growth of foetus's, whose cells are dividing at an extremely high rate, with the potential for mutation also increased as the foetus has absolutely no choice but to use the fats consumed by its mother. This damaging aspect of PUFAs is also applicable with hormone production, interfering in an infinite number of ways with optimum hormone manufacture.

The consumption of PUFAs has also been implicated in the inability to learn, depressing both mental and physical development as well as with mental decline, chromosomal damage and accelerated aging. When these incorrect fats are repeatedly and excessively consumed, which they are for the vast majority, damage to the intestines is also a likely outcome. When this damage is coupled with excessive consumption of the other damaging deadly whites of sugar, flour and dairy, there should be no surprise that the body reacts with a whole plethora of allergies, intolerances and auto-immune diseases. There have been numerous studies that have clearly shown that PUFAs stimulate the development of cancer, as these break down to cancer causing free-radicals, whilst saturated fats have been shown to not do this as they are far more stable, especially as saturated fat is the type of fat the body was expecting to be delivered to it to perform its intricate biological work. The Framingham Heart Study found that over the twenty years of their study, for those participants who increased their margarine consumption, heart attack incidence rose in line, but for those eating butter, heart attacks actually declined, although this was only noticeable after twenty years. This shows the importance of long-term human studies, which as we shall soon find out in the Canola case study in a couple of pages, have not been conducted on this refined rapeseed oil.

All this clearly demonstrates that the consumption of an unnatural and unexpected fat by way of these PUFAs for the body to deal with can lead to all forms of havoc on a cellular level, especially as the cellular level is the starting block for everything pertaining to life and health. It is no coincidence the field of medical cardiology didn't even exist until the mass production of polyunsaturated cooking oils. None of which would be apparent if the cooking oil industry was left to its own devices, left free to run all sorts of spurious marketing and health claims for their products, which of course it has been allowed to and done exactly this . . . Whoops!

Collective cholesterol confusion

Cholesterol was focused on by the margarine makers and still lingers in the mind because it was one of the only, if not the only word that could be lifted from the biological sciences to render the new margarine as being unique and different, being as it was dietary free from cholesterol. As margarine comes from a vegetable origin it has no cholesterol, as this is only derived from animal sources, so this word was the one targeted and used as some form of panacea for well-being. This is ridiculous, it's worse than marketing an apple as being vegetarian or gluten-free. The fact that the body produces cholesterol as a defence mechanism from margarine consumption, elevating bodily cholesterol went conveniently unmentioned by the margarine producers.

If the confusion the public is caught up in wasn't complex enough surrounding the fats: Which are the essential ones? Which ones cause human adipose fat? and a thousand other bogus claims, the real biological facet that gets continually shoved from pillar-to-post has to be cholesterol, whether it is high or low, whether the diet has too much and from where it comes from. The only straightforward answers appear to be coming from the margarine makers and the pharmaceutical corporations, and their answer is to get as many people as possible onto their products and drugs that help to lower choles-terol. So what on earth is this cholesterol stuff and why should it be low?

Primarily, cholesterol is blamed for atherosclerosis, strokes, heart attacks and high blood pressure, this is because it is a waxy lipid (which means fatty) substance and it's easy to imagine this substance causing blockages throughout the bodily system.

Cholesterol is made in the body by breaking down sugars, fats and proteins, there is no need to actually eat cholesterol rich food and here begins the confusion, as in many instances dietary input has little affect on the production of cholesterol. The fact that our present diets are super rich in sugars and fats is clearly an easy target to say that we are eating too much cholesterol inducing foods, which is kind of unarguable, but it hardly scratches the surface of what we need to know about cholesterol.

Cholesterol is used to maintain membrane fluidity and each cell has the ability to control its own membrane fluidity, so important is this steroid alcohol, cholesterol. Cholesterol is also used for the production of sexual steroid hormones such as oestrogen, progesterone and testosterone and the anti-inflammatory adrenal corticosteroid hormones, Vitamin D and the bile acids, as well helping with the breaking down of the fats. The skin also uses cholesterol for protection from the elements and growth, as well as it being used as a vehicle to transport antioxidants around the body, a task impinged by there being a dietary deficit of such antioxidant nutrients as vitamins A, B3, C and E and the minerals selenium, zinc, copper and sulphur, whilst being excessive in the foods that produce cholesterol. As the modern diet is deficient in these antioxidants, cholesterol is perpetually forced to do a job it should only be doing as a last resort, hence why there is constantly an elevated cholesterol count within the arteries and blood. Another job that cholesterol does as a last resort, is that it is used as a bandage to help heal damaged arteries, which are regularly put under strain from the constant acidosis and osmotic pressure from sugar and salt and the processed foods, cigarettes, lack of exercise and excessive animal protein in the diets. This was clearly and meticulously researched and reported in Dr Campbell's 'China Study'. Epidemiological research reveals the stark truth about cholesterol, showing it is low cholesterol levels which have a direct association with mortality; a sentence the makers of statins, the world's number one sold pharmaceutical drug, certainly don't want to be reading or hearing, even if it's the truth.

I know loads of people who have high cholesterol counts, who also claim their diets are low in cholesterol foods, and so are somewhat puzzled, although of course as just mentioned, serum cholesterol is not dependent or necessarily caused by dietary cholesterol. Just being stressed causes more cholesterol to be produced naturally, with stressed in this instance including mental, physical and dietary stresses. The biggest damage caused daily by many adults is the consumption of alcohol, which when drunk (even a pint of beer or a glass of wine) dissolves the fluidity of the cell's membrane, causing cholesterol to be produced, used to re-stiffen the membranes. As the alcohol blood levels return to normal (i.e. none) this cholesterol is ejected from the membranes by essential fatty acids (EFAs) and taken to the liver where it is turned into bile and can be allowed to pass through the digestive system. This natural process is inhibited severely by too much fat consumption, too little fibre, the wrong balance of EFAs and not enough vitamins and minerals to make the bile. This is why even vegetarians can have high cholesterol, because of alcohol consumption, as dietary cholesterol is only present in meats, egg, fish and dairy (although many vegetarians do eat plenty of dairy and eggs). As these foods rich in cholesterol are eaten excessively today, the body produces less cholesterol naturally to compensate, although without the full compliment of vitamins and minerals (notably the antioxidants) this is inhibited and the liver cannot cope and too much bile is produced (acid indigestion), and/or not enough fibre is eaten (processed foods have none or very little) to push it out, meaning the cholesterol is reabsorbed, hence why fibre is so important as it constitutes a vital component of cholesterol levels.

All that is needed to be understood from this chapter regarding cholesterol, is that cholesterol consumed via the diet is not necessarily linked to such diseases of civilization as CHD, of more importance is there being the correct nutrients to absorb cholesterol, utilize it and eliminate it. It is no coincidence that a diet high in meat is deficient in the vitamins and minerals and fibre required, as the human body is not designed to eat a diet of mainly meat. The fact it can survive on one and adapt (such as the Inuit) is because of the versatility of humans, a factor that has insured our continuance on this planet, not because we have ever been carnivorous. As a rule (from present anthropological observation) when living in our preferred environment, such as a Mediterranean one, or even ones more marginalised such as the grasslands and jungle, our natural diet is 80% vegetarian, and being a vegetarian living in the wild does not mean endless salads made from iceberg lettuce, white spaghetti and soy mince and other nutrient depleted items the average vegetarian eats in Shoreditch or Brighton; a foraged diet means a diet of mineral and vitamin rich, deep green plants, berries, seeds, nuts and roots.

Double winner of Nobel prizes for Chemistry and Peace (the only person to receive two unshared), Dr Linus Pauling, states that it is Vitamin C that is crucial in many of the diseases of civilization, and as such with cholesterol it is a key antioxidant in its absorption and elimination. Vitamin C needs to be eaten as we cannot make it ourselves, and this is best sourced from greens and fruit. Pauling was very into vitamin C, perhaps a little obsessed, but his orthomolecular diet in particular and his intellect and views are definitely not to be derided, only admired.

Getting it all wrong

After wrongly attacking saturated fats, the makers of margarine, who had switched to using as much polyunsaturated fat in their margarines as possible, the epidemiological analysis came to show that when these margarines had taken the market share previously held by butter, lard and coconut fat, there was an associated increase in the incidence of heart disease that had already begun to rise with the increased consumption of the processed deadly whites. The one ailment margarine was touted as helping with, actually saw an increase in incidence with an increase in consumption of this product, in exactly the same light as the ascribed benefits of dairy, improving bones and teeth, actually contributes to a similar associated increase in the very diseases it was meant to help with, namely osteoarthritis and teeth cavities. Dare I say industrial hypocrisy? Oh, I just did!

With regards dietary cholesterol intake being blamed for heart disease, consumption has stayed roughly level for the past century, although cancer has increased 500% and CVD 300%, so its unlikely cholesterol is a direct cause of these. In relation to atherosclerotic deposits (atheroma), the general composition of these is actually made up primarily from polyunsaturated fatty deposits not saturated fatty deposits, which surely underlines the incorrect stance of the margarine and anti-saturated fat lobby. Another very important consideration to understand is that the total fat deposits throughout a fit and healthy human, especially those of the superlative specimens of humanness that are exhibited by many present hunter-gatherers, is the fact that the human body is comprised of 97% saturated and monounsaturated fat and only 3% polyunsaturated fat.

Types of fat and a very important point

Just a very quick word on what the difference is between a saturated fat, polyunsaturated fat and a monounsaturated fat. The differences are not essential to understand but will probably help a little if not understood already, particularly as we are too infatuated with the polar mechanisms of good/bad, black/white, rich/poor, healthy/unhealthy. It is all to do with how the molecule is formed for these fats, made up of chains; some have no more chains or bonds that can be added to, these are the saturated fats, and because nothing can be added to them they are considered stable, with no room for free radicals to latch onto and attack; those with bonds still available are the monounsaturated fats, with one carbon atom free to be attacked by free radicals and subsequently oxidized; whilst the polyunsaturated fats have many free bonds and as such are much more likely to be affected by free-radicals and oxidized (in the body, in the bottle or from processing). What these chains are made of and what changes them is too much information for the general readership (and for my brain to fully comprehend and to translate into simple English for you, sorry), if you are chemically minded no doubt you already understand the difference. With these fats it is not always possible to simply state that the entirety of one type is bad while all the others are good, this only adds to the confusion of this whole topic. Very simply, all that needs to be understood is that of all the fats, the human body is capable of making all of them from dietary sources, except the Omega-oils, which is why these are called the essential ones, so these are required to be eaten for the body to utilize them and make other acids (which is what the fats are, fatty acids) from these; the shorter the chain, especially of a saturated fat, the easier it is for the human organism to convert to other required fats and acids. The inference here is that we can turn the famous saying 'You are what you eat' on its head, as it is still applicable to say 'What we are made of is what we should eat'.

If the above statement is true, as there are no vegetable polyunsaturated fats naturally occurring in the human body, let alone hydrogenated ones, it makes sense that these shouldn't be allowed to enter the body as there is no biological use for them. A statement, which if you break it down is true for all dietary components from minerals to vitamins, whilst those we don't have any of are alien and dangerous, such as many types of protein and the heavy metals such as mercury and lead. So what are we doing eating over 35kg of PUFAs a year that are not a part of the natural human body? Particularly if one considers that half of the brain consists of saturated fats and cholesterol, as does the myelin sheath protecting all of our nerve endings, with saturated fats making cells more resistant to oxidation, whereas the polyunsaturated fats are easier to become oxidized and turned into cell damaging free-radicals. Consumption of saturated fat also increases the levels of high density lipoproteins (HDLs), whilst helping to lower the LDLs, notably the new baddie, LP(a). Many of these fatty acids are the basic building blocks of not just proteins, but all life, especially lauric acid, butyric acid, myristic acid, palmitic acid, stearic acid and caprylic acid, all found in good quantities in those food items attacked by the polyunsaturated fat oil producers, such as butter and coconut oil, which have seen a reduction in consumption, whilst the illnesses these allegedly were risk factors in have seen no change in incidence (apart from increasing in prevalence).

We as humans are fortunate that we can eat foods that are both extremely rich in nutrients as well as food that is extremely rich in calories. Problems arise from the food consumed that is energy dense, as once found less time needs to be spent grazing and seeking further food. A natural reward system in the human lets us know we have found an energy dense food by way of a pleasurable hormone release. This natural reward system is still part of our biological make-up today and sadly such carbohydrate and fat dense food now forms the majority of our diet with little to no education given that the energy poor food is actually what we should be today seeking, along with wholegrain bread, nuts and seeds which satisfy this energy dense aspect. The diet eaten by the caveman and the present hunter-gatherers should carry the flag as to what represents the optimum diet for us today, but even this has been buried under levels of confusion, and not helped by the plethora of diets claiming that the diet of the caveman or hunter-gatherer as being the embodiment of them, such as the Origin diet, the Atkins diet and the Paleo-diet, which claim a meat heavy diet is what our ancestors ate and avoided all grains and legumes and other foods grown since the agricultural Neolithic revolution. Which makes me as a caveman most angry, because we have been obviously eating and enjoying many of these plants for an enormous length of time, before environmental and or population pressures made it necessary to domesticate and control the quantity and availability of our staples. The archaeological proof is there, in every site dated before the agricultural revolution where pollen analysis has been carried out; there is ample evidence for wild wheat, barley, rye, oats and corn, all utilized long before they became part of our agricultural conquest. After all, it makes little sense to domesticate the plants and animals not already part of our diet, especially those ones that cause ill health; as repeatedly stated thus far, it is only the modern refined and heavily processed foods that have clear detrimental associations with their consumption, not the natural whole foods.

Monounsaturated fats must be the answer

The move of the government health agencies in the 1950s and 1960s, coerced by the makers of margarine and cooking oils, to believe that many of our ills in the west were because of too much saturated fat adversely affecting our cholesterol levels and ultimately resulting in deaths, notably from heart disease, didn't end too well with the transition to polyunsaturated fats. If an increase in the prevalence of the very disease it was meant to inhibit can be said to have not ended 'too well' is of course a massive understatement, as it proved to be a shambles (to clarify what incidence and prevalence are: incidence can stay the same as this is a measure of the percentage afflicted, whilst prevalence can increase as this is total number afflicted and as the population has almost tripled since the 1930s, so prevalence can rise massively even if incidence stays the same, these two words are frequently used interchangeably to distort statistics). So it was back to the drawing board. The only fats left to consider were the monounsaturated ones, such as the one found in olive oil, oleic acid (Omega-9), whose consumption has been enjoyed for millennium, with many stories about its consumption being a crucial part of the Mediterranean diet, partly explaining why heart disease is much lower for those living around the Mediterranean Sea. Olive oil is problematic because there simply is not enough of it to fulfil the world's demand for cooking oil and its price is far too prohibitive for the cost-cutting fundamentals of the food industry. Another monounsaturated oil that had enjoyed a long continuance of use without too many health problems attached to it was rapeseed oil, commonly used throughout Asia. Perhaps this monounsaturated rich oil could be the key? It certainly could be brought in line with the modern agricultural model of huge mono-cultural fields, pesticides, fertilizers, patented seeds and expensive machinery, sold by a few dominant American and European global corporations. So out went the PUFAs and in came the MUFAs.

A conspiratorial case study on Canola

Rapeseed derives its rather unfortunate and poor marketing name from its Latin name, *rapa*. The Canadians came up with one of the first GM crops (not so much the Canadians, but our caring sharing friends at Monsanto and Bayer). Allegedly managing to get the FDA to pass it as GRAS (Generally Recognized As Safe) in 1985 with a $50 million sweetener, research grant or backhander. Since then, it has become a major export for the Canadians, of which canola adds $11 billion to the Canadian economy annually, with the government leading a propaganda campaign on a par with the Milk Marketing Board. Canola obtained its GRAS status without even any tests on humans, with those that had been conducted on animals being far from positive.

Rapeseed oil is about 60% monounsaturated fatty acids (MUFAs, olive oil is 70%), 60% of which is erucic acid, which had been mistakenly associated with Keshan's Disease in parts of

Asia, although selenium depleted soils appear to be a far greater risk factor for this disease, coupled with a deficiency of saturated fats to deal with the high (10%) Omega-3 content of unrefined rapeseed oil. This 10% Omega-3 content made marketing this oil much easier to those who are more health-conscious (as Omega-3 has been seen as the healthy EFA for some time now), especially as the modern diet is severely excessive in Omega-6, which should be consumed more in balance with Omega-3. So without much other thought, plant breeders developed a variety that had a low content of this erucic acid, coming up with Canola, getting its name from CAnadiaN Oil Low Acid, the acid here being erucic, which studies on rats showed when fed as a significant percentage of their diet by way of rapeseed oil, left fat deposits on the heart and scar tissue when it finally cleared, leading to worries about the effect on humans. It was deemed unsafe for human consumption, so a low erucic acid version was developed to prevent Keshan's and heart lesions. Very responsible one might assume, until one understands that exactly the same test was done replacing the rapeseed oil with sunflower and safflower oil, with exactly the same result, so the erucic acid was not at fault. Part of the blame is that rats digest and metabolize fats very differently to humans, coupled with the excessive, unbalanced Omega-3 intake, but what the heck, after spending so much money and time on research it was deemed best to keep this quiet and hang on to the name canola, as it had such a good ring to it and it looked excellent on paper as a healthy option, why confuse the consumer further with the truth?

With the FDA approval of canola in January 1985, large swathes of the US and Canada were planted with genetically modified (GM) rapeseed. It took a few years of exhaustive marketing by the producers of canola, organizing scientific conferences, product placement and promotions to top taste setters and influential consumer personalities, plugging the monounsaturated Mediterranean diet's health benefits (even if it is olives not rapeseed that has positive results) with books such as 'The Omega Diet'. Meaning by the late 1990s the worldwide use of canola had soared, its growth as a cash crop has continued to rise, helped by its ease to grow in the more arid climates of Australia and Canada and much of northern Europe. It is even available hydrogenated for frying, which of course removes any beneficial nutrient content, replaced with detrimental risk factors for a number of diseases. With its rise there was a fall in demand for what had been the number one oil before, soybean oil, which provides for an even more intriguing and concerning case study, looked at next.

Relatively easy to grow, the rape plant acts as a natural insecticide, which makes growing it even easier. Rape is a member of the mustard family, *Brassica*, which includes broccoli, cabbage, kale and turnips, amongst others, all well known as being exceptionally healthy. Rapeseed oil's main use was as a lubricant, fuel, soap, rubber-base and as the glossy sheen on magazines, before the drive to push monounsaturated fatty acids as the new health food. It has fantastic penetrative qualities, which might be great for an engine or machine but in the human body it manages to penetrate just a bit too much when it gets refined and the essential nutrients and antioxidants are removed. Of course there is no 'proof' for the following, because the human studies have not been carried out, although it appears on what can only be termed hearsay evidence so far, that so good is this oil at lubricating it can strip away the myelin sheath that protects all nerves, which is similar to stripping all the insulation from the wires in your home, leaving the wires bare. This loss of the myelin sheath has recently been associated with multiple sclerosis, arrhythmia, palsy like shaking, memory loss, blurred vision, hearing loss, lack of coordination, incontinence, an increased sensitivity to electromagnetic radiation, food and clothing allergies, shortness of breath, nervousness and a numbness to the extremities. Symptoms that have been repeatedly witnessed since the introduction of canola to the food chain, that coincidentally stops, when consumption of refined rapeseed oil ceases. Such allegations have been largely ignored, because just as with aspartame, canola has been awarded a GRAS and until extensive, expensive, long-term studies prove otherwise, the use of rapeseed oil will continue unabated. What has been established, is that this loss of the myelin sheath can take up to ten years to occur, within which time all manner of other detrimental entities could be blamed, rightly or wrongly. Rapeseed oil has even been linked with Mad Cow Disease, with cows becoming blinded and turning crazy, symptoms closely associated with this loss of the myelin sheath, as it leads to serious communication failure down the nerves, adversely affecting not just mental faculties, but also motor messages to move and chew etc. When rapeseed oil was removed from the feed, the disease ceased. Coincidence? Jury's out.

Canola appeared to easily float above all this, as the propaganda was shouted so loudly and expensively about the oils apparent health benefits, especially its monounsaturated fats, Omega-3 and vitamin E content, with any of the negative results from scientific research also being easily brushed aside. Any health benefits obtainable from unrefined rapeseed oil are irrelevant when it is refined, heated to over 350 degrees Fahrenheit and mixed with hexane, as these nutrients are destroyed and mutate to less healthy acids, even detrimental ones. Studies on piglets have also shown canola to actually deplete vitamin E within the body; when the piglets were fed canola, vitamin E deficiency occurred, even though vitamin E was added to the diets at adequate rates, there was also a decrease in the platelet count and an increase in the platelet size (both not good), changes that were mitigated when saturated fats from cocoa butter or coconut oil were added to the piglet's diet. The growth retardation problems associated with canola are well established, which accounts for the FDA still not allowing canola oil to be used in infant formula drinks (I can't associate the word milk with these nasty drinks for our little loved ones, as already shown in the Milk chapter). All studies tend to agree that the high levels of Omega-3 and the low levels of saturated fats appear to be the problem with unrefined rapeseed oil, not erucic acid (there are no independent research results that flag erucic acid as a danger, go check out Lorenzo's oil if you haven't heard of that or seen the film with the same name), not that this made any difference with the promotional machinations for canola. Even Omega-3 consumed excessively when done so with saturated fats helps the body convert the Omega-3 into longer chain omega-3 fatty acids, such as EPA and DHA, a conversion that is adversely affected with less saturated fats in the diet and more Omega-6 (Omega oils will be looked at after this canola, or is that, con-ola story). Animal research from the very late 1970s and still continuing, seriously undermines the health claims espoused by the canola producers, certainly about any heart-health benefits. Studies tend to enforce the notion that saturated fats are protective against heart lesions, whilst high levels of Omega-3 correlated to high levels of heart lesions.

Chinese studies have linked lung cancer in women as being caused by the high temperatures rapeseed oil achieves in a wok. Which after such heating contains the carcinogenic and mutagenic compounds, 1,3-butadiene, benzene, acrolein and formaldehyde. There is no mention if there has been a switch to refined oils from unrefined ones helping to account for this incidence of lung cancer. Historically and epidemiologically, it is near impossible to substantiate, but it appears that this increased incidence of lung cancer is only a recent phenomena and more than likely is determined by the use of refined oils not the traditionally unrefined oils. Also by switching to rapeseed oil from traditional ghee, butters and coconut fats, the diet has become deficient in saturated fats which would have acted as a protective agent against lung damage. So swapping to rapeseed oil from saturated fats is the ultimate cause of the lung cancers, not the rapeseed oil *per se*. Studies have also shown a higher consumption of monounsaturated fatty acids in preference to saturated fatty acids can lead to an increased risk of breast cancer. Rats fed monounsaturated fats in their diet had a higher incidence of atheroma than those fed saturated fats, totally undermining any heart-health association the cooking oil industry is trying to establish with refined monounsaturated oils, exactly the same as with refined polyunsaturated oils.

Multinational corporations behaving like colonialists

Moving onto some very serious industrial involvement by multinationals, putting the health of a whole country into jeopardy, not just a small country, the second most populous one in the world, India, with over 1.2 billion inhabitants. The story is incredible, in both what has happened and the fact that in Europe we are totally ignorant to what has gone on. All I can do is briefly outline it here and direct you to any of the writings of Shiva Vandana if you want more detailed information. Shiva is the Noam Chomsky (and much more) of the Indian subcontinent and I can only feel total sympathy for her as she witnesses her country being sold off to the multinationals for the best price, with absolutely no consideration for the health of her people. Digest this and then tell me I'm just being conspiratorial, as this story involving cooking oil is beyond belief.

The timeline is incriminating by itself. It all began in July 1998, when there were announcements that one million tons of soybean was to be imported from the U.S. This news was met with anger from locals, being not only unnecessary as India was self-sufficient in cooking oils and the last thing the Indians wanted was American genetically modified soybeans, especially as Europe had refused to import any. Monsanto was desperately looking for a new market-opening for their GM soy and RoundUp pesticide package, particularly as canola had taken over from soybean oil as the number one cooking oil in the US. One month later, in August 1998, there was widespread poisoning, centred in Delhi, where at least 41 people died and over 2,300 were taken seriously ill. The cause of this poisoning was attributed to several oil manufacturers who had adulterated mustard oil to an astonishing and unprecedented level. As much as 30% by volume of the oil had been adulterated with diesel and industrial oil wastage and argemone seeds, with no attempt to make this adulteration in anyway subtle. In the past, adulteration had been fairly common, but never by more than 1% of total content, usually involving just crushed argemone seeds, with it only being the occasional small-scale manufacture implicated. This time the adulteration was too blatant and centred on the capital where it was bound to receive extensive press coverage, which of course it did, with even the Health Minister at the time, Harsh Vardhan, claiming this poisoning had to be a conspiracy involving the international corporations, words echoed by the Rajasthan Oil Industries Association and Shiva Vandana. In September 1998, just two months after the plan to import the soybeans, the Indian government banned all sales of unpackaged cooking oils, outlawing the production of domestically produced cooking oils.

Before this ban, the cooking oil demand was supplied by hundreds of thousands of small artisan oil producers, each producing small quantities with no more than a small hand-held press, sufficient for households for a few days, allowing the poor oil producers to earn a few rupees and the poor households to only buy small quantities of fresh, unrefined oil at a time. The ban immediately made these artisan producers unemployed, whilst opening the door to the massive international soybean oil producers from America and the palm oil producers from Malaysia. Up until this ban, the domestic market had been regionalized, with the North and East predominantly using mustard oil, sesame oil in Rajasthan, with Central India and Gujarat using groundnut oil and the South using coconut oil, all predominately unrefined. A quick look at the forecast pages of commodity brokerage firms from Wall Street and the Stock Exchange today shows that soybean, palm and mustard oil (this oil only contributing a small proportion) make up 70% of the market for India now, the second largest market for cooking oil in the world. Considering that there was almost no palm or soy oil in India before 1998, this can only be seen as a huge victory for the foreign cooking oil producers. To cap it off, Monsanto now also own the patent for mustard oil. This clearly demonstrates a blatant example of imperialism, exactly the same as that done by the colonial empires of the eighteenth and nineteenth centuries. This is how the model of globalization takes over, criminalizing all local manufacture whilst making the country dependent on imported produce, in this case cooking oils. It doesn't end with the economic impact either, as the health ramifications of this change from unrefined oils to refined oils is only just starting to hit home, as the health apocalypse from this shift in cooking oil will be catastrophic for millions, if not hundreds of millions. Previously, the cooking oils comprised an essential part of the diet, much of which is vegetarian, providing essential fatty acids and nutrients. Now the refined oils, as we have just seen, provide nothing but a whole plethora of nutrient deficiency problems, which will see diseases that were previously rare, such as heart disease and cancers becoming forever more common in India. It would be naive to assume that there had been no collusion (which is the same as saying conspiracy) between the global corporations and high-ranking Indian officials (if you want to know more read any of Shiva Vandana's incredible books, especially 'Stolen Harvest', 2000). This international theft of the world's agriculture by a few companies can only end in catastrophe, particularly if the motive remains profit and not health. Apologies if I'm sounding a bit evangelical or angry, but

156

the truth is I'm completely pissed off and unbelievably angry, especially by the monstrous Monsanto poisoning every facet of the food chain. Aarrghhh!

Deep breath . . . Completing a full circle, from saturated fat to polyunsaturated to monounsaturated fats and back to saturated fats, it is clear that there is never going to be any change in health indices with the consumption of any processed refined oils, especially when these are consumed in excess and completely out of balance. Health will only ever come from balance, and as long as the modern diet remains the same, dominated by processed foods, what these are cooked in is never going to make much difference. Particularly as already mentioned, it is these fats that are a critical component of the make-up of the cell; the very start of any consideration of attempting to explain where health begins, the cell has to be a vital foundation block. The problem with humans is that we are predominately reactive, trying to fix what is broken, when the best way is not to break it in the first place, i.e. to be preventative. We need to ignore all the confusing hyperbole and rhetoric that filters down as flawed cultural and medical knowledge, espoused by those whose only interest is in maintaining and establishing new profits. It all has to be taken with a pinch of salt (a somewhat ironic and dodgy saying, particularly as salt is the next Deadly White to be looked at).

Coconut Oil

Let's move onto coconut oil, as this at least has a positive message attached to it and it will help me step off the soapbox. Coconut oil has enjoyed use in tropical environments for thousands of years, but is obviously not naturally occurring in the colder environs of Europe, so coconuts would not have been enjoyed by our European caveman ancestors, although this is no reason to exclude them today, as they represent what can be a very healthy addition to the diet.

As disease treatment, the use of high fat ketogenic diets are once again being looked at. Developed in the 1930s to treat childhood epilepsy, it is also proving to be effective in other areas as well, such as dealing with insulin resistance as we age, allowing the body to produce ketone bodies to serve as energy and food for the brain and nervous system, A commonly misunderstood fact is that carbohydrates do not solely make energy, in fact they only make about 45% of the energy we produce, with fats providing a similar amount. Saturated fatty acids (SaFAs) are the best for this as these are easiest to burn in the mitochondria furnaces of the cells, with short chain ones being the best, such as those found in butter and coconut. Pork and beef are the hardest SaFAs to be converted, often just stored as fat or worse, clogging arteries and requiring minerals and vitamins to carry out this energy conversion task, which is impeded due to dietary nutrient deficiencies. A ketogenic diet (this high-fat diet is not to be confused with the acidosis, arthritic causing Atkins meat diet) is also being looked at for the treatment of Alzheimer's, Parkinson's, MS, drug resistant epilepsy and where there is insulin resistance for those with either Type I or II diabetes, even helping prevent cancer as the cold-pressed virgin coconut oil has anti-carcinogenic effects. These health benefits will of course be seen as a direct threat to the food and pharmaceutical industries and it is expected that as more positive research results swing towards coconut as being exceptionally beneficial health wise, there will be detractors in these industries in an attempt to control the potential lose of income and shareholder dividends, irrespective of what the truth may well be. Millennia of constant use by many Asian and Pacific cultures, who also had little incidence of the diseases of civilization, is worth bearing in mind when negative literature and industry financed pseudo-scientific research results are marketed about negative associations with coconut consumption.

Coconut oil is 90% saturated, 7% monounsaturated and 3%

polyunsaturated, which is not too dissimilar to the proportions of the human body's natural fat make-up, fitting in perfectly with any notion that we are what we eat and we should eat what we are. Other benefits from a whole range of scientific and nutritional papers involving coconut oil consumption include: It increases metabolism, aiding weight loss; improves insulin secretion and utilization of blood glucose; improves heart health; supports thyroid functionality and the immune system; it is anti-fungal, antiviral, antibacterial and an antioxidant; promoting tissue repair; improves nutrient bio-assimilation; hydrates the skin and prevents wrinkles and aging; reduces eczema and psoriasis; improves hair and scalp; it is an easy energy source and reduces sugar craving; decreases symptoms of chronic fatigue syndrome, pancreatitis and prostrate enlargement; reduces epileptic seizures; protects kidney and bladder from infections and more. Much of this positivity comes from coconuts' very high lauric acid content, nearly 50% of its fat content, converted in the body to antifungal, antibacterial and antiviral monolaurin, which has been shown to also help with measles, Candida, athlete's foot, influenza and hepatitis C. These antibacterial and antiviral properties come as no surprise when one considers another excellent source of monolaurin is human breast milk. See the coincidence? It's all about eating all the things that we are already made of, in as close a relationship and proportion as possible, whilst the further we stray from this balance the less we achieve homeostasis (equilibrium = health). Babies make the monoglyceride, monolaurin, from the lauric acid in breast milk, preventing viral, bacterial or protozoal infections. In terms of infection fighting, the monoglycerides are active (unlike the diglycerides and triglycerides commonly found in processed oils), inactivating on a cellular level viruses, for which it has been shown to be effective with HIV, measles, herpes simplex virus-1, vesicular stomatitis virus as well as many more.

Another advantage of the saturated fat of coconut is that it is comprised of medium-chain fatty acids (MCFAs), and these MCFAs are made of smaller fat molecules and are metabolised by the liver, being immediately made available for energy, similar to what glucose does, but without the need for insulin, therefore not only good for diabetics it is more importantly good as a preventative measure to ever getting Type II diabetes, which is predominately caused by the over use of insulin and other dietary factors that attack the beta cells in the islets of Langerhans of the pancreas. Other saturated fats found in meats and trans-fats have much longer chains of fatty acids and larger molecules that are not as readily broken down and are simply deposited as fat. Coconut oil with its propensity to increase the metabolic rate encourages the body to use fat as energy, accentuating fat and weight loss – an all round winner.

Coconut oil is perfect for cooking with, it has a very high smoke point, although of course food should be cooked as low as you dare, to retain maximum nutritious content, not as high as to burn. It is an excellent alternative to butter, margarine and the vegetable cooking oils, as whatever they can do, coconut can do better. Cookbooks of the nineteenth century in England, and more popularly in the US, advertised and recommended coconut oil as shortening, as it has long been known by bakers as the best for this, as well as being preferred for confectionary purposes, where its lower melting point than the hydrogenated vegetable fats and lard meant it has the best texture and taste at room temperature. Unfashionable nowadays, coconut in its desiccated form was once liberally used in many cakes, both home-made and commercially bought, even though some refined beneficial lauric acid would remain. Sadly, coconuts' relative cost compared to the heavily advertised other oils soon turned the tide, and it could never compete with the super cheap but super unhealthy polyunsaturated and monounsaturated fats of soy, sunflower and rapeseed.

Coconut oil also makes the best face and body moisturiser, bath oil, soap, deodorant, toothpaste, being ideal for oil-pulling, where a teaspoon is swashed and pulled through the mouth and teeth for a few minutes, providing much better results than toothpaste and brushing; it heals sunburn and can even act as a barrier from the sun with an SPF4 rating; improves cellulite; can be used as a baby lotion and general skin aid for many ailments; promotes healing with added antibacterial antifungal properties; is an ideal vapour rub with eucalyptus and rosemary oils and aids healing of cold sores and Candida. It truly is amazing, although as just mentioned it's only downfall is the cost, which can't be looked at too negatively because the extra expense today will save much more expense in the future by its preventative capabilities.

From the research on coconut oil thus far conducted, any negative results have only been established from the use of hydrogenated coconut oil (although in a few instances, positive results were even established from the use of this denatured oil as well). When eaten as a significant percentage of the dietary input it is already well established knowledge that this would be damaging, as coconut oil is particularly rich in Omega-6, and if no Omega-3 is included to balance out the Omega-6, the result is an increase in cholesterol and atheroma, occurring whatever oil is used. Any experimental negative results from hydrogenated coconut oil when repeated using other hydrogenated vegetable oils always had the same negative results, as that is what excess Omega-6 causes, cholesterol being used as a healer of the last resort. Raised serum cholesterol appears to act as a protective agent when sourced from coconut oil, where rats bred to get cancer show less tumour growth when fed coconut as opposed to those fed polyunsaturated fats. As already mentioned, there isn't even any rationale in the medical sciences as to why it is unquestioned that high cholesterol is bad and low is good, especially as incidences of cancer and CHD are more prevalent amongst those with lower serum cholesterol levels.

EFAs are where it's at

A brief look now at the final component of these fats and oils, the essential fatty acids (EFAs), namely the Omega-oils, which have been mentioned a few times already and can only be sourced from the diet. The best known is perhaps Omega-3, as this is the one that has been targeted by the food industry with it having beneficial health capabilities. In our dualist world, Omega-3 is the good one and Omega-6 is the bad one, which is far too simplistic, especially as we have already seen a diet too rich in Omega-3 causes heart lesions as well as causing terribly dry skin, amongst many other ailments. It's all down to balance, because indeed Omega-3 is an anti-inflammatory and Omega-6 an inflammatory, although sadly there is no balance in the consumption of these essential Omega oils. The best ratio to be consuming these two essential oils lies somewhere between 1:1 to 1:3 (Omega-3 to Omega-6) where in fact the average ratio of the modern diet is more like 1:10 and approaches in excess of 1:25 for many. Omega-3 is easily damaged and destroyed, being a shorter chain fatty acid, whereas Omega-6 (which Omega-3 can convert to) is made of a longer chain and can be found in many processed oils, so is easily excessively consumed.

An excess of Omega-6, also known as Linoleic Acid (LA) and a deficiency of Omega-3, also known as Alpha-Linolenic Acid (LNA), is well known to have multifarious detrimental effects. Importantly, the conversion for biological utilization of these EFAs requires certain nutrients, especially Vitamins B3, B6 and C as well as magnesium and zinc. There are a number of dietary deficiencies in the western diet, notably amongst these very nutrients that act as co-factors (helpers), and it is these deficiencies and imbalances that are beginning to manifest as an increased prevalence of the diseases of civilization. It is getting the balance right that is crucial, when very often the worst approach is to consume as much as possible of a deficient nutrient with little consideration to the balance that is required for other nutrients to bio-assimilate it. This Reductionist approach adopted from science has not helped with the steady decline in health, in some instances only exacerbating the problems. Reductionism is the breaking down of whatever is being studied into its smallest constituent elements; this is the antithesis of a whole-food plant based diet, which has the ability to deliver all nutrients in the balance expected by the body for utilization. Reductionism always looks for there being only one or two beneficial ingredients and treats these in isolation, never looking at the bigger picture, as holistically it is true to say that the whole is greater than the sum total of its parts.

EFAs are required for intra-cellular messages around the entire body, brain cell function, hormone, glandular, immune and nervous system operation, as well as passing oxygen and nutrients into cells and assimilating nutrients. These EFAs are destroyed when the food they are found in is refined and processed, as they are sensitive to both heat and light. EFAs also stimulate metabolism and speed up the rate our bodies burn fats and glucose. These EFAs are crucial in maintaining health and could well be argued as being the first stage in ascertaining health. Admittedly all minerals and vitamins need to be consumed in a certain balance for them to be effective, and considering that it is these oils/fats that produce human made nutrients and do the balancing work, if these are eaten out of balance the system has been compromised before it even begins its job of making other very important nutrients. The book by Udo Erasmus 'Fats that Heal, Fats that Kill' is an extremely good introduction to the importance of these oils, as well as offering an excellent overview on general health, very much along the same lines as this book, although his area of expertise is very much focused on these essential fats, unlike the holistic approach adopted by the Culinary Caveman (me).

Another source of confusion and a weapon used by the anti-vegetarian lobby (meat and fish industries predominately) is that fatty acids such as Omega-3 can themselves be found with varying names from different sources, all providing different benefits. A prime example is EPA (Eicosapentaenoic acid) and DHA (Docosahexaenoic acid), both of which in their raw state can only be effectively sourced from deep-water cold fish. They are a crucial part of every cell, helping with cancers, atherosclerosis, blood pressure and the like, and as these are fish sourced, they are used as proof that the vegetarian diet is incapable of achieving real health. However, the truth about EPA and DHA is that they are not essential, as they do not need to be eaten, as the body can and does make them by breaking down alpha-linolenic acid (LNA, 18:3w3, AKA Omega-3), which is best sourced from flax and hemp seeds. So if the diet has sufficient Omega-3 in the right balance, the body will never require fish sourced EPA or DHA, particularly as the body makes fresh EPA and DHA at a higher quality, as well as being free from any of the contamination increasingly found in seafood, such as PCBs (polychlorinated biphenyl) and other deadly chemicals found in seawater from plastic, agricultural and industrial pollutants. It's only because we are deficient in unrefined seeds that this problem ever arises and supplements are required. The co-factors of this conversion of vegetable sourced Omega-3 to EPA and DHA are zinc, magnesium and the vitamins B3, B6 and C, which are of course usually deficient, as is 95% of the western population deficient in Omega-3. The best sources of Omega-3 are the seeds from the flax and the hemp plants, with flax oil being particularly rich in Omega-3, whilst hemp oil provides all the Omega oils in the perfect ratio for human utilization (Omega-3, 6 and 9, of which only 3 and 6 are essential).

Another key role of these EFAs is the production of what are known as Prostaglandins (PGs), which regulate cellular functionality. There have been about 30 of these PGs identified so far, with

PGE1 shown to help with atherosclerosis, arthritis, cholesterol and the production of insulin and the immune system's T cells. As with the Omegas, some PGs are seen as bad, especially in the predominately sedentary state of modern life, causing clots and inflammation such as PGE2. PGE3 has been shown to inhibit PGE2 and this PGE3 is made from the conversion of EPA (hence the importance of dietary Omega-3). All PGs require EFAs to be made, with similar co-factors being required in PG production, notably zinc, magnesium, vitamins B3, B6 and C.

Beware of any processed foods that claim to be a good source of Omega-3, as more often than not this means that the food item is actually predominately rich in Omega-6, with only a limited amount of Omega-3 added. If a processed food item needs to promote and advertise any alleged beneficial results from its consumption it is invariably just a ruse, exactly like the addition of the words 'balanced diet'. Which brings us nicely to another confusing and basically erroneous term 'low-fat'.

This phrase is only ever used to lure those concerned about any associations with fat consumption and body fat, which brings to mind an excellent quote by Uffe Ravnskov, MD,PhD. "Saying we become fat by eating fat is like saying we become green by eating green vegetables."

I trust the message conveyed in this chapter is that well-sourced, healthy fats, especially the saturated fats, actually do the opposite of making us fat, they stimulate the metabolic rate, help with producing energy and can be extremely effective at helping with weight loss and general health. In most instances it is the consumption of carbohydrates (especially the deadly whites of sugar, flour and dairy) that is much more closely associated with weight gain and increased fat deposits around the body. Research clearly shows that fat intake is not a risk factor for the biggest killers, cancer and heart disease, in exactly the same way that fat intake has not been linked with obesity (unless of course it involves a couch potato eating crisps, cakes, candy and ice-cream, such a link is blatantly obvious, not so for an average weight, active adult, who does not put on adipose fat around the body merely by eating extra butter or coconut fat). If any food item claims to be low in fat but is actually comprised of white flour and sugar, then it is just a play-on-words to get you to buy it, skewering the truth to distort its detrimental attributes.

This rise of products proclaiming to be low-fat, directly plays on the consumer's insecurities and the erroneous assumption that successful weight loss and health can be found by avoiding fats. Also weight loss has been focused on the 'calories in-calories out' theory, all based around the fact that a gram of carbohydrate has four calories, whereas a gram of fat has nine calories. Which might be true if the diet was comprised of healthy calories from whole food and healthy fats, but its not, its predominately derived from processed carbohydrates. A simple comparison of those countries with the least fat intake actually shows the highest rate of obesity because so much carbohydrate is eaten (increasing diabetic rates in the process), whilst those countries with the highest fat intake have the lowest incidence of obesity. This apparent paradox is because when food higher in fat is consumed, the body far more readily triggers the satiety hormones (primarily leptin, as we saw in the Sugar chapter), meaning we stop eating; when food is eaten that is high in sugar, starches and carbohydrates, these satiety hormones are not triggered until more food is consumed. This is only appropriate to natural food containing fat, processed food containing fat is of course far lower in nutrients and this fat is not dealt with biologically. Simple observation tells the story: the population is eating more carbohydrates whilst at the same time it has gotten fatter, obviously not from the fat that hasn't been eaten, apart from an increase in the long chained animal fats that the body has trouble in bio-assimilating (chicken consumption for instance has risen by 400% in the past 30 years as has its saturated fat content, rising from 2% to 22%), laying it down as adipose fat deposits, whilst the shorter chain fats from natural whole food, such as nuts, seeds and unrefined oils are easily broken down, although these are of course under-eaten in the modern diet.

Healthy saturated fats are essential for the absorption and storage of vitamin D, whilst those on low-fat diets have been observed to be deficient in vitamin D, connected with bone thinning and initial onset symptoms of rickets. Fats are also associated with mental health and depression, where those following a strict low-fat diet have a much higher incidence of depression and even suicide. The scientific literature also tells us that children fed a low-fat diet and where processed vegetable oils have been substituted for unrefined oils, there is a general failure to grow tall and strong, combined with learning disabilities, increased susceptibility to illness and infections and behavioural problems. Teenage girls who stick to a low-fat diet have many reproductive problems, and if and when they do manage to conceive there is a much higher risk of birth defects and a smaller baby.

Low-fat as a shambolic marketing exercise

Low-fat food, or those labelled as 'light' and 'healthier' are simply used as a tool for marketing, especially as they often have detrimental health associations attached to their consumption, as these products just have more added salt and sugar to improve taste – it's a complete con. As we saw with HFCS (and also sugar), which is often used to replace the removed fat, this suppresses the production of many hormones, leptin amongst them which tells the brain to stop eating, as this is not produced from eating sugared and HFCS processed foods (as well as a general diet deficient in other hormone producing nutrients such as iodine and selenium), the individual will quite happily continue eating more and more, wrongly assuming that the food is low-fat and healthy, when all they are doing is eating more and more food that is detrimentally affecting their mental condition and increasing their chances of falling victim to obesity and diabetes. If less polyunsaturated fat is used in the cooking of crisps, extra sugar and salt is added to compensate for any loss in taste, so the food item may well be lower in dietary fat but is actually higher in ingredients that cause bodily fat. Even selling a smaller packet than previously can lead to boasts of the product being lower in fat and healthier, when in fact the ingredients haven't been changed at all. Avoid all low-fat and fat-free foods, especially low-fat dairy foods and skimmed milk, here's why, (if after reading the Milk chapter didn't make you think twice before eating any dairy).

There has never been any evidence that the fat in milk or cheese actually makes you fat when consumed in moderate quantities, it's just the word fat and the all too easy conclusion to jump to that it will make you fat, although of course eating a kilogram a day will probably lead to fatty deposit, especially if sedentary, although certainly nothing like as quickly as a kilogram of crisps and chips everyday. In full-fat raw milk (obviously the raw grass-fed variety not the pasteurized rubbish from the supermarket) there are excellent quantities of palmi-toleic acid (Omega-7), shown to help protect against insulin resistance and diabetes, whilst the conjugated linoleic acid (converted Omega-6) lowers the risk of certain types of cancer, especially bowel cancer. In the early twentieth century, raw, full-fat milk was used by Dr Crewe at the Mayo Clinic to successfully treat a wide variety of illnesses from cancer, urinary tract and skin problems, anaemia, chronic fatigue, hypertension, tuberculosis and more. Any benefits from raw milk are of course not going to occur from modern pasteurized milk as we saw in the Milk chapter, even if pasteurized milk does have any benefits, when it is skimmed of the fat there is no chance of there being any benefits, especially from those nutrients that are fat soluble, such as vitamins A, D E and K. Skimmed milk also has none of the fatty acids such as caprylic, lauric, palmitic and stearic and therefore none of the health benefits these might bring (if of course full-fat pasteurized milk has any of these still within it, which is unlikely, particularly as homogenization will detrimentally affect any remaining). Also the helpful bacteria prevalent in raw milk are destroyed by pasteurization, all of which feeds the intestinal flora and benefits the whole immune system.

The only winners with fat-free or skimmed milk are the milk producers themselves, because previously when the cream was removed the rest was just thrown away (a good mnemonic is 'the whey is thrown away'), so now with skimmed milk they can sell the milk twice. In fact a common use of this skimmed milk, after the cream had been sold for human consumption, was to feed it to pigs to fatten them up prior to slaughter. That's right, farmers used it to fatten them up, but of course humans aren't pigs. Pretty similar though, being higher mammals like us, although not as fussy about their food and drink (as they have no choice), as this skimmed milk (whey) is most unpalatable and is actually a slightly bluish insipid liquid, which needs to have powdered milk solids added to make it white and thicker. This powdered milk is made by forcing milk through miniscule holes at high pressure that causes the cholesterol in the milk to oxidize, allowing toxic nitrates to form as well as contributing to the atheroma in arteries. The proteins found in powdered milk are so denatured that the body doesn't recognize them and they contribute to inflammation, which is the exact opposite of the role played by the cholesterol in raw full-fat milk. Skimmed milk with this added powdered milk also still contains a proportion of the antibiotics and other pharmaceuticals that dairy cows are regularly given, with none of the nutrients that may help to eliminate the adverse affects of these chemicals, as well as often being fortified with synthetic vitamin D2, which research has proven to be a useless, if not a harmful addition.

Some heavy figures and statistics

It appears that a very rough average for fat consumption is somewhere around 35kg a year, a figure I believe to be much too low for many people, more realistically 50kg a year would be more reasonable. As many authorities have already established that the average citizen on a western diet is consuming 150grams a day of fats, which makes just over a kilogram a week, 55kg a year is a more realistic figure for yearly consumption. For many obese people this 50kg will be much too low and they will be looking at figures nearer 100kg to 150kg a year, if not more. Most people have no idea how much detrimental fats are added to processed foods (just as with sugar and salt), for instance a bag of crisps can have as much as 40% by weight of added cheap cooking oil saturated in the potato. Even what many think of as a healthy food item, such as a supermarket's hummus, can have 40% cheap oil added (traditional hummus is made with only virgin olive oil). Almost all the oil consumed is from eating out of home, particularly processed foods. Most of the public use a little sunflower oil at home for roasting and frying and assume this constitutes a significant part of their daily oil intake, when it is just a fraction (which reminds me of friends who are proud of having no sugar in their tea, whilst dunking several biscuits into it!).

This makes our yearly total for the four Deadly Whites so far encountered, for the lower average (for those cautiously bracketed as having a healthy diet) at 125kg flour, 100kg dairy, 60kg sugar and 50kg fats, totalling 335kg or a third of a ton of unnecessary and detrimental dietary input. For those nearer the worst end of the scale, this total is more like a staggering 275kg flour, 225kg dairy, 150kg sugar and 150kg fats, totalling 800kg, with many of those considered as morbidly obese easily topping a ton of unnecessary food every year. It makes the mind boggle how there can be any confusion as to why the health index of the western world is getting worse. If we all ate a ton of fresh vegetables, whole grains and fruit in a year what do you think the health situation would be like?

Consumption rates of certain food has also changed drastically over the past century, if not the past 50 years, even just 30 years for many so-called food items. There is therefore little reason to look as far back as prehistory to try to replicate a diet free from the diseases of civilization, a 100 years is more than sufficient. At this time there was no refining of healthy staples, and if we had continued on this path, taking into account the massive boost to the diet from worldwide refrigerated fast transportation, the diet of today would be superlative as would health, with only a miniscule fraction of the degenerative diseases being allowed to take hold.

Cancer in 1900 accounted for 1 death in every 30, today that figure is somewhere between 1 in every 3 or 4 deaths, whilst the increase in CVD deaths has risen from 1 in 7 deaths in 1900 to 1 in every 2 in 1980, and has since fallen to 1 in 3 (to much hysterical self congratulations by the medical industry, although this drop according to Dr Linus Pauling is that since 1980, millions of people are aware of the role of vitamin C and take supplements, this would have to be coupled with slight improvements in post surgery care and diet).

Dairy consumption has seen an increase in cheese, low-fat milk and ice-cream, with a drop in whole-fat milk and butter. In fact butter consumption has dropped to about 20% of its consumption 100 years ago, whilst margarine use has increased 900%, so it's illogical to level much blame on the rise in the diseases of civilization on the saturated fat of butter, whilst the rise in diseases has been in line with the increase in margarine and vegetable oil usage, which have escalated from near zero in 1900 to as much as 50% of total fat consumption today. Cholesterol consumption has remained roughly similar over the same time frame, so again it's hardly the candidate for heart disease the vegetable margarine and oil industry claims it to be.

What I believe to be most significant about the changes in consumption is the huge increase in Omega-6 oils (at least 200%, if not much more), whilst Omega-3 has dropped to about 17% of the consumption 100 years ago. The figures say a lot, but as with all statistics they can be interpreted in any number of ways. However, from reading the literature from all sides of the arguments, the two figures that really shout out the loudest are the massive increases in margarine and vegetable oil consumption and the sharp decrease in Omega-3 oils, both of which are definitely correlated to CVD and cancer. Omega-3 and saturated fats could very well be what could be termed a golden key to health, although its vital to realise it requires co-factors (helpers), and these are the vitamins A, B3, B6, C and the minerals zinc, sulphur, iodine, selenium and magnesium, especially as these are commonly deficient. Although of course regarding co-workers, all 50 essential nutrients play a vital role in achieving and maintaining proper health and longevity, (13 vitamins, 21 minerals, 9 amino acids, 2 EFAs, carbohydrate, fibre, water, light, oxygen, see Appendix for this list with the best sources for each), particularly as deficiency in only one nutrient can cause serious adverse long-term health defects.

Now hear this

To end this chapter I feel it is necessary to reemphasis that it is almost certainly the excessive consumption of the wrong type of fats and oils that makes this chapter a critical one in under-standing the recent rise of the diseases of civilization. Health begins from its basic foundation at the cellular level, and if this is compromised then so also is general health. The proliferation of vegetable cooking oils throughout the modern diet most definitely adversely interferes with our cells' production, division and functionality, as well as the movement of nutrients to the cells and the elimination of unwanted inputs and dead cells. This last sentence should be flashing, if not screamed from the rooftops. Without initial cell health there is no point in addressing a person's cancer, heart disease or even ADD (attention deficit disorder). If the basic foundational cellular stage is left compromised and unbalanced, then illnesses will always manifest again and again, until the background cellular homeostasis is established. This cell health and production is completely dependant on the fats and oils eaten. If these are not the best, then neither will general health be the best, it will be the worst.

This is why the Deadly Whites have appeared in the current order through this book, as the first three (Sugar, Milk and Flour) create a severely compromised organism, and instead of the Fats/Oils acting as a saviour for the previous ills to the diet (which they could), this one is made deadly by its refinement and unbalanced consumption.

With no further to do, let's move onto salt and as to why perhaps it wouldn't be best to take the information or your food with a pinch of this.

The Fifth Deadly White

Salt

" . . . all of us have in our veins the exact same percentage of salt in our blood that exists in the ocean, and, therefore, we have salt in our blood, sweat, in our tears. We are tied to the ocean. And, when we go back to the sea . . we are going back to whence we came.
(John F. Kennedy)

I really fancied getting a JFK quote in the book. It's the sentiment that's more important than the actual quote, as he's a bit off with his math, as human blood is about 0.9% salt, whereas seawater is nearer to 3.5% salt. I trust by the end of this chapter you will see why it was pertinent to include this quote.

Of the little nutritional knowledge shared by the general public, it is well known salt is unhealthy. It makes up a triumvirate of information of what most people know concerning food and health, alongside too much sugar being bad for us and also too much fat, especially the saturated one. Hopefully it is now clear not all saturated fats are ruinous for us, with some being exceptionally healthy, for instance the saturated fat content of a coconut or organic, unpasteurised, grass-fed butter. There is no doubt that refined sugar remains bad for us; although the public has been fooled recently into equating sugar and fat content with calorie intake, when the dangers of refined sugar, flour and fats far exceed any concerns that may arise from calories alone. There is also the exceedingly worrying industrial move, backed by the government, of offering an alleged healthy outcome from swapping sugar in drinks for calorie-free sweeteners or HFCS, a move that is absolutely guaranteed to end with disastrous consequences.

As much as I would love to say that salt can be dealt with

quickly as we all know how bad it is for us, this barely begins to lift the veil of ignorance surrounding this little white grain, as we open yet another can-of-worms. However, our mantra of a natural unprocessed version eaten for millennium being healthy, whilst the modern processed version is unhealthy, still most definitely rings loud and true. Deafeningly and ear piercingly so in fact for this particular deadly white.

As with the other chapters, we will look at the history of this deadly white, its biological function and the adverse affect of modern salt in an attempt to establish where the actual problem lies with salt, especially as it is claimed to be an essential ingredient that has to be consumed via diet, whilst at the same time it is bandied about that its consumption has to be reduced. Is it a case of too much of a good thing? Or should it be avoided at all costs? All will be revealed after we first get to grips with where salt comes from, as well as a brief history.

Where does all the salt come from?

Salt, as most of us probably remember from basic junior school science, is the residue left after seawater is evaporated. In hot countries this process is still ongoing naturally, whilst in other more temperate countries, salt can be found in massive quantities from the ancient geological processes of shifting plate tectonics, sedimentary rock deposition and polar movements, over a huge length of time. Britain may be relatively cold today (not to mention wet) but in the deep past it enjoyed an equatorial, or tropical environment more conducive to this evaporation, as proven by the vast underground salt deposits still exploited for commercial gain from Cheshire, where Liverpudlian merchants got rich long before the slave trade by exporting salt from these Cheshire salt mines.

Rock salt is a mineral called halite, it is made-up of roughly 40% sodium, with the chemical symbol Na and roughly 60% chloride, whose symbol is Cl, giving us NaCl. This rock salt, halite, is mined across the world and used in various industries, with about 160 million tonnes of salt being produced globally every year from rock salt. Figures vary, although on average about 80% of salt produced globally comes from rock salt either directly mined and removed as rock, or it has water pumped into seams and this is removed as a brine with roughly 26% salt saturation (called solution mining). Within this mineral, halite, there is a varying degree of other chemical elements and compounds, which determine the colour that can range from white, grey, blue, orange, pink, purple, red or yellow, usually in a cube crystal shape (isometric) found in vast sedimentary beds, which are the result of the evaporation of the water it was once suspended in. The world's largest salt mine is in Goderich, Ontario, Canada, situated on the east side of Lake Huron, part of a gigantic salt deposit that extends as far as Detroit, where massive salt mines can also be found. The Khewra salt mine in Pakistan is the second largest salt mine in the world with about 385,000 tonnes of Himalayan sea salt mined annually, with enough to last another 350 years at present extraction rates. The Himalaya is hardly the first place that springs to mind when thinking of sea salt, this deposit is literally older than the hills (mountains in this case) being about 250 million years old. With salt making up roughly 3.5% of the content of seawater, every litre therefore has roughly 35 grams of salt in it, with a cubic kilometre of seawater weighing in with about 26 million tons of salt. There is reputedly enough salt in the world's oceans and salty lakes to cover the earth with a 35 metre thick, salty crust.

The remaining 20% of worldwide salt production (40 million tons) comes from solar evaporation, where the sun is used to separate the salt from seawater or salty lake water. Along the coasts, seawater is often diverted into large clay lined depressions where it is left to evaporate naturally from exposure to the sun and collected when the salt reaches the desired thickness, usually once a year. This method has been employed for at least

2,000 years on the coast of Brittany, NW France, where Celtic sea salt is still harvested today using these traditional methods with only wooden tools employed. Then there are inland salt lakes where salt is often harvested, where large shallow inland lakes subject to reasonable rates of evaporation have the salt continually gathered into mounds. These lakes gradually become saltier as the water evaporates, eventually leaving just a vast saltpan, such as Bonneville Lake, an ancient Pleistocene dried up lake near to Salt Lake City, USA. Lake Bonneville's salt is currently being extracted at about 1% of its volume per year. In 1963 the salt covered 90,000 acres, it now only covers 30,000 acres. The Bonneville Salt Flats are famous for hosting the world land speed record attempts, where Malcolm Campbell's Bluebird reached 301mph in 1937.

Each salt has its own unique flavour dependent on the composition of the other minerals in the salt, whereas refined table salt has the same taste wherever it is produced. There is of course a multitude of different locally produced salts from across the globe, employing different methods to get at the salt within the water, from small mines, solar evaporation, or other novel methods such as Korean bamboo salt, where salt is evaporated inside bamboo lengths over a fire and plugged with mud at each end, adding minerals absorbed from the bamboo and the mud to the salt. This is not too dissimilar to the method of traditional salt production from across Europe, where seawater, usually already partially evaporated with concentrated brine, is put inside clay containers and heated until all the remaining water is evaporated, the clay container is then broken open to reveal the salt, a process known as briquetage. The rough clay remains from briquetage have been extensively found in the archaeological record from the Neolithic to Medieval periods throughout Europe. There is also what is known as Kosher salt, which can be found in many local stores and delis and used in the preparation of dried kosher meats; it has a larger crystal size than other salts.

This is certainly not a definitive list, only a very brief outline.

History and trade routes

Regardless of salt's immense ancestry, being as old as the water it was suspended in (and older than the mountains), there is no proof of salt being utilized by humans much before 6,000BC, with the earliest evidence of briquetage coming from the Poiana Slatinei site in Romania, dated to 6,050BC. Early Chinese documentary evidence suggests Lake Yuncheng in the province of Shanxi had contemporary salt works to those found in Romania. However, from ethnographic analysis, it appears hunter-gatherers and many tribal peoples have little to no use of salt, surely a clear paradox if salt is essential to all life. This apparent paradox will be answered after some more historical, etymological and cultural information about salt.

There is no question that salt has been an extremely important trade item since civilization and agriculture began in earnest, with salt being a precious commodity. As civilizations grew and expanded, so the trade in salt increased in tandem. It could well have been this trade that elevated the position of salt in the first place, not its biological essentialness, which as we will discover is highly questionable.

The ancient Egyptians aggressively held onto salt routes that traversed the Mediterranean and Aegean Seas, trading it with the Phoenicians for wood and dyes. A very popular early salt route traversed Morocco across the Sahara to Timbuktu in Mali. One of Rome's most heavily trodden roads was the Via Salaria, the Salt Route, following the River Tiber from the saltpans at Ostia on the Adriatic Sea to Rome. Celtic tribes of northern Europe traded salted fish and meats with Rome for luxury goods and wine. Venice became rich from trading salt, notably with the traders from Constantinople, with whom they traded it for their spices brought from across Asia. In the sixth century Moors were reputed to trade salt ounce for ounce with gold, indeed salt slabs were traded as currency in Abyssinia in Ethiopia and some parts of central Africa. The Maya produced salt using solar evaporation, as well as filling large ceramic bowls with salt water and boiling them, as done extensively at Salinas de los Nueve Cerros in Guatemala, from where it was traded throughout the interior to the Lowland Maya.

Salt is a neglected source of immense power and prestige, or at least very little thought is given to its position in the past. Perhaps because we are repeatedly being told to eat less of it, it is hard to imagine what a central role it would have played for many communities throughout history, which of course beggars the question that if its consumption played a pivotal role for millennia, why should it be included as a Deadly White? There is after all, little to no folklore that suggests that it is a poison responsible for a whole host of deadly diseases.

Somewhat surprisingly, contrary to our view of salt today, one of its earliest uses would have been as a medical aid as well as a dietary supplement, with its role as a meat preserver and a flavour enhancer only being of secondary or later importance. Perfect for cuts, wounds and abrasions, used on the skin for its anti-bacterial and antiseptic qualities, it is also ideal as a mouthwash for clearing abscesses and ulcers, as well as eaten in small concentrations for digestive and kidney ailments. It is only twentieth century man that has once again successfully managed to turn a health-promoter into a life-taker. Exactly the same story as with the other Deadly Whites we've come across: as soon as modern, economic and industrial man gets his grubby fingers on it, all notions of health, sustainability, goodness and longevity quickly slip through his meddling fingers.

Salute to Salus and other salty words, phrases and places

A good way to highlight the importance of salt to communities in the past is from the legacy of words and sayings derived from salt that have been passed down to us today. Salt names many towns and cities throughout the world, such as Salzburg, Hallstatt and English towns that end in wich and wych, such as those from Cheshire, where below Northwich there is a salt seam over 400 metres thick, and Middlewich with seams over 280 metres thick, as well as the salt marshes in the flatlands of East Anglia near to Norwich and Ipswich, where salt was obtained from the briquetage method. Also towns ending in saal and lick, would once have been important salt trading posts, located on salt marshes or near to salt mines.

Sal is Latin for salt, which is where the English word salary derives, from the phrase *salarium argentum*, meaning 'salt money', where salt was either given as part of the Roman soldier's wage, or they were expected to buy their own salt with the money. Salt also has many health associations, not least its antiseptic properties, being no coincidence that the Roman Goddess of health, *Salus*, was named after salt, which is where the word salubrious derives, meaning 'to give health'. As a form of greeting, perhaps after journeying to meet someone, custom dictates it was welcoming to offer the guest some water, bread and salt, no doubt to replace any nutrients and fluid expended during the journey, with words such as salem and salaam (meaning peace) and salutation being used as a greeting, with a salon or saloon being an appropriate venue for meeting, with the words salut, salute or salue said before having a drink to bestow health on those present. Salvation probably comes from salt being used for preservation and as an anti-septic, whilst the word salad comes from the Roman *salata*, where it was common to have a salted dressing on vegetables, a *'herba salata'*. Finally the word sale, indicates salts worth as a trade item in times past. The Greek for salt is *hal*, where the name for rock or crystal salt, halite, derives, as well as the words halal, as in meat prepared in accordance with Islamic law. Hale and hail are forms of greeting and of course Halloo (hello). Haler was the currency in Bohemia,

Moravia and Slovakia. A halidom is a holy place, as hol shares a root with hal, just as sol shares a root with sal, as of course it is the sun that gives life in the same way that it is salt that gives life (as shown later), hence halo pertaining to the sun as in sol (Spanish for sun), then there is the hall and the expression Hallelujah. There are of course many, many more, although I trust these reflect a few more significant and common uses.

As for the phrases, there are also many, such as 'worth ones salt', which has been given different connotations but ultimately it means whether one is worthy of their salary. From the Bible we find in Leviticus 2:13: "With all thine offerings thou shalt offer salt" due to its use as a preservative and a symbol of permanence, whilst in Genesis 19:1-29 Lot's wife whilst fleeing Sodom is instructed to not look back – she does and is turned into a salt pillar. In Matthew15:3, in Jesus' Sermon on the Mount he called his disciples 'the salt of the earth'. Muhammad said 'Salt is the master of your food. God sent down four blessings from the sky – fire, water, iron and salt.' 'Rubbing salt in...' has to originate from salt's antiseptic and healing capability, although corrupted today to mean being antagonistic, whilst a 'pinch of salt' means to take advice with some precaution.

Then there is a whole world of cultural practices involving salt, from the Romans placing salt on an eight day old baby's lips, adapted by the Catholics to ensure purification, by putting salt in water and calling it holy water. Salt was a common funeral offering in ancient Egyptian tombs in the third millennium BC, no doubt influenced by the fact that their art of mummification used natron, a particular type of salt found at Wadi El Natrun, also known as Natron Valley, located in the north of Egypt, uniquely composed of sodium carbonate, sodium bicarbonate, sodium chloride and sodium sulphate. Both Homer and Plato called salt a divine substance (we shall see later why this is the case). In many cultures of the Middle East, salt is and was used to ceremonially seal an agreement, as with the ancient Hebrews who made a 'covenant of salt' with god. Shinto Buddhists in Japan use small piles of salt at entrances to ward off evil and attract patrons, whilst Sumo wrestlers throw salt into the ring to sanctify the arena and ward off evil spirits before a contest. Chinese Buddhists would throw salt over their left shoulder when returning home from a funeral to prevent evil spirits from entering the house, a practice also done in England and possibly elsewhere, as the left side in some cultures is seen as the side where evil lurks (hence the persecution of left-handed people as recently as the 1970s, being forced to write with their right hand, also why the right-side is called right, as in the opposite of wrong). In Jainism salt is sprinkled before a cremation and in Hinduism it is used as a house warming, at weddings and other ceremonies. Due no doubt to its previous relative rarity and worth, the spilling of salt is considered ominous, hence in Leonardo da Vinci's Last Supper painting, Judas is depicted with a knocked over saltcellar in front of him. In Europe, the saltcellar was often an elaborate silver table ornament, with those sitting above the salt towards the head of the table being seen as more distinguished than those who sat further from the salt.

One negative aspect of salt, which has nothing to do with negative health aspects, is its taxation by the rulers. The tax on salt has always been an important levy to finance armies, conquests and other imperial tendencies, whilst the repealing of such taxes has commonly been a sure sign of revolution and anarchy. The tax on salt in France was said by Cardinal Richelieu to be as important as American silver was to the Spanish, needless to say the overturning of this tax was one of the main objectives of the 1789 French Revolution, although successful, the tax was soon reinstated by Napoleon after becoming Emperor to pay for his frequent military expeditions.

The twentieth century's most famous revolutionary act involving salt has to be Gandhi's 23-day salt march in 1930, the Salt Satyagrah, carried out as a protest because Indians had to buy salt via the British, who taxed it heavily as a result of the 1882 Salt Act, where the Indians were even prohibited from producing it themselves irrespective of its natural abundance. In early April 1930, having reached the sea at Dandi, drumming up support as he walked with a growing entourage, Gandhi picked up a handful of salty mud and proceeded to evaporate it to make salt, proclaiming as he did: "With this, I am shaking the foundation of the British Empire" and indeed he was, after being jailed for about eight months, along with up to 60,000 others. As the leader of the Indian National Congress, Gandhi was committed to non-violent, civil disobedience in order to achieve independence from a country whose only interest in India was to make profits for the Empire. The last thing on Viceroy Lord Irwin's agenda was to stoop as low as to listen to the indigenous plebs, even if this one thorn in the side was educated in law at University College London. Independence still took 17 years to achieve but there is no doubt the salt march unified the country against the greed of the British overlords. One has to ask where is the modern day Gandhi to protect the Indian people from the imperialism of the global corporations? Particularly with the legislation and banning of home-made cooking oils, as we saw in the last chapter, the words of Shiva Vandana are easily muffled and corrupted today, but she is certainly one of a few who have the proclivity and determination to stand up to the food, chemical, pharmaceutical and agricultural corporations, all presently ruining her country.

Little catch-up

After the undisputable historic and linguistic preamble, it would be here, as has been the case with the previous chapters, the dangers of excessive consumption and constant irregular practices from industries and government agencies are introduced, showing why salt is hazardous. With salt, we have been told our entire life that it is bad for us, with its inclusion as a

Deadly White fully expected, particularly the refined, processed variety used in the food industry and sold in the stores as table salt, although it is not as straightforward as this. From here on in it is imperative that salt is analysed, as there is a very clear distinction between what we think we know of as salt, be that refined table salt or unrefined sea or rock salt and what salt is in the human organism. There is quite literally a world (if not a universe) of difference between these entities, all going under the guise of salt, so it is imperative the differences are made as clear as possible to ascertain what kind of salt is a deadly white and why it is so and what salt, or part of salt, is essential.

The deadly whites of sugar, milk and flour began the book, as these are quite visibly being eaten in completely excessive quantities with significant health implications, an association that is relatively easy to appreciate. Fats and oils followed; these are also eaten in ridiculously excessive, detrimental quantities, especially the wrong type of oils, but as these oils are soaked into the food items it's not as easy to see and appreciate this excessive erroneous consumption. The Fats/Oils chapter also introduced the real source of the danger posed by all the deadly whites, which is on the cellular level, a more personal and microscopic danger, as it is these fats that are used by the body to make the membrane of each and every cell. Regardless of the quality of the fats eaten, the body has to use them as it has no other option but to use the dietary inputs it is presented with (we shall delve further into the world of the cell toward the end of this chapter). Only for a miniscule proportion of time on this planet has the human body been faced with the inclusion of detrimental fats (and of course all the processed foods made from the deadly whites) and it is this interruption to proper cell manufacture which results in significant health ramifications. So, with fats/oils we have compromised the very structure of each and every cell and so it is with salt that this blunder in diet is having an even more sinister consequence at the cellular level.

Wrong type of salt

Salt, or at least its ionic nature (in that it holds a negative chloride ion and a positive sodium ion), gives life to each cell, providing the electrical charge that enables all communication to happen, from nerve messages to hormonal production, muscular action and thought processes. It is on this most basic level, the foundation of all life – as the cell is the smallest living organism – that we have started to interfere with nature and seriously compromise the health of every cell, from not just the nutrients required for the cells to be built but also how the cells generate their own energy to perform their tasks and move to the desired location within the body. We are not only eating the wrong type of salt, we don't even need to eat salt for the body to make the salty solutions that fill the spaces between the cells and within every cell (the cells aren't actually filled with any NaCl, another salt is used and here lies the crux of another serious related and dangerously neglected problem, which we'll get to later, a clue is to note how often the mineral potassium is mentioned). It is no coincidence that humans managed to evolve over millions of years and then for *Homo sapiens* to survive for over 100,000 years with absolutely no use of salt, certainly not the salt we know today.

It's not from drinking blood, that's just wrong

Modern day hunter-gatherers have no use of salt, nor do they seek it out or pay much attention to any that is naturally occurring. The real problem with salt lies with 'balance' again, as it has nothing to do with salt as such being an essential ingredient, it isn't. If salt was essential, how could we have evolved without it being readily available and consumed? It wasn't. Arguments state that salt was obtained in the past from drinking the blood of killed animals, which it would have been to some extent, although it is too easily imagined when looked at through our twenty first century spectacles, as we have been indoctrinated into believing our past was one of violence and carnivorous blood lust, it wasn't. This argument is only given any credence, as there is more salt available from eating animals than there is from the same quantity of vegetables. The Maasai of east Africa (Kenya and Tanzania), who are well known for drinking the blood of their herds by nicking an artery and siphoning a bit of blood from a living animal, are used as the singular example to prove this continuum of blood drinking globally. However, the Maasai cannot be used as a pertinent example of what the whole human race has done since eternity, as the Maasai have only been herdsman (pastoralists) for no more than the past few centuries, having been displaced from the north-west (Sudan), moving to their current location as recently as the nineteenth century. Today they struggle to survive from their herds and most eat maize meal and cow's milk, as they gradually become progressively marginalized and the pressure to assimilate with an agricultural world exerts an increasing force.

There are more domestic animals alive today than ever before and there is little compulsion to drink their blood, even if some is used in black puddings and the like, with about 450ml of blood, almost a pint, needed to be drunk daily to get what many health authorities state should be our daily salt intake of 4.5g (with blood's salt concentration of 0.9%). If we only got our essential dose of salt in the past (or present) from dead animals (before animal domestication) how do vegetarians get their salt? I can't keep arguing about our past diet (you'll have to wait to read about it in the final instalment of the Evolution to Devolution series of books), there are vegetarian (even vegan) foragers and tribal peoples today and in the past, even those omnivorous hunter-gatherers obtain most of their meat from small mammals or fish, admittedly large game is killed occasionally although the fat and skin of these is of far more importance than the blood. From ethnographic analysis, these people don't suffer from diseases brought about by a lack of salt, because, and here's the crux of this chapter, there are no diseases associated with a lack of salt. What there are, are diseases associated with the deficiency (and imbalance) of sodium or chloride and the minerals that act as co-workers with these two.

Salt just happens to be the most convenient medium for these two nutrients to be consumed in, especially when the diet of today is deficient in so many essential nutrients; although it still begs the question, how do vegetarians who eat no processed food get their salt, or as just mentioned, sodium and chloride intake? Well believe it or not, it was never exclusively sought out, it was just a happy coincidence it was available from eating a varied, whole food diet, which provided all the essential nutrients in the best balance possible of not salt but sodium and chloride, with the added bonus of all the other minerals and vitamins as well. If this isn't the case, then there is a huge paradoxical nutritional conundrum to solve, about how it is anyone can survive without salt, whilst at the same time we all know that salt is deadly. "Oh it's all so confusing" as the little girl said in The Poltergeist, "the windows are where the doors should be and doors are where the windows should be"!

It just underlines how completely out of touch the human race is in the industrialized world as there is such confusion about the stance of salt. Salt we do not need, but sodium and chloride we do and to make it even more confusing, we also need other nutrients to be eaten in balance, such as potassium and calcium. There is also a whole chain of other nutrients that also need to be eaten in balance with these for the body to bio-assimilate these nutrients, such as magnesium. Without this balance (homeostasis) achieved from all nutrients, the foundations for ill health are established on a cellular level, allowing any number of diseases to manifest. A balance established by humans living as nature intended, as gatherers of wild food, providing the full spectrum of nutrients to guarantee our survival. As soon as civilization reared its head by way of agricultural dependence, this balance in the intake of nutrients obtained from varied wild plants was broken and the easiest way to correct in some small way this dislocation from nature and its natural source of sodium and chloride was to eat salt – in exactly the same way consuming raw, unpasteurized milk provided nutrients that became missing once existence on a few agricultural crops became the norm, such as the saturated fat butyric acid and the minerals iron and calcium. As we became 'civilized', instead of having all of nature's food at our disposal (as is the case with hunter and gatherers), our larder became, just as with Mother Hubbard's, bare.

Some definite health issues attached to salt

Moving onto health implications and why it is that refined salt plays such a negative role in our daily lives, as opposed to the role played in Roman times when salt named the Goddess of Health herself, *Salus*. Something's gone on, if not wrong, unless the ancient Greeks and Romans were either totally mistaken or there is indeed an adverse health reaction associated with the excessive consumption of a different type of salt today.

The human body is one comprised of small oceans, with around 50,000 miles of waterways, arteries, blood vessels and capillaries, where salt acts as the electrical medium for everything to manifest within a self-regulating mechanism. All we have to do is feed our amazing bodies the correct basic nutrients and it does it all for us, it's all laid on, leaving us to enjoy life on this incredible planet. However, we haven't been left to our own devices. The basic nutrients are deficient and economics has manipulated our whole existence, to the point today where our bodies are no longer self-regulating and disease has become pandemic. Salt plays a phenomenally more complicated and pivotal role than is currently understood by the vast majority, even if we all know it should be reduced.

Salt is the intermediary in the planetary oceans that initially provided the energy for life to begin, just as salt is still today the intermediary for the whole animal kingdom to carry out all thoughts and actions. It is no small matter that we have irreparably altered this intricate salt balance within our own internal oceanic bodies. Most people know of the importance of maintaining an electrolyte balance within the body, with salt and other substances such as coconut water helping to restore this electrolyte balance. If again it looks as if salt plays a positive role, here are the alleged, adverse health-affects, associated with the consumption of salt:

Even a very small intake of raw salt will trigger thirst, which is why salted snacks are widely available in bars, even given away free, to get you to drink more. When salt is abundant in a meal, the body will be insatiable in its desire to drink in order to dilute the excess salt; sadly for far too many people this craving is satiated by a sweetened water, milk or alcoholic drink. The body craves dilution as it considers sodium chloride to be a toxic substance, requiring immediate dilution.

Salt has long been known as being a cause of stomach cancer, causing irritation and inflammation in the stomach, encouraging cancer growth. Plain and simply, this makes salt a known carcinogen in the same way cigarettes can cause lung cancer, salt can cause stomach cancer, which must therefore implicate it as being a major risk factor for many other cancers as well. Stomach cancer was far more prevalent when salt was more widely used in the preservation of meat and fish, being number one in the cancer charts 100 years ago. This is because of the very high osmotic level of salt, drawing water from the tissues, causing localized inflammation and if repeated it causes irritation and lesions on the tissue membranes of the digestive system. This cell damage is a definite risk factor in encouraging cancer cell growth at these locations (with the cancer cells being further encouraged to grow from its favourite foods, glucose and growth hormones, constantly coursing through our systems). Refrigerators caused a massive decline in stomach cancers, a definite health benefit from a consumable, a rarity so worthy of a mention. As we are still eating too much as well as the wrong type of salt, which as we've just seen is a carcinogen, cancer is always going to be a possibility. The Scandinavian cultural cuisine involves an assortment of salted fish and meat and as a consequence they endure a higher rate of stomach cancer than the rest of Europe today.

Excessive dietary salt creates an acidic environment within the body, with this acidosis preventing homeostasis. It is only with homeostasis that the conditions are correct for optimum cell health, which is the ultimate foundation block of general health. The acid environment encouraged by excessive salt intake is rectified by the body removing calcium from the bones and teeth, further compounded by the fact that the excessive dietary sugars, dairy and flours are also acid inducing (and inflammatory), requiring even more calcium, which is sadly not just deficient from the diet to begin with, the massive deficit in magnesium and other co-factors (helpers), means efficient biological calcium absorption is never possible, even if the diet is abundant in calcium rich foods. That's a very important point, which is why osteoporosis, or varying degrees of brittle bones, has to be the only logical outcome if the bodily systems are kept acidic, which is of course also an ideal environment for some types of cancer, if not all types of cancer to flourish. Without an acidic system, cancer has real problems in proliferating. Enough said on that for now.

Blood pressure is said to be raised by salt in a number of ways, partly due to the acidosis from above, where cholesterol is released due to salt's inflammatory and acid inducing nature, being used to repair the damage caused to arteries and capillaries. This atheroma (which as we saw in the last chapter is today comprised of predominately polyunsaturated fats due to the excessive dietary input) constricts the arteries and increases blood pressure. If the arteries that are damaged lead to the heart or brain and the delivery of nutrients is hampered, this could potentially result in cell death, with it being only a matter of time until the entire organ is starved, areas become hypoxic (absence of oxygen) thus allowing cancerous growth to be initiated, that's if the organ doesn't just switch off. With damage to the arteries leading to the heart, heart attack and stroke can occur, and if the arteries supplying the brain get affected this can be a significant risk factor in the development of dementia, as cells die within the brain by receiving no oxygen and other essential nutrients. This is all preventable by cutting out refined salt (which would mean 99% of all processed foods, whilst slashing the other deadly whites as well), which should facilitate an increase of natural whole foods rich in sodium and potassium being consumed, helping to restore homeostasis and health.

Blood pressure is also raised more frequently from a less obvious source, the kidneys, probably with far more negative consequences. Excessive sodium out of balance with potassium hinders the osmosis performed by the kidneys, making drawing water from the blood to the bladder more difficult, thus causing there to be more water in the blood, which is retained elsewhere, causing oedemas. This extra water in the blood causes, if only fractional, an increase in blood pressure. If this condition is left unchecked, which it generally is, what with at least 10 grams of refined salt eaten each and every day (where the kidneys can at best cope with only about 7 grams), the result is kidney disease, for which dangerous pharmaceuticals will be prescribed with many adverse side effects. One of the first drugs given will be a diuretic, which makes the kidneys remove more fluid from the bloodstream. After what has probably been years of punishment, the kidneys have lost much of their ability to filter the blood, so the toxic waste is not expelled and allowed to build up internally – this will ultimately lead to kidney failure and or death. This accounts for many diseases, particularly those alleged auto-immune diseases, where the unrefined salt has been the catalyst that compromised the kidneys, leading to the failure to expel toxins and other unwanted products that are left to circulate repeatedly, building up internally. This might take a long time to manifest as a diagnosable disease of civilization, many of which coincidentally also have a long incubation period. If the sodium imbalance was addressed to begin with, the kidneys would not run into problems and the toxins would not have built up. The result of too much refined salt therefore leads to kidney disease, a life long dependence on prescription drugs and a toxic build up that can result in any number of deadly diseases from cancers, cardio-vascular disease (CVD) and dementia. As kidney problems are one of the most common diseases, to avoid most of these and the much more deadly diseases that poor functioning kidneys can lead to, it's worth promoting a preventative approach and insist a balanced intake of sodium and potassium is established.

Worryingly, as with Ancel Key's work managing to get international news coverage and becoming a cultural fact (regardless of its real truthfulness or any links between fats and CVD), there is the same situation with salt. With salt, it is quite possibly the work of Lewis Dahl in the 1970s that got erroneously used as a tool for marketing with its scientific credentials blown out of proportion, with it being often repeated in respectable publications it began to be seen as a medical and cultural truth. Dahl's study involved feeding rats the equivalent of 500 grams of salt (if the rats were human sized) and noted increases in blood pressure, concluding salt intake was a determining variable into looking at causative agents that could increase the blood pressure of humans, although not very relevant or scientific when looking at daily consumption by a human of 12 grams a day. Many studies since have failed to find any association between salt consumption and blood pressure. The answer is never straight-forward.

How much salt do we need and what the Salt Institute say

What is commonly referred to as salt is comprised, as we know, of two main ingredients, roughly 60% chloride and 40% sodium (this is not strictly accurate, as described in a few pages). The reason salt has this ratio is because of the different atomic weights of chlorine and sodium, where an atom of chlorine is about 50% heavier than a sodium one, with one sodium atom bonding with a single atom of chlorine. There are plenty of other salts in the human body and in nature, although our view of salt is somewhat blinkered to just sodium chloride (NaCl), of which there is about 0.15% of total body weight of each of these in the human body, meaning an 80kg adult will have about 200g of this NaCl within them, which is quite a lot, particularly as salt itself can be fatal at an ingestion rate of 1g per kilogram of bodyweight or less, with a teaspoon being potentially fatal to a baby or small infant.

As far as the biological sciences go, the average human body under normal day-to-day conditions requires about 1.5 grams of sodium a day. Health authority recommendations from varying countries give a preferred range of intakes of sodium from between 2g to 4g (5g to 10g of salt) a day. The Foods Standards Agency (FSA) in the UK has attempted to initiate a traffic-light colour coding of foods, displayed on the packaging; spanning from less than 0.3g of salt per 100g of a food product being designated a green light, with 1.5g of salt per 100g being given a red light and anything in between getting an orange one. Unsurprisingly, the Salt Manufacturers Association (SMA) is particularly unhappy with this scheme and even less happy with another one titled 'Salt – Watch it' with a cartoon slug as its avatar. To reduce salt in America, Nestle has agreed to cut salt in their prepared foods by 10% by 2015 (2015 has nearly ended as I edit this and there is no indication this insignificant goal has been achieved so far) and General Mills will try for a 25%

reduction in 40% of their foods (a little better), whilst Pepsi have formulated a new super fine salt that will hopefully cut salt by 25% in their crisps (so they say). The American equivalent of SMA, the Salt Institute, has begun a campaign to promote salt use and create increased confusion about the logic of reducing salt. This would occur whether or not salt was healthy – it's what businesses do, it's called marketing and protectionism, although if refined salt were really healthy, it shouldn't take quite so much effort and money to spread the message. With considerable money behind them, the SMA and Salt Institute do market their product extensively, irrespective of the truth or the danger of their trade in a Deadly White.

How much salt is in food and average consumption

Salt can be found in all processed foods as well as those not considered as being processed, such as there being at least a gram in three slices of whole wheat seeded bread, to the more obvious, such as the processed ready meals that contain on average 2g to 5g of salt per portion. Supermarket pizzas have up to 4g of salt in a couple of slices; whilst a pot noodle has fractionally less; three chocolate digestive biscuits will contain a gram; cheap sausages (a word that is derived from *sal*) will have at least 1g per sausage; with many sweetened cereals having at least 1g per serving; whilst amongst fast food, chicken is one of the worst offenders, with every piece of thigh or breast from KFC having well over a gram and a BigMac having at least 2g of salt in it. So, with a diet high in processed foods, which is the norm, it is unrealistic and basically wrong to state that the average intake is between 7 to 10 grams of salt a day, it isn't, it is much higher than this, with many consuming over 20 grams a day, which is most definitely a toxic level.

This means the salt intake for the majority of people is constantly excessive. The average in the UK is said to be falling slowly, presently at just under 9 grams a day, although as just mentioned, it is much more than this for many people. As with sugar consumption, most estimates are severely underestimated, where the actual average salt intake figure probably lies nearer to 15 grams daily. 10g of refined salt a day equals 3.65kg a year of what has been hailed by many nutritionists and doctors as the most poisonous substance in the food chain (I'd argue it was aspartame). In an ideal world we should consume none of the refined industrial table salt and no more than 1.5 grams of sea-salt or unrefined rock salt daily. The rest of the sodium requirement the body requires should be obtained from the rest of our diet, not industrially derived salts, which even contain waste products from other industrial sectors (we haven't even seen what salt's real purpose is in the modern world yet, which might come as a bit of a shocker, if not an eye-opener, in a couple of pages).

There are so many other factors to consider when looking at appropriate levels of safe salt intake. Everyone's salt require-ments are different, depending on where they live in the world and what work and activity levels they sustain; those with more perspiration and heavy activity schedules require more salt to be replaced, whereas sitting at a desk all day, then a sofa all night requires less salt. We're all different. The World Health Organization with their recommendation of 2g of sodium a day have found that an intake any lower than this shows no beneficial effect. In a cruel twist of irony, when a low salt (sodium) diet is advised by a health professional, sodium deficiency can easily occur, especially because dietary sodium from fresh vegetables is not a common part of most people's diet. Heart patients showed a greater rate of mortality when salt levels are reduced below the WHO recommendations. Sodium deficiency can result in hyponatremia, with symptoms ranging from spasms, cramps, irregular heartbeat (arrhythmia), increased risk of heart attack, swelling of the brain and sudden death (loss of electrolytic connectivity).

There has even been in some instances a situation where a low salt diet increases risk of heart disease with no change in blood pressure (as reported in the Journal of the American Medical Association). Irrespective of this little trifling matter of the truth, all health associations globally follow the belief of calling for salt restrictions, without understanding why. Although I concur that salt should be restricted, although not for the dogmatic notion of salt's main danger being associated with heart health. Before this is explained let's finish with looking at what modern refined salt is all about.

Refined salt and its fortification

Refined salt isn't just sodium and chloride. Other chemicals are added for convenience, as well as attempting to improve health. Refined salt has a natural tendency to clump together, so to help with the way the salt flows, anti-caking ingredients are added to the extent of 2% by weight, such as potassium or sodium ferro-cyanide, ammonium citrate, aluminium silicate and dextrose (a sugar, used as a stabilizer). Industry says these chemical additives are inert, a statement which has to be taken with the proverbial pinch of their own product, particularly as the inclusion of these inert chemicals includes forms of cyanide, ammonia and aluminium, three ingredients that most definitely do not have any positive health associations and certainly don't sound inert. These additives have only been used for the convenience of the food industry, whose inclusion has been ascertained by scientists whose brief was to find the cheapest and best chemicals that are fit for the purpose of aiding the flow of refined salt; health or nutrition was never an objective or part of their brief.

Chemicals have also been added to salt in attempts to improve the general health of the population, as dietary deficiencies have been recognized for many years now. Salt was one the mediums chosen to attempt this, as most homes had salt in them, with only a minority using unrefined salt. With most people genuinely assuming there is little difference between the two there is little point in the added cost of the unrefined varieties (a terrible deduction as we'll see when we get to look at the unrefined salts in a few pages). Regarding fortification, it became a common practise in the US to add iodine to table salt from the 1970s and has been a legal requirement in Canada from as early as 1949. No doubt the general public is deficient in this crucial mineral, which determines much to do with wellbeing, from thyroid health, essential for proper hormone production as iodine is essential in the production of thyroxine; it's also an antioxidant and is especially important for pregnant women and foetal development. A deficiency in iodine has many symptoms, amongst the most common is cretinism and developmental retardations in children and enlargement of the thyroid gland (goitre). The RDA of iodine is in the region of 150mcg, and fortification in the US is set at about 100ppm (parts per million) which works out to about 100mcg per gram, so just a couple of grams of iodized salt will provide the RDA of iodine; in the UK and much of Europe only 10-22ppm is added. The success of this strategy is very hard to gauge, especially because iodine's co-worker selenium is still deficient, which inhibits bio-assimilation of iodine. Goitre (swelling of the thyroid gland) being uncommon is seen as a sign of success of this initiative, although whether cretinism, hormonal and behavioural dysfunctionality has seen any reduction is certainly open to debate.

As there has been much mention of potassium already, there is firm evidence that it plays all the roles mentioned throughout this chapter. The medical and commercial world realise this, as potassium salts have been available for some time. Potassium chloride is added to sodium chloride in varying proportions, producing a salt that is lower in sodium and higher in potassium (which has a more metallic, saltier taste). However, as potassium is a relatively easy nutrient to find in a range of food, such as nuts, bananas and deep green leafy vegetables, caution has to be attached to any recommendation that advises the ingestion of a refined salt in preference to a natural whole food. An extra bowl of kale or broccoli a couple of times a week is definitely a good thing, providing potassium and balancing out the sodium disequilibrium instead of exasperating it.

Magnesium chloride can also be found added to refined salt. Just as with potassium, a diet that includes a good amount of dark green vegetables and nuts and seeds will also be rich in not just magnesium but also potassium and several other essential nutrients. Iron has been added to refined salt in the form of ferrous fumarate in some countries to alleviate iron deficiency anaemia, which can cause mental development disorders in developing countries. Again the uptake and efficiency of this strategy is questionable, with much new research indicating that fortification of iron in flours and cereals could well be a contributing factor to various auto-immune diseases, forms of dementia and osteoporosis.

Folic acid is also added to salt in several countries, as unarguably vitamin B9 is deficient in many diets and is especially crucial for proper foetal development; the inclusion of folic acid often taints the salt a yellow colour. A much better source of folic acid than a fortified salt would be plenty of fresh parsley, spinach and sunflower seeds, as these are also full of other nutrients, all enabling better bio-assimilation of vitamin B9. It has been shown that only a minority of expectant mothers take heed of this advice to consume more B9, with part of the blame for this being that health advice only extends to stating that folic acid can prevent spina bifida, an unknown disease to most people. Folic acid is actually essential for proper cell division and much more, it is certainly far more important than solely helping to prevent spina bifida.

Sodium fluoride is added to 35% of table salts in France as a preventative measure to alleviate the formation of teeth caries in areas where the water is not already fluoridated. All bad science, especially as there is absolutely no indication that all this fluoridization has had any affect on caries (it is also stated in much literature that calcium fluoride should be added as this is less toxic, if toxic at all; sodium fluoride sneaked in as it is part of the economics of making profits out of industrial wastage. American health authorities have recently admitted they have over-fluoridized the population, weakening teeth . . . oh! it's a bit late now).

There is the obvious glaring problem with fortifying table salt, inasmuch as it still requires refined table salt to be consumed to provide a level of iodine, or any of the other fortified nutrients. This will not help to reduce refined salts intake and can easily draw the consumer into a mistaken sense of security, with the false assumption of consuming a healthy product. Adding nutrients by way of fortification proves there has always been the understanding that minerals and vitamins play an enormous role in health. It is no secret after all, even though recent legislation is geared towards removing this health provision from small independent providers of nutritious ingredients making it illegal to claim any health associations from their products.

The Codex Alimentarius

To see how the law is changing it's worth having a peek at the Codex Alimentarius (The Food Book) set up in 1963 with the honourable intentions of improving food safety, standards and information across the world. As is the case with many websites, it's very hard to see the obvious flaws in this international organization fronted by the WHO (World Health Organization) and the FAO (Food and Agriculture Organization of the United Nations), so its worth doing a Google search for the dangers of this Codex. As with all rules and laws, after over 50 years there has been more than enough time for the larger corporations of the pharmaceutical, chemical and food industries to apply continual pressure with their substantial financial leverage to not only bend the rules but also to make new ones in their favour, especially those protecting the market share of their products. The Codex has enabled this, as slowly it is becoming impossible to market a food product and associate this with any health claims. The Codex will legislate and make it financially unviable for small health practitioners who claim health is possible from food and herbs, whilst at the same time the Codex will allow large corporations with their processed, patented products, free reign to make such health claims. The initial intention of the Codex was to increase global food standards. After half a century it has become a platform for the large pharmaceutical and food corporations to monopolize the markets with their version of food and health, whilst at the same time making it illegal for anyone else to make such health claims. It's the same economic model as that laid down by colonialism (with the salt taxes etc.) and international global corporations (legislation against domestic cooking oils in India). There is a very real business ethos, fully supported by governments, that wants to funnel all power from a diversification of industrial sectors into the board-rooms of only a few global mega-corporations.

As a brief aside, the manipulation of the Codex Alimentarius has a very similar history to that of the FDA (US Food and Drug Administration). The FDA has already been mentioned several times and perhaps it may appear that to constantly disrespect them is merely conspiratorial anti-establishmentarianism. This would be an erroneous conclusion. The history of the FDA is the same as the Codex: an official body originally established with only the public's best interests at its heart, which in time has been thoroughly manipulated and corrupted by big business. The FDA began life as the Bureau of Chemistry, founded by Dr Wiley who pushed through the first Pure Food and Drug Law in 1906 as a measure to prevent the sale of adulterated, processed and demineralized foodstuffs. Wiley even brought lawsuits against Coca-Cola to protect the American public from this diabetes inducing sugar and chemically laced, filthy drink. This was to be his undoing, as this merely unleashed the machinations of the food industry to get him removed from office and allow free trade of all deleterious produce. He was duly replaced in 1912 by a Dr Nelson who saw no correlation between dietary input and ill health (I kid you not), whilst the Bureau of Chemistry was renamed the FDA. As the saying goes, it's been downhill ever since.

Alternatives to salt

There are many alternatives to salt, although salt is often added as many of the processed foods have little other flavour. Home cooked food should not require any extra salt, if it does there is something wrong with the ingredients and preparation. If your food tastes of nothing and the flavour of salt is preferred to that of your food, the first step would be to get used to adding a handful of fresh herbs to dishes. The flavour of the herbs will deter salt addition, also with more herbs eaten the more nutrients that are consumed, as herbs have a fantastic range of nutrients, especially when compared to the food consumed in the modern diet, which is so rich in carbohydrates and fats, with little, if any nutritious content left in them.

In many cuisines worldwide, especially in Asia, the use of salt is minimized, replaced with salty condiments, with soy and fish sauces being very popular, some of which are fermented, such as miso to bolster nutrition. An old traditional method of food flavouring, no doubt practiced around the world, was using dried seaweed as a flavouring. This practice also included throwing into the drying process fish eggs and unused fish parts such as bones and heads, all of which when crushed together gives not only a salty taste, but also is extremely rich in many of the minerals currently deficient from the modern diet, such as iodine and zinc. The minerals from dried sea-food provide a greater concentration of many of these minerals found in unrefined salt, without the concentration of chloride and sodium.

The real purpose of refined salt

Having established the significant role played by salt in civilization, both linguistically and culturally, and that too much is bad and that not enough also has problems attached to it, what is often not realised about salt is that it plays a critical role in allowing the cogs of industrialism and capitalism to turn. In fact, without salt the world of consumerism and industrialism would be a very different and smaller place. There is over 200 million tonnes of salt produced every year, of which only about 6% (12 million tonnes) ends up in the food chain. Of the rest, 12% ends up being used for water treatment plants, where the chlorine is processed for sewage facilities, domestic water and swimming pools and the like. 8% is used for road-de-icing and grits, with a further 6% being used in the agricultural sector, being processed as an ingredient in fertilizers or being used directly on some agricultural crops, such as asparagus. This leaves roughly 68% to be used predominately in the chemical and manufacturing industries, where a considerable proportion is used to make chlorine (and its derivatives) and hydrochloric acid.

Hydrochloric acid was a crucial ingredient in bringing the Industrial Revolution to fruition. A revolution which sugar and the slave trade might well have financed, it was hydrochloric acid that enabled this revolution to be so diverse and unstoppable, being used to make all manner of substances and chemical reactions. The annual production today of hydrochloric acid is around 20 million tonnes (with Dow Chemicals producing about 10% of this, we'll become quite familiar with Dow by the end of this series of books, if for no other reason than they and Monsanto were responsible for the Agent Orange and napalm that rained down on SE Asia during the Vietnam War in the 1960s and early 1970s). Hydrochloric acid's old name gave a clue as to its provenance, 'spirits of salt', which when mixed with nitric acid was known as Aqua Regia (royal water) due to its ability to dissolve gold and platinum. Hydrochloric acid has unique properties that make it so useful in industry because it is the least likely of the strong acids (nitric, sulphuric, perchloric, hydroiodic and hydrobromic) to undergo an undesirable oxidation-reduction reaction, whilst also storing well and retaining its pH level, as well as being the least hazardous.

Without salt, all the following industries would be either impossible or at the very least, considerably inconvenienced: petrochemicals, explosives, metal production, notably aluminium and steel, where it is used as a cleaning agent for steel and as a flux in aluminium (where rather surprisingly the waste is reused in items such as bathroom products, toothpastes and food additives and even goes full circle as an anti-caking agent put into table salt). Chlorine is a major component of cleaning fluids, detergents, caustic soda, bleach, soap and glycerine. Salt is also used in the manufacture of dyes, an emulsifier in the production of synthetic rubber, leather processing, paper pulp, ceramics and glazes, glass manufacture, plastics such as polyvinyl chloride (PVC) and the very contro-versial bisphenol A (BPA), which is a failed female hormone replacement from the 1930s adopted by the plastics industry to soften plastics for use in baby bottles, nipples and the lining of cartons and cans. And the list goes on, with hydrochloric acid being imperative in the production of sweeteners such as aspartame and saccharin, ascorbic acid (falsely named as vitamin C), fructose (HFCS) and hydrolysed vegetable protein, gelatine, medicines, the illegal drug manufacture of cocaine, heroin and crystal-meth, as well as pharmaceuticals, where the chloride is used to make calcium chloride, magnesium chloride and potassium chloride, all of which are also used in the cement industry. As industry demands 'pure' salt, with its 'impurities' causing adverse reactions, such as the magnesium attracting moisture, all of these 'impurities' have to go, amounting to about 2% of halite (rock salt) by weight, this totals a huge 4 million tonnes of unwanted minerals (which is what these impurities actually are). These are sold onto the supplement industry (not all the 4 million tonnes is moved on this way, although a proportion definitely is) at an enormous profit, reaping more than the profit from the salt itself. This is another example of clever economic management, with a previous waste product now being resold at vast profits and re-branded as a health supplement, where research is now proving these supplements are far from being healthy, they are probably detrimental to human health in many instances.

Without getting too embroiled in conspiracy, this is a fact (this movement of wastes to alleged health products) and it is exactly the same as the flour industry selling the vitamins and minerals removed from the processing of white flour – just as for the rice industry, as we will see in the next chapter. This processing/removal of the nutrients hasn't been done to make the population dumber or sicker, as many conspiratorial commentators argue, these are just unexpected coincidences and results from economic rationality creating more profit from a raw material. It's not possible or fair to blame those governed by economics to make the best of the economic world, just as it's not possible to blame those governed by a certain religious belief to live their life by those religious beliefs.

The industrial uses of salt makes for a somewhat surprising list. This list reflects the real role of salt in the modern world, as a raw material for almost any industry you'd care to think of. I hope now the picture is becoming a little clearer as to why refined salt is a dangerous product, because it's an ingredient in the chemical and manufacturing industries, which is where refined salt should stay. It most definitely should never have been allowed to become a ubiquitous ingredient in the food chain.

The industrious body and the role of chloride

Incredibly, the production plants within the body, making
hormones here, delivering nutrients there, regulating temperatures, viscosity, pressures, acidity, changing electrons and
making vitamins and other chemical reactions, all share similarities with many of the industries that use chemicals. With salt,
where its prime use industrially is in the production of
hydrochloric acid, the human body also makes this acid from the
chloride bit of salt, or whatever food items that have been
consumed with chloride or chlorine in them, forming a part of
the gastric acids in a biological process that has only changed
minutely in the past 100,000 years. However, the food consumed
manufacturing gastric juices has changed enormously in only the
past 50 or 60 years, and we have yet to recognise or understand
what health implications this change has had.

There has been a distorted bias with sodium dominating our
view of salt, when in fact by weight there is 50% more chloride
than sodium in it, although this is largely ignored. The
conclusion from this bias toward sodium would indicate that the
chloride part is practically inert. Without wishing to sound
argumentative (I like to call it one-way discourse), could this
possibly have something to do with the fact that by not
mentioning chloride, industry has hoped attention will be
always focused on the sodium, not least because the negative
affects of chlorine are clear to see? The chloride in salt is made
after some natural chemical magic, as chlorine is actually a
greenish yellow gas, becoming a chloride by the shifting of
electrons when it comes into contact with water (changing from
a halogen to an anion – a negatively charged ion). Chlorine, the
gas, is lethal after only a few breaths, coming to prominence as
one of the deadly gases initiated in the horrendous waste of
young lives that was the First World War. Chloride is not much
better, being a severe irritant to the respiratory system,
damaging and depleting the mucous membrane and increasing

acidosis and causing reflux.

The amount of chloride in the body is monitored and controlled by the kidneys, which of course requires the kidneys to be fully operational, which is rarely the case when homeostasis is seldom obtained for the majority. Chlorine is an incredible chemical; apart from it being one of the first chemicals in the primordial soup at the beginning of life on this miraculous planet, it readily forms many other derivatives with other chemicals to make some odd sounding anions, such as tetra-chloroaluminate and perchlorate. The actions of chloride within the cells are an absolute necessity in the body's utilization and biological transport of oxygen, carbon dioxide and proteins – its importance is at the most fundamental level of health. This means that its balance is of paramount importance when not just considering an abstract term such as 'health', but also life. All the chemicals are of course required, especially those essential ones, although without the basic preliminary ones of chlorine, oxygen and hydrogen, life as we know it was a non-starter well over a billion years ago.

In the digestive juices, hydrochloric acid forms a major component of acidifying this gastric acid. The role of hydrochloric acid is to break down and unravel proteins (chains of amino acids) and expose the peptide bonds enabling absorption, as well as acting as an antibacterial agent destroying unwanted organisms, preventing infection. The stomach is protected from the gastric acid by a thick layer of mucous, which when damaged leads to acid reflux or heartburn. Another important part of gastric acid, playing a vital role, is potassium chloride, but as we are discovering potassium is either deficient or severely imbalanced in the diet of today, compromising the production of this potassium chloride.

There is no room in this book to become submerged in the digestive juices, particularly as this subject is immensely confusing, with far too much contradictory evidence from competing scientists. All that needs to be understood is the fact that these digestive juices are not human, being composed of archaic bacteria up to a billion years old, and it is this primitive digestive system we have within us that is quite possibly as crucial as the health of a cell in determining overall wellbeing. Without optimum cell health, as we have clearly seen throughout this book, overall health of the organism is impossible, a situation that is just as true with regards the stomach flora being healthy and capable of doing their job. The stomach flora and its array of bacteria is a critical element determining health, which is a somewhat new science, the continuing study of which will no doubt unlock several doors for optimizing health. That said, it is already well understood that a diet dominated by meat, sugar and processed foods severely depletes good bacteria, whilst a predominately vegetarian diet comprised of unprocessed whole foods is the best way to encourage and maintain a healthy balance of the good bacteria. It should be blatantly obvious that cells and bacteria, which are millions of years old, would have significant difficulties when confronted with the industrial types of food that have predominated in the diet of the past 60 years, contributing towards the host of dietary intolerances and allergies that are becoming forever more frequent.

This is the difference between salts

Which moves it finally along to having a look at the unrefined salts. What needs to be appreciated about unrefined salts is that they are mined from the same places as refined table-salt. Both start off as identical halite, only one goes off to be refined, with the 'impurities' removed to make it more useful for the chemical and manufacturing industries, whilst the other is merely crushed to the desired grain size, packaged and sold in a health store for a premium price.

From analysis of Himalayan sea salt, 87 chemical elements

have been detected. There are 98 natural chemical elements found in the periodic table, 84 of which are primordial (being here since the formation of Earth), whilst the remaining 14 are as a result of the decay chain of these 84. In fact there are 117 chemical elements in the periodic table as of 2014, although the other 19 are either laboratory produced or highly contentious. Of the 87 found in Himalayan rock salt, some are certainly not at first glance (or second or third glances for that matter) obviously fit for human consumption. Take for instance, the presence of uranium, plutonium and polonium, detected at levels below 1 part per million (ppm – a very rough approximation of a part per million, would be a cup of water in a swimming pool); with some bizarre sounding ones such as europium, tantalum and iridium also found at only 1 to 2ppm. Of the other minerals with suspect health claims there is aluminium at 0.661ppm, fluoride at less than 100ppm and lead at less than 10ppm. Others that could well turn out to be very beneficial after future research include strontium at less than 14ppm, lithium at 490ppm and vanadium at 0.06ppm. Of those with definite health associations, there is chloride at 590,000ppm, sodium at 382,000ppm, magnesium at 160ppm, sulphur at 12,400ppm, potassium at 3,500ppm, iron at 38.9ppm, calcium at 4,050ppm, manganese at 0.27ppm, copper at 0.56ppm, zinc at 2.38ppm, selenium at 0.05ppm and iodine at just less than 100ppm. This provides a similar proportion of iodine as that found in iodized salt, although unrefined salt has the clear advantage of having all the other co-factor minerals present to aid with biological usability. All the trace minerals are present in Himalayan sea salt, in, as their name suggests, trace amounts, miniscule quantities that are unlikely to be consumed from any other food source, not only because the majority of people eat predominately denatured processed foods, but more importantly because the agricultural soils are infertile, virtually barren in many instances, only managing to support the crops grown on them with the addition of fertilizers, which definitely do not contain a broad spectrum of minerals, being dominated by nitrogen, phosphorus and potassium (NPK). It's incomprehensible to understand where even a ppm of the essential micronutrients of say selenium and iodine can be found in food if the soil of today is barren.

Disappeared without the trace minerals
Mineralization of vegetables can only occur if the minerals are present in the soil to begin with, which today is not the case. Iodine was very rarely deficient until as recently as the 1970s due to most farmers using a seaweed compost on their soils to fertilize the soil, which also added other minerals more commonly found in seawater food, such as zinc, selenium, chloride and sodium. When this practice of seaweed fertilization became phased out in favour of the NPK mix, another chip was taken out of the immune system of humans who depend on produce from the soil for their own mineralization. The soil today does not have the same nutrient profile it would have had 20, 100, 1,000 or 100,000 years ago. With the present practice of monoculture (one crop covering vast fields) we have put the earth to slavery, producing unnatural crops and quantities of them, with the produce flown 1,000s of miles away. The natural feedback is lost; with the diverse organic vegetative cover replaced, no longer do all the minerals get recycled through the plants, worms and all local flora and fauna, no recycling whatsoever, as everything is obliterated and a single crop planted with deadly agricultural chemicals sprayed onto it. The soil today is a weak reflection of the soil of old, it has become demineralised, as has everything that depends on it, which equates to all life. This is a vital consideration, although one which little to no thought is given when attempting to understand health and proper reproduction. The soils of old, before agriculture, would have been superlatively rich in all nutrients, being the result of thousands of years' worth of sediment

deposition, shifting sea levels and glacial erosion. Agriculture, significantly its modern model, has stripped all these nutrients from the soil, replacing them with NPK and a range of agricultural toxic chemicals. Compounded by the diet being dominated by processed foods, there begins to be no avenue for these essential minerals to ever become part of the diet. This deficiency of the soils is a definite positive argument for the consumption of unrefined salts, as these unrefined salts provide a source for the majority on a western processed diet of, what will undoubtedly prove to be with future research, essential trace minerals. As we saw earlier, iodine was deemed so crucial it was added to table salt in an attempt to restore the consumption of a vital nutrient, fortified to a level of sufficient iodine to prevent illness from its otherwise deficient intake. This beggars the question, that if iodine has to be replaced and coincidentally is fortified in refined salt to a similar amount as found naturally in rock salt, would it be so ludicrous to assume that all the other trace minerals removed from salt also play a critical role in determining human health? As can be seen from the breakdown of the composition of Himalayan salt, there are 87 elements, or 85 other than NaCl, and if the amount of iodine found naturally is sufficient to stave off disease and growth retardation, are the infinitesimal quantities of trace elements also staving off disease?

This demineralization of salt, the Roman Goddess of health, *Salus*, has to be a contributing factor as a reason for the increase in the diseases of civilization. This is not just another coincidence, it is a catastrophe caused by the use of industrialized refined salt as opposed to unrefined rock salt. If the food industry had used unrefined rock salt in its processed foods the demineralization of the human organism would not have escalated to such an extent where the diseases of civilization have reached such epidemic proportions. This may appear over simplified but it's the truth; the soils have been robbed of their nutrients by improper agricultural practices, leaving it to salt to provide these essential trace minerals, which has in turn been bastardized into not only a poor reflection of its former healthiness, but into a toxic refined product not fit for human consumption . . . oops!

Celtic Sea salt and Spas

A modern variant of an unrefined salt goes by the trade name Celtic Sea Salt, harvested from the Brittany coast of NW France, channelled through clay lined ponds, left to evaporate and removed with wooden tools when the thickness is sufficient, usually once a year, employing a method at least 2000 years old. The mineral analysis is fairly similar to Himalayan salt, although not such a comprehensive list is available. Ignoring the sellers' spurious claims, both Himalayan and Celtic salt have a wide spectrum of trace minerals and as knowledge of these increases, the health benefits of these minerals will undoubtedly broaden their appeal. A somewhat different use and type of salt is the continuous human use of mineral spas and natural springs throughout the world, which due to the porosity of human skin, by soaking in them, a small portion is absorbed. Budapest In Hungary is famous for its spas, as is of course Spa in Belgium, Lourdes and Vichy in France, the numerous German cities and towns containing the word Bad, usually as a prefix, sometimes as a suffix or even in the middle, as with Wiesbaden, Germany's biggest spa city, there is also Baden in Switzerland. There are thousands of spas throughout Europe, all attesting to the healing attributes of the waters and salts within them. Spas can have any combination of mineral salts and compounds within them, from sulphur and iron to hydrogen sulphide, calcium hydroxide (lime) to lithium salts, with sodium, calcium and magnesium amongst the commonest components of salts found. The variety and number of spas and springs considered to have healing qualities is a formidable endorsement of their healthy attributes, as opposed to a warning of their use. Even those springs with radioactive material such as uranium and radium can be healthy, as these also only have positive folklore attached to them.

What and where are all the elements from?

We are more than three-quarters of the way through the chapter and there has been little reference to the actual processes that made salt what it is. We all think we know what salt is. I've elaborated somewhat already upon what salt is, what salt is used for, and what it does. We come into contact with it every day although there is an aspect that truly makes this a processed deadly product, when originally it was essential for life due to the whole range of minerals in a readily useable format for animals and plants to utilize within it. How did these minerals get there in the first place? An answer which really opens a cosmic door; for instance, how did the sodium get there? If you were to put sodium in its raw state as a white soft metal into water, it would react extremely violently. As for chloride, what is chloride anyway? And those other 85 chemical elements found in Himalayan sea salt, how did they get there? Complicated chemistry, that's what has gone on. In nature the chemical elements rarely appear in isolation and have gone through any number of reactions that have left these elemental chemicals mixed with other chemicals to form what is called a compound. This is why sodium found in water is not a metal but a compound that makes it stable in water. When consumed by a human or plant the sodium can be utilized for biological purposes. What actually occurs with salt, or at least the sodium and chloride part, is that when chlorine and sodium come into contact with one another, the sodium atom gives an outer electron to chlorine, leaving both atoms with a secure outer shell of 8 electrons. The stable compound formed is known as sodium chloride. The chlorine has become a chloride by this borrowing of an extra electron – this is how all chlorides are formed. There was a time in Earth's history when there was far more chlorine and methane in the air, obviously a time when delicate creatures like us requiring in the region of 78% nitrogen and 21% oxygen to respire could not have survived. Another common reaction would have been when nitrogen and oxygen are heated by lightning and a chemical reaction occurs that makes nitrogen dioxide, this dissolves in water and falls to earth as nitric acid, which will then further react to create more compounds. When methane and water react, the result is carbon dioxide and water, a process that would have helped to create some of the water on Earth along with that brought by comets all the way from the Oort Cloud found at the edge of the solar system. With the billions of years that Earth has been impacted by galactic flotsam and jetsam by way of universal chemical elements, these chemical reactions have been ongoing and it is here the narrative gets even more cosmic.

For the chemical elements of the periodic table (and for that matter those 87 found in Himalayan sea salt), their origin is a fascinating tale, even more amazing perhaps than how all these chemical elements can now be found within a grain of salt. The ultimate origination of the chemical elements is a huge matter of debate amongst scientists, although what is agreed upon is that the chemical elements have arrived on Earth from across the universe as a result of stars exploding (going supernova). As stars go through the process of exploding they get progressively hotter and expand, where different elements are formed. With the subsequent explosion, these elements are scattered across the universe as a fine coating of space dust; with each star exploding at different temperatures, different elements are sent floating through space, varying proportions of which eventually came to be deposited on Earth where they began to go through reactions with the gases already present on Earth, as well as water or sunlight and these in the great wheels of creation eventually finding themselves as compounds that are suspended in water. As this water evaporates it's left as salt deposits in thick seams such as halite. So a grain of unrefined salt comes from a completely cosmic beginning, the age of which is not the vast 250 million years for Himalayan sea-salt, laid down as a sedimentary rock when the vast sea was displaced at the time when the Himalayas pushed up as continental plates collided. The elements in a grain of salt are already billions of years old by this time, having travelled across the universe to merge with other elements that have come from other parts of the universe. Some of the chemical elements (notably those ending with 'ium') are reputedly to be the end result of elements undergoing more than one supernovae event before finally alighting on Earth.

Unimental – all of time and space in a grain

Plato and Homer were quite right to bestow divine qualities on salt; it is nothing short of miraculous and modern industrial man has been so disrespectful as to swap this incredible universal gift for money, power, profit and industry. We've taken salt, ripped out the tiny important parts, the trace elements and kept the gross body (I've a theological analogy in my head about ripping the soul out of the goddess, although I don't know how you'll perceive this, but now that thought is in your head!). It is this deficiency of trace minerals in the soil and in the human that is the root cause of our present illnesses, and it is with these trace minerals where unrefined salt plays an essential role. Just the same as with processed foods constituting the main part of most people's diets, these also are de-mineralized. These heaven sent mineral elements underline the major difference between food today made of the refined deadly whites and food of the past, the unrefined natural food; food today quite simply is demineralised and as such is no comparison to food of old. So extraordinarily different is refined salt to unrefined salt they hardly warrant sharing the same name. A better name for unrefined rock salt would be 'unimental', as it is comprised of the UNIversal eleMENTAL chemicals. Unimental (a single grain of unrefined rock salt) is an accumulation and a reflection of all the universe and all of time – now if that isn't unimental, what is? Unimental holds within it the story of creation and all modern man has done with it is desecrate it, use it to make deadly chemicals and pollutants in a selfish quest for profits.

5 Elemental Chemicals

To focus on just a few of the elemental chemicals repeatedly mentioned throughout this tome thus far, let's have a very quick look at calcium, sodium, potassium, magnesium and chlorine. Whenever a nutritional breakdown of a food item is included on the packaging, if the mineral calcium is mentioned, it is not present in the food item in its raw white metallic form - calcium would be present as a compound, such as calcium carbonate. We cannot eat raw metals for nutrition, although without consuming these elemental minerals as biologically useable compounds we would die, indeed every mineral has an essential role for all life on this planet. How these elemental chemicals become useable is when they take on a form known as a colloidal. In this form they are negatively charged, are non-toxic as well as being biologically digestable. This explains why miniscule parts of radioactive chemicals are often actually inert, certainly in comparison to their refined use in the nuclear power and weapons industries. Plant colloidal is the smallest size chemical elementals can be broken down into and as such give colloidal particles special properties that are not available to the same chemical element if they were presented to the body as a positively charged much larger metallic particle. Being negatively charged, the colloidal minerals stay in solution, being absorbable when required and non-toxic; iodine in colloidal form is healthy, in its raw state as iodine it is deadly and this is true for other minerals, so when found in salt these minerals have the propensity to return to this colloidal state they were in when suspended in the water. This state is easily mimicked within the body where required minerals can be utilized at will.

A similar process, utilized by the supplement industry, is to chelate minerals for better absorption. When a mineral supplement tablet is eaten, only about 8% to 10% at best is bio-assimilated. When it is chelated, up to 50% has the potential to be utilized. Chelation copies what occurs naturally within a plant, which enables the minerals to be useful for those that consume that plant. In the soil elemental minerals are present in minute quantities, these become even smaller when they mix with ground water (becoming colloidal). Plants absorb these and incorporate it within their structure, becoming joined as an amino acid complex; it is this process that is called chelation (wrapped in amino acids) and it is via this route that elemental chemicals become bio-available, whether from the plants being eaten by a human or the herbivore being eaten, or its milk drunk.

Without consuming salt, as would have been the case before agriculture, our ancestors still needed to find essential nutrients for their diet. To venture down an avenue the Codex Alimentarius is trying to block, what types of food would need to be eaten to get the recommended daily allowance (RDA) from natural foods? (A glance at the essential nutrients in the appendix will give a brief overview of some of the superlative sources of the essential nutrients).

With a diet of agricultural food there is little chance of ascertaining the RDA of a spectrum of essential nutrients. For sodium, even when consuming the crops richest in sodium, 3 kilograms of broad beans or carrots (depending on the fertility of the soil it was grown in of course) would need to be eaten to provide the RDA of 1.5g of sodium; with only 2mg of sodium per 100g of wheat, rice and oats, about 75kg of either would have be consumed to get the RDA, neither possible or advisable, so salt is indeed a quick fix. To get the RDA of our ancestors through their foraging diet this level is achievable, although it requires a lot of dark green leaves to be consumed, with the greens of beets providing about 220mg per 100g – nearly 700grams would have to be eaten.

Ethnographic evidence shows that excellent health is achievable with an intake as low as 50% of the western RDA, as is the case with calcium. Calcium as mentioned in the last chapter needs to be consumed in an equal ratio with magnesium, and when it is, the RDA is easily achievable from the deep green leaf vegetables, nettles, nuts and seeds. For magnesium, it is the deep green vegetables and nuts and seeds again that easily provides the RDA and more, with 30gram of sorrel providing the RDA of 300mg, 70g of pumpkin seeds or 100g of nuts also providing this RDA. With potassium it can be seen that the range of food is quite broad for getting a good intake, from nuts, fruit, seeds and deep green vegetables, avocado and the staples of yam and taro, potatoes and sweet potatoes, with a 100 grams of yam, avocado, banana and 50g of pumpkin seeds providing the RDA of 2g of potassium. Chlorine consumption would also have been significantly lower before the widespread use of salt.

All the types of food from the above paragraph constitute some of the staple food types of our ancestors, whereas today none are eaten in any quantity, or at best very occasionally. This nutrient analysis also shows that the accepted RDAs are fairly nonsensical and as previously mentioned we can achieve homeostasis from consuming only a fraction of the RDA of sodium as long as sufficient potassium (and magnesium) is consumed. These five critical mineral elements (sodium, potassium, magnesium, calcium and chlorine) are just the tip of the nutrient chain, with their deficiency being avoided when our staples were foraged greens, nuts and seeds. As soon as our staples became wheat and rice the balance changed and sodium for instance was suddenly not available (especially for those without easy access to water borne food, such as fish and seaweeds), so salt became the solution, not an ideal one because of its mineral imbalance, but an easy one nonetheless.

From unimental to the really mental: The cell

As the above indicates, unimental (unrefined salt) is a fairly accurate representation of the universe and all of time, which amounts to a pretty gigantic macro overview; the antonym of which is also true, namely that unimental also represents the microscopic overview of cell biology. Science currently knows more of the macro-view than the micro-view, although a better picture is being painted year-on-year as our understanding of how the cell works and the role played by all the universal chemical elements within it and its constituent parts improves.

The cell is the smallest unit of life, being the building block of all larger organisms, as well as each of the 200 or so cell types (each gland and organ has different cells) all forming the four tissue types (epithelial, connective, nervous and muscle) that in turn make the twelve organ systems of humans (digestive, respiratory, endocrine, skeletal, cardiovascular, which includes the blood and heart. Integumentary are the skin, hair and nails, urinary/ excretory, reproductive, sensory, muscular, immune and lymphatic). Smaller than the cell are the genes, of which over 35,000 can be found along with over 100,000 proteins (all made from combinations of the 20 amino acids) combining to make the cells. The cell is a remarkable feat of minute nanotechnology, looked at by itself it contains a whole world within its phospholipid membrane. Quite how such a complex microscopic phenomenon ever came about is mind blowing, particularly when one considers an adult human body is made up of about 50 trillion of these cells (estimates range from 1 to 100 trillion, with a consensus of agreement nearer to 50 trillion), each about 10 microns diameter (a micron is a thousandth of a mm) and weighing about a nanogram (a billionth of a gram).

Cells are the most incredible entities, constantly performing amazing acts of DNA replication, moving electrons from here to there, splicing amino acids and making their own energy source. This brings to mind what Francis Crick, the first person to identify the DNA helix had to say about the state of the evolution of the cell. Crick believed that cells arrived on this planet as they are today, via what is known as panspermia. He assumed it could even have been via spaceships, which is a little out there, as ice from comets is a much more acceptable transport mechanism for this panspermia. This might sound a bit out of place here, but I only mention it because the deeper I got into studying cells the more apparent it became that plant and animal evolution is only a secondary phase of evolution, building upon what was already here, the cell. The cell is not just a miniscule thing that happily splits to become two cells, then splits again to become four cells, until eventually we have a tree, rattlesnake, polar bear or human comprised of up to 50 trillion cells. Not at all, on the cellular level, each and every cell is a tiny civilization in its own right, the complexity and functionality is truly stupefying, and it is this complexity of just a fraction of the cell, a strand found within a part of the cell, the nucleus where the DNA can be found, which if unravelled is 6 miles long. This truly beggars belief. It was this that led to Francis Crick stating that it is impossible for this level of complexity to have just miraculously evolved from a primordial soup to suddenly become this intricate cell, which has remained unchanged for as long as a billion years – admittedly there has been extensive evolution outside of this cell, with agglomerations of these cells forming together to make the whole multitude of living things on this planet today, but still the cell has remained unchanged and it is this that is the miracle of life. This miracle of life is totally dependent on just a few basic nutrients to continue quite happily, although unfortunately modern Man (and I mean predominately man not woman in this case) has changed these basic ingredients, denatured them and turned them into poisons, with salt, the most primordial of all ingredients, one that contains most of the elements from across the universe being reduced to a taker of life and a halter of health, when it could so easily be the other way round. Crick was himself somewhat of an enigma and from reading his biography by Matt Ridley there is no indication about where the source for his revelation stemmed, apart from hard work. Rather surprisingly, Crick's eyes were opened (or rather he was tuned in) by ingesting LSD, he experienced elucidation through hallucination, just like a shaman, he had to lose his twentieth century spectacles in order to focus correctly on the problem at hand. Crick definitely enjoyed this drug on many occasions, although his scientific credibility would have been severely tarnished if he publicly announced he was partaking of mind-altering drugs to further his scientific understanding.

Where health begins and refined salt ends

Remember that health begins with a healthy cell, if the cell can properly receive and get rid of nutrients transported across its oily membrane, then the system as a whole has an extremely good chance of being healthy also. When the cell is compromised, then in turn so to is the whole organism, and with the wrong diet, dominated with the wrong fats and overloaded in sugars and animal proteins, the cells themselves take on this erroneous ingestion as the body still has to make new cells and repair damaged tissue and remove alien and detrimental proteins. It only takes a short while, when armed with the knowledge of how a cell works, to see how it is that modern humans are significantly stressing this incredible and delicate balance from its most fundamental micro-level (cellular) all the way to the macro-level of each of the twelve bodily systems, or the body as a whole. It is critical, if one is to gain some insight into why it is we are getting ill, to have some understanding that it is at this microscopic level where the foundation blocks for the present rise of the diseases of civilization begins. It's necessary to picture in the mind's-eye your body from the cellular level up, imagine if you can, exploring the inside of the human as in the film Fantastic Voyage.

Removing refined salt and the rest of the Deadly Whites would be the quickest way to expedite the disappearance of the diseases that have become ingrained in our society, resulting perhaps to the illumination of our health crisis within a generation, it truly is this simple. It's not going to alleviate obesity or cancer over night, it has to be a generational long-term strategy, but as long as there is a negative economic price tag attached to health and the quagmire of legal ramifications of culpability, there will be no ascension to a healthy way of life.

The food industry is ultimately responsible for the level of unhealthy food they provide, it is not the consumers fault as they have been unwittingly manoeuvred into the present health predicament through lifelong propaganda via advertising and product placement. Recent news reports of a 15 stone 11 year old boy's parents being arrested for negligence, or a 10 stone, 5 year old being put into care, underlines this dilemma. Whose fault and responsibility is it anyway, the ill-educated, misled parent, or the propaganda and indoctrination espoused by the food industry? Clearly the source for an interesting debate, and as such, further discussion of this topic is elaborated upon in the final chapter of this book on White Lies. The food industry is making very small steps in the right direction, although often less salt just means more sugar or fats are added. The only real answer is to raise food awareness and to become personally responsible for what you eat, whilst seeing the food industry for what it is, a huge money making enterprise that has neither any incentive or legal requirement to make the food they provide healthier. As an industry (as for all industries, be that health, manufacturing or banking), its only legal requirement is to service the dividend payments to its shareholders. Any changes are only made when consumer pressure threatens profits and then industry makes a PR fuss that they are being responsible and altruist to make us all healthier.

Let's move onto the last of the food derived deadly whites

before what could be seen as some comparative light enter-
tainment and personal philosophy of the last deadly white. We're
nearly there . . .

The Sixth Deadly White

White Rice

"Give a man a bowl of rice and you will feed him for a day. Teach him how to grow his own rice and you will save his life."

(Confucius)

Rice is a staple for over half of the world's population today and it is by far the single most important crop, having fed more people over the past 10,000 years than probably all the other staples of wheat, corn, the tubers of potato, cassava and yam put together. That said, in Europe it languishes somewhat behind wheat and corn as the most economically important food crop, predominately because it can only be successfully grown in the warmest climes of Europe. Rice provides somewhere in the region of 50% to 60% of the calorific input for much of Asia, whereas for Europe and North America it provides only somewhere in the region of 2%. As we have seen, it is the deadly whites of processed sugar, dairy, wheat and the fats and oils which provide as much as 80% of the calorific input of the 'western' diet, although for many of those who eat a healthier diet in Europe, rice will invariably be eaten a couple of times a week.

As rice provides the majority of the food eaten by such a massive swathe of the human population, we are presented with an exclusive opportunity to observe a critical food source consumed in many instances almost solely, with direct observation of the mantra that an unrefined food, eaten for millennia is healthy, whilst its modern refined variant, eaten for only a couple of generations is unhealthy. Uniquely in this case, because there is very little that interferes with this observation, there is not the excessive consumption of all the other deadly whites, or in some instances, little industrial pollution. For many of those still getting the mainstay of their food from white rice, this singularity of just one deadly white being consumed is indeed unique and should provide clear and objective epidemiological analysis. Annoyingly, the bias in medical research toward matters European and North American makes this study a little harder than it should be, although with some digging it has been possible to get to the bottom of this deadly white, so without any further ado, let's smash this last deadly food related white.

The history of rice

The English word 'rice' appears to date back to the thirteenth century, derived from the Old French *ris* or the Italian *riso* and probably referred to the rice that had been grown for a couple of centuries in southern Europe. These words originate from the Latin *oriza*, which itself comes from the Greek *oruza*. There is some speculation about where the Greeks got this word, although a likely source could be the Old Tamil *arici*, as it is almost certainly from the Indian subcontinent that rice spread across Iran and into the Middle East and finally into Europe.

The rice we eat today goes by the Latin name *Oryza sativa*, be it either the sticky *Oryza japonica* (usually grown on dry land), or the longer grain and predominately non-sticky *Oryza indica* (usually grown in wet paddies), both originating from the wild variants, *Oryza rufipogon* and *Oryza nivara*. It is currently agreed amongst palaeo-ethnobotanists (those looking at the food eaten by humans long ago) that these wild progenitors underwent the process of domestication in China, sometime between 8,500 and 13,500 years ago in either the river valleys of the Pearl or Yangtze. *Oryza nivara* was more important in the development of rice in India and parts of SE Asia and could have been the catalyst for a separate domestication there, whilst *Oryza rufipogon* was used in China. Further intricate archaeological excavations and investigations on pollen and grain analysis throughout the whole of Asia will no doubt provide further evidence, painting a clearer picture on the dating and the route rice took during domestication. Countries such as Thailand, Vietnam, Indonesia, Korea, India and the Philippines all have a tremendous number of cultivated varieties as well as wild varieties, and these countries could unearth evidence that runs contrary to current understanding of this domestication process. What often confuses the archaeological record is the unexpectedly long preponderance of collecting wild grains before domestication takes place, as with wheat. It's naturally going to be the grains that formed an important part of the wild foraging diet that would have been chosen to become the domesticated species, usually when the wild harvest became compromised from either climate fluctuations, over-gathering, or population pressure, so as to guarantee a stable supply of the desired food source.

Both Africa and the Americas have wild rice species as well. The African rice, *Oryza glaberrima*, was first cultivated about 5,500 years ago around the Niger River delta and by 3,500 years ago it had extended its range as far as Senegal. At some time thereafter it lost out to the hardier and higher yielding *Oryza sativa* varieties. The wild varieties from America are from the genus *Zizania*, which although still a grass is unrelated to the *Oryza* genus. The species *Zizania palustris* was a fairly important food source for various native Indian tribes from the Great Lakes and into Canada and can still be found growing in relative abundance. Asiatic rice was taken to the Americas by the enslaved, uprooted Africans, being an important staple for them back home, where it thrived in some of the southern-most states in America.

Rice was grown by the ancient Egyptians from where it spread to Ancient Greece, with the Romans extending its range as far north as Germany. The Moors introduced Asiatic rice to the Iberian Peninsula in the tenth century and by the fifteenth century it had become an important crop in Sicily. Soon after fields were planted throughout Italy and France, weather permitting, as rice requires an average of about 75 degrees Fahrenheit and sufficient rainfall or irrigation throughout its growing season.

Rice varieties and the Green Revolution

Today there are a massive 40,000 varieties of rice with what is known as 100,000 accessions (variations or steps between varieties) held in the secure Rice Genebank at the International Rice Research Institute (IRRI) in the Philippines. Found in a number of colours in its unrefined form from brown to red, black and purple, this chapter is of course chiefly concerned with just the refined, white polished variety, be that the white fragrant jasmine, basmati or simply white rice, as it is these that have been refined with just the starchy endosperm remaining. Rice is classified into four groups, either *Oryza indica*, *Oryza japonica*, fragrant and glutinous (glue-like), with the main distinctions between varieties being whether a grain is short, medium or long. The shorter ones tend to be more 'sticky' or glutinous, which has nothing to do with the gluten protein found in many grains. There is a very low incidence of intolerance or allergy attached to rice, unlike wheat and corn, both of which contain gluten, which is a contra-indication to wheat's use as a staple that has seen intolerances and allergies rise in number since the processed white version has dominated the food chain within the past couple of generations. Rice, with so few inherent problems to its consumption, could be viewed as a 'better' food source for the general population than wheat, although (as with the other grains) it still needs to be consumed with other plants to achieve a full spectrum of the essential amino acids, minerals and vitamins required for optimum health. Its relatively small impor-tance to the European and American cuisine and hence economy has meant there has been a bias in excluding it from much dietary debate in the west until very recently, where the rise of diabetes and rice's poisoning from agricultural chemicals has brought it more to the fore of the general public's gaze.

It was from the International Rice Research Institute that the first seedlings of the Green Revolution were established, with a higher yielding rice plant being developed (IR8) in 1966. The general perception of this Green Revolution is that it was initiated to benefit the poorer nations by giving them greater harvests to alleviate starvation. Sadly the reality is that it was pushed through to benefit the developed world by guaranteeing food stocks, and more crucially, it freed up a vast labour source, shifting them from living a rural, self-sufficient, small-scale pastoral life to becoming urban, dependent industrial workers. Very rapidly, within less than a generation, where the land once provided for all the families, the implementation of western agricultural models of monoculture, large machinery and agricultural chemicals, meant only a fraction of the workforce could survive from the land and hence a massive translocation to cities began, using this workforce for the benefit of the emerging western global corporations as cheap labour in their factories. This displacement has continued ever since the late 1960s and with it a huge surge in the global population has resulted. With this urbanization there has been a global rise in the diseases of civilization, as more and more people become compromised from increases in pollution, poor diet and a forever increasingly sedentary existence.

The global increase of rice production since the Green Revolution in the 1960s has been impressive, from about 160 million tons being produced in 1960, rising to 480 million tons by 2012. It was in 2012 that China, the largest rice producing nation, produced 143 million tons (mt), India which has more land devoted to rice growing than China produced 99mt, Indonesia came in third with 37mt, then Bangladesh with 33.8mt. All the other major rice growing countries are Asian apart from Brazil, coming in ninth with 7.8mt (China, India, Indonesia,

Bangladesh, Vietnam and Japan between them produce and consume about 90% of the world's rice harvest).

As we saw in the Flour chapter, the global grain production is currently enough to supply every person with nearly a kilogram every day if distribution were fair. Even after allowing for the 80% of the global grain harvest that gets diverted to other uses such as animal feed and bio-fuel, there is still 200g for everyone everyday. So why is starvation still so rife? This inequality is driven home by the fact that for every extra person born in the world there is a person who dies of starvation, usually in the developing world (world population grows by about 81 million every year, whilst 80 million die each year from starvation and diseases caused from malnutrition). This dilemma, short of disputes and warfare disrupting food supply, could have been alleviated over a generation ago. Although of course it is common knowledge that capitalism only thrives when there is inequality and warfare (see Chomsky et al for a discourse on this).

Although rice is the third largest crop harvested, the major difference between rice production and the other grains is threefold (there are loads of others but there's only three here). Firstly, nearly all the rice harvest is used exclusively as food for humans, with up to 50% of the world's population eating it daily, the majority of this as a refined grain, the same as with the other grains. A small percentage is used as an ingredient in animal feed pellets for cows, sheep, pigs and dogs, although rice bran is usually used for this, which is cheaper and more nutritious, as well as being a waste product after the refinement of white rice. Secondly, there are no significant industrial uses for rice, unlike corn which has a thousand other uses. Thirdly, about 92% of rice produced by countries is used internally to feed their own nationals, which means China keeps nearly all its harvest, whilst India, Vietnam and Thailand accounted for 70% of all rice exports, with China and Nigeria being the largest importers as of

2012.

An FAO (Food and Agriculture Organization of the United Nations) study claims that somewhere in the region of 8% to 26% of harvested rice is lost in developing nations from various post-harvest farm losses, poor transport and improper storage. The study went on to state that in India alone the losses could feed anywhere between 70 to 100 million people over the course of a year. Also in India, if it were to adopt the knowledge and technology used in China (where more rice is grown from less land), 100 million tons of extra rice could be grown, enough to feed about 400 million people, as well as earning the farmers an extra £35 billion in revenue. However, much of this loss has to be as a consequence of the recent industrialization of rice production, irrespective of how 'backward' the FAO and others may want to tarnish Indian production as being. Before massive mono-agricultural farms became the norm, most farms were no more than a hectare in size (many smaller), producing about four tons of rice a year with the vast majority of this being used and sold fairly quickly and locally with minimal wastage, as well as being unrefined, nutritious and reducing starvation.

Some Asian rice dishes

As to be expected from a continent eating so much rice, there is an abundance of dishes made from it. In some of the languages throughout Asia the word rice is the same as the word for food; in China, its meaning is synonymous with the word for 'meal', as in Thailand, where the word 'eat' is the same as 'eat rice', clearly inferring the central role rice plays in the diet of this continent. Each country has its own unique way of cooking and eating rice. A very quick dip into the various uses of rice globally should give some indication of the importance and versatility of this little grain.

The Japanese are of course famed for their sushi, using a short grain *japonica*, which thanks to the excellent fresh fillings in it, such as raw fish and seaweeds, a good semblance of health can be obtained from its consumption, which is more than can be said for the fermented alcoholic beverage sake, which uses varieties of rice not used for eating (although in moderation well brewed sake, like beer has little ill effect). The Indonesians also make a similar alcohol, arak, as do many nations across Asia. Boiled and pounded to make the Japanese rice cakes, known as mochi, these are traditionally used as an offering at Shinto shrines. Conventionally brown rice was used, although today this is seen as old fashioned and has been superseded, with associated health consequences, by the use of polished white rice. A similar rice cake is made in the Philippines called bibingka. Rice can also be turned into flour and made into noodles or used as a batter, giving a crispier and puffier texture than a batter made from wheat flour. This flour is also used to make rice milk; in India a type of bread is made from the flour, called akki rotti.

When the rice is fried for a brief period before cooking the result is a less sticky rice dish, as with the Indian and Pakistani biryani dishes, as well as Italian risotto and Spanish paella and pilaf. Short grain rice is used to make rice puddings, white rice is often used but there are also plenty of Asian versions that utilise black sticky rice for this purpose. A type of porridge can be made from rice, where it is saturated with water to form a near glutinous mass, known as congee, another Tamil word – it can be found throughout Asia, although Hong Kong is renowned for it, served either plain or with any number of fillings from different types of meat to fruit. This has been traditionally used throughout much of East Asia as a food during convalescence. At the other end of the continent, popular in Arab cuisine and around the Mediterranean, is dolma, where grape leaves are wrapped around rice and other savoury fillings.

Brown rice can also be soaked and sprouted, which takes between one to three weeks to achieve and is by far the most nutritious way to eat rice. This is known as gaba rice, or germinated brown rice, with the process activating certain enzymes that allow for a more complete nutrient and amino acid profile to be bio-assimilated when eaten. Nutritional benefits can also be obtained from soaking brown rice in warm water for just 24 hours, as this will initiate germination.

Rice is also well known as the breakfast cereal Rice Crispies, which has virtually no nutrient content, irrespective of its popularity. There's obviously a whole world of different uses, this is not the place to exhaustively look at them, all that needs to be said is that the vast majority of cultural cuisine involving rice today utilises the white variety and for this alone they all have one thing in common, they are made from a deadly white, instead of the traditional and healthy unrefined brown or other coloured rice.

The emergence of white rice

The transition to eating white rice as opposed unrefined brown rice has been a gradual shift. For most of those in Asia born after 1970, there is little recollection that it was white rice that was once a novelty. This has now been reversed and brown rice is seen as a novelty, only recognised by some as a food for the poor or sick, as is the case in the Philippines where brown rice is prescribed for diabetes (we'll get on to this diabetes aspect in a few pages, as it is this disease that holds one of the keys to unlocking the door to the diseases of civilization, as already mentioned in this book and fully covered in Book 3, with its own dedicated chapter). This shift to white rice is a fascinating study, if for no other reason than there appears to be so little infor-mation readily available on the transition – it's as if the knowledge has been wiped from the culinary cultural memory banks, making it easy to come to the conclusion it has been forever present and eaten. It's very similar to the mainly forgotten fact that until just over a 100 years ago the entire Japanese population (exception being the ancient Ainu of northern Japan) were predominately vegetarian Shinto Buddhists, as the first Buddhist precept can be interpreted as to not take the life of anything that breathes air, which did allow fish to be eaten. This preponderance to vegetarianism is no doubt where their legendary longevity stems from and the continuance of this cultural legacy is what has given them an advantage in the lifespan stakes, although such practices are rapidly becoming eroded with their switch to white rice, meat and now dairy consumption.

White rice, requiring extra preparation, was as with white bread, once the preserve of the ruling classes. Innate snobbery within most humans always desires that we have some of what the rulers have, as this is somehow perceived as being better, as is the case with the view of brown rice in Japan being only fit for the lower classes (which is as ridiculous as Henry VIII not wanting to eat vegetables as he saw them as only being fit for the plebs, a view that rather ironically more than likely foreshortened his own life by at least a decade or two). With white rice, the beginnings of its rise to eminence could have been that early traders were offered white rice, as this was the more valuable commodity and trade item, being what the rich ate. Rice mills were implemented soon after to produce more of this white rice, only being in operation from about 1860 (with most regions of the world having followed suit within 80 years). Exported rice further favoured the white variety as it has less chance to spoil, as the oils within the bran and germ in brown rice can go rancid relatively quickly with poor storage. Also due to its lack of nutrients, white rice is far less likely to get eaten by vermin such as rats, mice and weevils, so it more readily survives months at sea.

An export item, preferred by the ruling elite of rice producing countries, this 'posher' version and this distorted philosophy soon caught on, meaning the healthy alternative gets relegated to the ranks of a 'dirty' undesirable product. As this traded white rice became more desirable amongst the locals, at first the wealthier and as time went on gradually filtering down to the less wealthy and finally to the poor, a slow but steady shift over a few generations (predominately taking place throughout the twentieth century), everyone has ended up eating white rice. In the Philippines white rice was known as 'American rice', and of course it's not hard to imagine that the whole of the developing world wanted a slice of the prosperity associated with the American Dream. It's worth bearing in mind that the wealthy would have always been able to afford to eat a varied diet, so the health ramifications of this shift to white rice were less noticeable for some time, which is not the case for the poor, who eat little else but white rice today and as a consequence suffer far more readily from malnutrition. This has led to a significant rise in the diseases of civilization (the risk of malnutrition is exasperated by the legislation in India banning artisan seed oils in favour of imported processed oils, with none of the nutrients available from the traditional cold-pressed oils and only white rice consumed, with associated deficiency related diseases increasing in incidence).

It is certainly somewhat depressing to consider that the health of a whole continent has been compromised solely due to economic reasons, beginning with the fact that white rice was easier to transport. This is of course the case with the food industry in general as we have repeatedly seen throughout this book, with the modern definition of economics dominated by profits, always winning over the original definition of economics, *oikonomia*, good household management, in exactly the same way that the wealth of the corporation is more highly esteemed than the health of the individual. It is somewhat surprising that with such a rich heritage of rice from Asia, it has been so easy for the vast majority to disregard this and happily swap the traditional brown rice for white and thus lose all the health benefits, the very rationale for why it had been so esteemed for many thousands of years. White rice (along with a slow transition to a western processed diet) has within merely a couple of generations seen a rapid decline in the overall health of rice-eating nations. This has not been headline news in Europe and North America because quite simply it's not a part of our culture, but considering it affects over half of the human population it is far too serious an issue to simply ignore or brush aside just because it doesn't directly affect our ethnocentric life.

Epidemiological evidence is surprisingly somewhat hard to come by, especially from the larger rice consuming nations such as China, Indonesia and Japan. Campbell's 'China Study' makes no mention of any correlation between an increase in white rice consumption and any associated rise in the diseases of civilization, unfortunately he focuses almost exclusively on the rise in dairy consumption being the major causal factor, an unfortunate bias because he himself was raised on a dairy farm. There has indeed been a significant rise in the consumption of dairy and an associated rise in the incidence of these diseases, although dairy has not been the only change in diet. This makes the China Study a very useful piece of epidemiological evidence on a massive scale, but it has to be appreciated that it is also somewhat flawed because of this bias in blaming just dairy (he also tentatively blames all animal proteins, although his research tends to focus on dairy). A more holistic approach would have considered the nutrient deficiency of this switch to white from brown rice causing the diet to become lacking in all the nutrients that are available from brown rice. Not to disrespect Campbell's outstanding and exceptional study, it's just a little too narrow in its vision.

Indonesian chickens, stricken with beriberi

Rice is refined in very much the same way as wheat. When only the husk is removed, also called the chaff, this is termed as brown or unrefined rice, whilst further milling removes this outer casing, the bran and the germ, leaving just the starchy endosperm. This is the refined result, and as with wheat, most of the nutrients are found within the bran and germ.

Knowledge about the dietary deficiencies that can result from the eating of this refined grain is not new. In 1929 the Nobel Prize for Medicine was awarded to the Dutch physician Christiaan Eijkman, in recognition of his earlier work showing the association between the disease beriberi and white rice. Dr Eijkman was posted in Indonesia in the 1880s where he noted that the local chickens often became ill in his laboratory with beriberi symptoms when fed solely the military rationed white rice. When they were fed unrefined rice they either regained health or didn't get ill. Fortuitously this was what Eijkman was looking at in humans, so he instantly recognised weight-loss, vomiting, trouble with walking and mental confusion in the chickens as probably being related to the similar symptoms of human beriberi. He didn't know that it was the deficiency of vitamin B1 (thiamine) that caused this to occur, as this had yet to be isolated, although he guessed it was a dietary deficiency of some sort. It was the Polish biochemist, Casimir Funk, who upon reading Eijkman's report a few years later finally isolated a whole group of what he called 'vitamines' in 1912. By 1936 he had found most of the vitamins we know of today (the 'e' was dropped when it was discovered that vitamins didn't need to be amines that contained nitrogen). Funk perhaps has been somewhat under-appreciated for his work, which not only included his work on vitamins but also diabetes, cancer and hormones. He was not only a visionary, but a possessor of what must be one of the coolest names in the history of science.

It isn't just vitamin B1 that is heavily depleted when rice is refined, a proportion of every nutrient is lost. White rice has on average only 10% of the Omega-6 and magnesium that can be found in brown rice; 15% of the fibre, phosphorus, potassium, manganese and sodium, 25% of vitamins B1, B3, B5, B6 and zinc,

30% of the vitamin E and Omega-3, calcium, copper and selenium, 50% of the vitamin B2, 60% of the iron and 75% of the protein (the breakdown analysis varies from source to source, these are a general average of available figures, although all agree that there is a significant loss. Some of the losses may appear small, but if rice constitutes the bulk of the diet then such a deficiency over a length of time will have serious ramifications). It is not just the vitamins and minerals that are lost in refining brown rice to white rice, there is also a loss in the entire spectrum of amino acids that are found in the bran and germ, notably lysine. There is no reliable analysis on specific amino acids and other micro-nutrients (also called phytonutrients = minute plant nutrients) lost from this refining, but it goes without saying that the loss is substantial and in no way is the nutritious content ever bolstered by refining. There has been an attempt to add some nutrients back into rice after it has been refined, notably vitamins B1, B3 and iron, although these are easily washed off during rinsing or cooking, and if the rice is not thoroughly washed there is the added complication of arsenic and other pesticides being inadvertently consumed.

As with salt and wheat refining, the nutrients are not simply thrown away, they are sold, often to a pharmaceutical company for the manufacture of drugs or supplements; this is where a good proportion of the 75% of the B vitamins lost in rice refining end up. Rice is a well-known cure for high blood pressure and the healthy parts of the resold refined rice 'waste' often finds its way into this class of heart drugs. Not that supplements necessarily have to have natural vitamins in them; products such as the massive Centrum supplement company (owned by Pfizer) make all their supplements artificially in a laboratory, which will be explored in the next book in this series on Pollutants, in which we will discover that most recent scientific evidence indicates that supplements in many instances achieve detrimental health affects.

Medicinal uses of rice

This depletion caused by the refining of rice is made all the more significant when one considers the medicinal uses that rice is and has been used for across the world, a very small selection of which includes:

Whole grain brown rice, its bran and the oil have all been used for treating skin ailments, constituting one of the most universal traditional remedies using rice. For this, the rice is often boiled and moulded into a ball with or without other ingredients added, such as comfrey or tea-tree oil, to give additional benefits, this is used to treat boils, sores and swelling of the skin. Crushed rice can also be used for the skin and is particularly useful to alleviate nappy rash. Sticky rice is used to treat indigestion and other stomach ailments, whilst extracts from brown rice have been used to treat breast and stomach cancer, as well as warts. The water remaining from the boiling of rice (known as the broth), has been used as an anti-diarrhoeal, a demulcent (used to treat the irritated or inflamed skin and internal parts of the nose, mouth or throat) and for stomach ailments from pancreatitis and gastritis, (this is a a popular Ayurvedic method of treatment). The rich concentration of potassium in rice helps alleviate oedemas and high blood pressure (as we saw with potassium in the last chapter on salt) and aids with many general problems involving the kidneys. During WWII, American prisoners of war interned in the Philippines managed to ward off beriberi by convincing the guards that all they needed to alleviate them of their symptoms was the bran that had been removed from the rice.

A major component of rice bran oil, is the plant sterol, gamma-oryzanol, which has been shown to help lower the LDL cholesterol. Whilst raising HDL levels and diminishing triglycerides, it can be found in a variety of health supplements promoting health for the heart, skin and even as an anti-carcinogen. An increase in the amount of brown rice consumed will see a natural rise in the amount of this phytonutrient oryzanol. Dr Michio Shimabukuro from the university of Tokushima states that as well as the cholesterol lowering potential, it is also anti-inflammatory, anti-carcinogenic, anti-diabetic and an antioxidant. Not being present in white rice these are clearly five important benefits of brown rice over white rice, as well as of course the fact that white rice is more than a likely contributory factor, as well as a risk factor, in all these conditions that brown rice can help with. Oryzanol has been sold in Japan since 1962, originally to help with anxiety and menopausal symptoms and despite clinical trials since the 1960s, there has yet to be any negative results or side-effects resulting from its use, unlike the reams of evidence stacked against pharmaceutical medicines for these same ailments. Rice bran has also been effectively used in Japan to eliminate and prevent kidney stones, although caution needs to be applied here as rice bran can interfere with the absorption of calcium. If ones diet is already deficient in calcium its best to avoid, or at least don't eat calcium rich foods at the same time as rice bran.

The story for refined white rice is the same as for the other refined deadly whites, where cancer, heart disease, obesity and other degenerative diseases are more likely when the diet is dominated by refined rice. For instance, the risk of certain cancers in equally impoverished regions of the world is 50 times higher in areas where refined rice and other refined grains are consumed as opposed to brown rice and wholegrain wheat and corn, as demonstrated by a 1996 study by S. Rensburg, whose results showed that the risk of oesophageal cancer amongst those eating a diet low in micronutrients (a typical diet dominated by the deadly whites) was 50 times higher than for those of an equally deprived economic status who ate predominately unrefined rice. A study in Korea showed a 19% increased risk of breast cancer for every 100g of white rice consumed, whilst wild brown and black rice decreased this risk of breast cancer by 24%

for every 100g consumed.

Purple rice has many properties completely absent from white rice that are only just beginning to be appreciated by modern science when looking at associations between health and nutrients, such as the free radical scavenging antioxidants found in relative abundance in black, purple and red rice, the anthocyanins and the various tocols (vitamin E precursors). What has currently been established is that coloured rice reduces and prevents atherosclerotic plaque development. With further research more benefits will undoubtedly be discovered. So esteemed was black rice in the times when China was ruled by an Emperor that it was reserved only for his consumption, being called 'Forbidden Rice'.

Cases of anaemia are also much higher when refined rice is a staple, as much of the iron is lost. Just as is the case with the missing vitamin E, giving the immune system no help whatsoever to combat illness. Brown rice is also far less constipating than white rice and there is ample evidence to show that healthy gut biota and the beneficial faecal micro-flora, also known as probiotics, have been shown to flourish far better when presented with the extra fibre from brown rice (and its full compliment of nutrients) and all whole grains, as opposed to their refined, denatured, poor cousins. For those eating brown rice there is a positive increase in beneficial bacteria and less of the harmful bacteria, with a fourfold association in protecting against diverticular disease, co-rectal cancers and other diseases, all achieved from the extra fibre available from brown rice. These benefits are enhanced by a phytoestrogen called lignan, a free-radical scavenger and antioxidant that is converted by bacteria in the intestines into enterolactone which has health promoting properties. On-going research into lignan will uncover far more health bonuses, which it must be said is found in much higher concentrations in flax and sesame seeds, although a bowlful of unrefined rice is certainly a good source, particularly as sesame and flax seeds are rarely eaten in large quantities.

The nutrient content of the rice, whether it be brown or white is also totally dependent on the soil it was grown in. With the common, modern practice of large mono-cultural fields for rice as opposed to the traditional small hectare farms, fertilized naturally, the soil has become increasingly depleted, which in turn yields a crop that is also depleted of minerals and vitamins. So, brown rice may be potentially more nutritious than white rice, although if the brown rice has come from a field heavily sprayed with agricultural chemicals it is quite possible that this actually contains less nutrients and more toxins than a white rice organically grown in a small farm using rich natural fertilizers. Caution needs to be used every step of the way in the minefield that is food and its nutrient content – nothing is black and white or set in stone.

A meal that includes rice in the west is often a healthier one as it will invariably not be eaten by itself and will include a selection of vegetables, possibly in a tomato sauce and usually with meat. This means that at least the right direction is being taken and it is not too difficult to steer a course to a meal that has brown as opposed to white rice, as at present only 1.3% of rice meals in the US are of brown rice and hopefully thereafter also include less meat, with an increase of the vegetable ratio.

White rice and diabetes

The association between white rice and diabetes has been a bone of contention for some time in Asia, although it has only recently been given newsworthiness in the west because it is being seen that a significant proportion of the American-Chinese community are being afflicted with Type 2 diabetes, and as a consequence research has been conducted which irrefutably points a finger at white rice consumption being a definite risk factor, a risk factor that has been associated in India for some time now. Diabetes is also now a worrying threat to many in the

Philippines, with a Harvard study showing that those who ate white rice five times a week as opposed to once a month were 20% more likely to develop Type 2 diabetes, with doctors even prescribing a switch to brown rice. Perhaps not conclusive, but as we shall soon see the evidence of the direct association between diabetes and white rice consumption gets more damning.

As is the case with the refined flours, the insulin response time is more elevated with refined rice as opposed to the whole grain, raising concerns connected with obesity, diabetes and heart disease. As with oat bran, rice bran lowers blood cholesterol, as well as helping with lowering blood pressure. Brown rice has been shown to actually help in the prevention of diabetes, as it releases insulin at much slower rates, meaning there is no sharp rise in blood glucose levels. Brown rice has a lower glycaemic index, meaning less insulin is required, making it far more suitable for those with diabetes to eat, with studies showing that white rice is actually a significant risk factor in developing diabetes. As mentioned, in some countries brown rice is either prescribed for those with diabetes or is actually tarnished with the reputation that it is a health food, only necessary for those already suffering from diabetes. So the association is fast becoming a cultural fact.

The glycaemic index (GI) of white rice has been variously measured around the world as ranging from 48 for Australian Doongara white rice (not readily available in the supermarket that's for sure), 75 to 109 for white basmati rice, with up to 121 for Thai white jasmine (white bread is 100). Brown rice averages 55, although some varieties are much higher. Even if brown rice has the same GI as that of white rice, it is established that the insulin response for brown rice is significantly lower than for white rice, without any sudden spikes and a slower steadier release. Surprisingly, women have been found to be more prone to diabetes from white rice consumption than men. For Japanese women this risk rose 65% and for Chinese women 78%; such risks were significantly lowered when brown rice was substituted for white.

From the Indian Journal of Medical Research (2010) it has been recognised that the prevalence of chronic non-communicable diseases has now reached epidemic proportions, especially considering that not so long ago these were extremely rare compared to the communicable diseases. India now has the most diabetic patients in the world (50.8 million in 2010, so today its probably nearer 60 million with there undoubtedly being significantly more undiagnosed but still suffering from the disease). Part of this surge can partly be accounted for by increased urbanization and a decrease in physical activity, although this only partly accounts for the increase. A more significant risk factor is that white rice is so heavily consumed, whereas as recently as thirty years ago it was very uncommon. There is a direct link between carbohydrate consumption and diabetes as we have seen throughout this book, with the refined deadly whites being almost pure carbohydrates. The carbohydrate input has remained constant in India with the only change being the input of refined carbs from refined rice, and as just mentioned the GI load of white rice is higher and causes significant spikes in the insulin response, a key factor in developing Type 2 diabetes. Diets high in refined carbohydrates also raise plasma glucose, insulin, triglycerides and non-esterified fatty acids, which all lead to insulin resistance, a direct risk to developing Type 2 diabetes.

From a 2001 study, India has an average daily rice consumption of 208 grams, China 252g, eclipsed by Indonesia with 414g, Vietnam with 465g and Myanmar tops the scales with 578g per day. Needless to say other studies have reached different average consumption rates, with one stating Indians ate 8.5 servings a day but failed to mention serving size. Irrespective of the actual quantity consumed, it should not be too surprising that such an intake of a denatured refined grain will lead to not only the rise in diabetes but also cancers and CVD. Indeed these diseases have a higher prevalence in southern India, where rice is more heavily consumed than the north, where wheat, other cereals and legumes form the staples of the diet.

Other studies have shown that simply replacing 50g per day of white rice with brown rice can lower the risk of diabetes by an estimated 16% and by replacing 150g per day the risk is reduced by 48%, whilst replacing all refined grains with unrefined grains the reduction is a massive 108%. A Harvard School of Public Health epidemiological study published in the British Medical Journal showed that for either Japanese, Chinese, American or Australian (the studies looked at over 350,000 people from these four countries) the risk factor of developing Type 2 diabetes increased a full 10% with each additional serving of rice consumed in a day. These results were backed up by Dr Mohan a leading authority on diabetes in India, who found a 400% increase in diabetes for those who doubled their white rice consumption from 200g to 400g per day.

It is interesting to look at Indian postings on various health websites on this topic, as it becomes clear that they are in somewhat of denial, refusing to accept that it could be rice causing this rise in the non-communicable diseases (diseases of civilization). It is mentioned on numerous occasions that rice can't be bad for them as its been eaten for thousands of years, completely missing the point that white rice has only been consumed for a couple of generations by everyone and in the recent past only unrefined rice was eaten. The Indian bloggers also tend to blame bias reportage by western researchers, when it's only comparative epidemiological research with absolutely no racist overtones. Although its clear many blame the increase in diabetes and obesity on the lack of exercise today, where many no longer walk to work, preferring to drive or take a bus/train and of course the type of work has changed from agricultural to industrial and office. This is also true in Britain, where the level of exercise has decreased considerably. Starting at an early age, for instance, when I was growing up I spent all my time outside, kicking and throwing balls, playing in the park, walking or cycling to school, whilst today children are ferried to school in cars, spending an increasing amount of free time glued to the omnipresent variety of screens. Childhood being the foundation stage for later health has unarguably been severely compromised.

It's not just the Indian bloggers who are in the main confused by the health implications of the switch to refined rice. In the Philippines and China there are many who refuse to accept the association that white rice is a direct risk factor to the development of diabetes. Arguments often rely upon opinions that white rice is easier to digest, the children only like white rice and even giving the excuse that brown rice is too hard to find. If they are missing out on nutrients they argue it would be easier to simply take a supplement tablet than it would be to switch to a different type of rice, or that brown rice attracts insects and vermin as these intuitively prefer brown rice for the very reason humans should be eating it, because it contains far more nutrients.

A major disadvantage with brown rice is that it does take twice as long to cook, and for those that truly are impoverished, not only is it more expensive, it requires more fuel. This is a seemingly irrelevant point when we can just put more water in a pan and leave it on the stove, although this is not an option for many who have rice as their staple throughout Asia, the Americas and parts of Africa. To cook for twice as long requires twice as much fuel and when this requirement is met by having to either buy fuel or chop twice as much wood, this is a heavy price to pay, so it is not an easy transition to make when the health consequences are not understood or taken into consideration.

If there was a shift back to consuming brown rice many of the poorest countries could alleviate themselves of the burden of trade deficits, just from the simple rationale that as brown rice is far more nutritious, less needs to be consumed, therefore less needs to be imported and as more of the people eat the nutritious brown rice there would be significantly less pressure on the health services and the reliance on imported pharmaceuticals. Although this underlines why this model of white rice is so controversial, it would lose the pharmaceutical corporations billions, which certainly is not part of their insidious economic model. Even if they accepted this as true they could not agree to it because, as we have seen repeatedly, the only legal requirement of a corporation is to guarantee dividends to share-holders, so any programme that narrowed profit margins is going to be either a non-starter or fought over aggressively because conscience and morality are not an economic consider-ation in the capitalist market place. Another consideration is that if all food aid sent to countries suffering from starvation was restricted to only unrefined, whole grain rice, the suffering and malnutrition could be alleviated more swiftly and completely.

Bacillus cereus

A negative aspect regarding both white and brown rice is the bacteria *Bacillus cereus*, some strains of which can have positive health affects, although it is the harmful strains that are of concern here. This bacteria is often the cause of what is sometimes known as 'Fried Rice Syndrome', as the spore is not killed from cooking at or under 100 degrees Celsius (requiring temperatures in excess of 120 degrees to kill the spores), allowing the bacteria to germinate and proliferate at a prodi-gious rate when this improperly cooked rice cools slowly and is left to sit at room temperature for a couple of hours. The simplest solution is to thoroughly soak the rice in cold water after it is cooked, this removes much of the bacteria and any remaining bacteria does not have the opportunity to grow when the temperature is suddenly dropped, which also has the added bonus of removing any surface starch that tends to cause the rice to clump together. The real danger therefore is to let the rice cool slowly, as this is what activates the growth spurt of the bacteria, it can also be caused by the failure to immediately drain with cold water and/or improper refrigeration. This bacterium is the cause of between 2% to 5% of food-borne illnesses: if presented as a diarrhoeal type with gastrointestinal pain, its incubation time is between 8 to 17 hours after consumption; when the illness presents in an emetic (vomiting) form, symptoms (i.e. vomiting) will occur 1 to 5 hours after consumption, although it is not the bacteria directly that causes this vomiting but the production of a toxin, cereulide. Often, people will blame the meat from the Chinese or Indian take-away or restaurant for food poisoning, when in actual fact it is just as likely to have been this bacteria in the rice. This *Bacillus cereus* has also been known to cause keratisis (inflamed cornea) although this is a very rare causal factor, as is a chronic skin infection it can cause. I mention this not to cause unwarranted concern, as this bacteria is not present in all rice and if properly cooked, rinsed and drained there should be no problem.

Bacillus cereus is just as likely to be present in white or brown rice. One health concern more likely to occur from brown rice rather than white rice is that brown rice has a greater concentration of phytic acid, so to give a little balance, it's not all positive associations with brown rice, there are some instances where its consumption could be toxic as opposed to nutritious. This phytic acid concern is most often exacerbated when the brown rice has not been adequately soaked or cooked, with complications arising with this phytic acid as it can prevent the proper bio-assimilation of nutrients being absorbed by the small intestine. With inadequate soaking or boiling the activation of the phytase enzyme can be prevented, and it is this enzyme that helps in the breakdown of the phytic acid, as well as aiding in the absorption of various minerals. The best way to activate this phytase enzyme is to create the gaba rice as mentioned earlier, by soaking brown rice for at least 24 hours before boiling (a common practice throughout Asia), if a portion of the water used for soaking is put aside and reused to soak the next batch of brown rice then the kept water becomes phytase enzyme-rich. This is not an essential precaution and is understandably a little laborious (particularly in the west where rice is rarely eaten as opposed to daily for much of Asia) but it does guarantee maximizing the full health potential of brown rice. After the soaking stage, the next step is to fully cook the rice in plenty of water as there is a further complication associated with rice, namely that it has the potential to harness arsenic, a recognised carcinogenic toxin with the ability to bio-accumulate. This is partly negated by cooking in the same way as it is with pasta: in plenty of water as opposed to cooking rice, as is often done, with just enough water to be ready when all the water has been fully absorbed. After cooking in plenty of water, drain thoroughly, as this will remove much of the remaining phytic acid. There will be a little nutrient loss with this but its better to be safe, whilst the draining will also remove some of the remaining arsenic, a totally unexpected chemical to find in white, brown and even organic rice.

"Arsenic with your brown rice and lentils sir?"

To put it bluntly, to get to this point in the book I have had to wade through a swamp of conflicting scientific research. How many points of view can there be based around the same topic? How can research led by one team reach a positive conclusion, whilst another team looking at the same topic reaches a negative conclusion, with all of them getting their results published? With science one would assume there was a single answer, but as with everything there are as many opinions as there are studies and as many studies as there are opinions, very rarely is there a consensus of opinion that points to a simple, single answer. Admittedly this is the part of science that makes it scientific, insomuch as it can be ever changing and as already mentioned, every decade 25% of all scientific fact is proven to be not factual at all. With rice and its arsenic content there are several key points that make little sense, and irrespective of the level of enquiry and alleged intellect of the scientists concerned, answers are never consistent.

Arsenic found in rice has been a hot topic for the past few years. The baton was picked up first by the UK's Food Standards Agency (FSA) in 2009, when warnings were issued to parents that rice milk should not be given to toddlers and babies as it would expose them to arsenic. It went quiet after this initial report, although the baton was firmly handed over to the American Consumer Reports magazine in 2012, which analysed over 200 types of rice and products with rice in them from around the world and found varying levels of arsenic in all of them, some well over the FDA and WHO safety levels (not that any level of arsenic, or any other carcinogen can ever be considered safe, as stated by the EPA - Environment Protection Society). Even Rice Crispies and organic baby rice cakes had worrying levels. Considering some of these baby products are a baby's first solid food, with arsenic not only bio-accumulating but also known to adversely affect later brain and physiological development as well as being a known carcinogen, this arsenic component that could have been avoided with some forethought in the past can only be viewed as a major fuck-up.

We all know that arsenic is deadly, made famous no doubt by the arsenic suicide pills carried by spies and secret agents, both fictional and real, to chew on when captured to preserve secrets and identity. Arsenic has also been blamed for the crippling deaths from exposure to it used in the production of fashionable deep emerald green wallpaper in the homes of the upper classes in the eighteenth and nineteenth centuries, with Napoleon Bonaparte being one famous example. Other deaths associated with arsenic poisoning are King George III (possibly also due to the wallpaper or his medication), Simon Bolivar, Francesco I de' Medici, The Emperor Guangxu, as well as it being a fairly commonly used substance to murder relatives to expedite inheritance. In the Middle Ages its symptoms were easily confused with those of cholera, allowing numerous common folk to avoid the gaze of suspicion, possible until the beginning of the twentieth century, as arsenic was freely available from chemists or could be soaked out of fly-paper for various nefarious activities.

Arsenic is indisputably best avoided, so when reports surfaced in the Consumer Reports that some rice regions have dangerously high levels of arsenic in their grain, found both as an inorganic or an organic compound – as part of the fabric of the grain itself – concern is naturally aroused. However, there is no reliable information about what to do next: is this inorganic form, which is the more dangerous of the two types (a definite carcinogen) of arsenic actually causing cancer? Is it flushed out of the system as the body can chelate it and allow it to be passed through the digestive system? Or is it chelated and actually biologically absorbed? Does it bio-accumulate with repeated ingestion, as the deaths of the past from something as innocuous as wallpaper demonstrate? The answer to all these questions, depending on where you look for answers, have conflicting opinions and answers. This has been a recurring problem I have encountered with every chapter so far. Especially as industry led research, which is where much of the information comes from, unsurprisingly often results in conclusions that ameliorate the paymasters, whilst independent research often ends with damning results at the other end of the scale, although this is not always the case, and to make it even more confusing, often it is not transparent about where, why and by whom the research has been conducted (Monsanto for instance employ scientists whose only remit is to disprove damning independent research irrespective of the truth, undoubtedly a policy employed by most large corporations).

As arsenic is a known carcinogen and developmental disrupter, it is listed amongst the most toxic and deadly of all substances (Class 1), so its presence within rice is no light matter that can be simply glossed over. It is often mentioned that brown rice is far worse than white for this arsenic content and as a consequence there are recommendations that white rice is superior to brown, which as seen from the rest of this chapter is blatantly rubbish. The only reason brown rice would have more arsenic in it is because there are far more layers within a whole grain where it can be stored, whilst the white rice has literally been scrubbed clean of both beneficial nutrients and adverse chemicals. That said, the extensive study by Consumer Reports conclusively showed that even if brown rice had more arsenic in it, white rice was only marginally better, with some regions of the USA, notably Missouri, Louisiana, Texas and Arkansas, having extremely worrying levels of the chemical, both in brown, white and organic varieties. The study also looked at rice from other parts of the world and many of these fared much better than the American rice, although some, such as those from parts of India and Thailand also had appreciable levels (although none as high as the American ones). The FDA were quick to reassure the consumer that rice was still safe to eat and unsurprisingly the American Rice Federation (a $34billion industry) was quite vociferous to not only rubbish the study but to also reassure consumers their rice was safe; whereas the conclusions from independent bodies clearly stated that it was best to either avoid American rice entirely or cut down on its consumption. Considering that the western diet incorporates little rice it's easy to avoid, but what about those nations we have already seen who eat little else but rice? And where did this arsenic come from?

Arsenic is found naturally within many bedrocks around the world and as a consequence can be found in small quantities in drinking water and soil, although the quantities found in the study are clearly far above and considerably more widespread than could ever be accounted for by it being a result of simply being drawn from natural deposits or from erosion. Much of the world's supply of arsenic had come from Devon and Cornwall in England, where it was contained within mined ores for tin, copper and sulphur and as a consequence much standing water and even natural streams in SW England can have exceptionally high levels of arsenic in the water and are unsafe to drink unfiltered or untreated, which were either contaminated from the mining industry or are merely naturally present due to its high concentration within the bedrock. In some areas of SW England it is even unsafe to grow root vegetables. Worryingly, regardless of where the arsenic was mined, much of this arsenic comes from agricultural chemicals, as arsenic was a key component of many herbicides and pesticides before most were banned in the 1980s (in fact they were lead-arsenate pesticides and it was the lead content that was banned, although there are still today some pesticides in use containing arsenic). America used more than the rest of world of these arsenic based pesticides, using as much as a million tons worth of arsenic in their pesticides from just the 1960s to today. Arsenic in rice today is predominately the legacy of this poisoning of the waterways and soils, which is nothing less than a clear catastrophe and indictment that the agricultural chemical corporations should never have been allowed to use such dangerous substances, particularly as its persistence is clearly evident and the illness it is reaping on generations to come is nothing short of what many commentators against the chemical businesses have said all along will happen, playing havoc with future generations and adversely affecting the very genetic blueprint of humans, our DNA, for the worse . . . oops! Professor Smith of the University of California for instance has shown from studies that arsenic from agricultural chemicals in public water in Chile and Argentina has already caused lung and bladder cancers, amongst other diseases. He urges that the time to act is now, not wait for evidence to arise from retrospective epidemiological studies, with the phrase involving horses and bolting coming to mind.

It gets no better, because arsenic was not banned from the entire industry, just those pesticides that contained lead, being predominately used to contain a boll weevil and other beetles. It's not just rice fields that have a problem with these arsenic based pesticides, worse are the cotton fields, which were more liberally sprayed with these poisons, however due to arsenic's persistence, when rice is grown in what were previously cotton fields the rice sucks up the arsenic used a generation or more ago for an entirely different crop. This partly explains why the southern states of America have rice with far more arsenic in it today, because these are the regions where cotton is also grown extensively, as is the case with parts of India. Not that its easy for the end consumer to know where their rice came from in their weekly shop, whether it was grown on land previously used for cotton, or for that matter even if it has any arsenic or other toxins within it, as there is absolutely no legislation that requires such information to appear on the product's labelling.

Making matters even worse, arsenic is not even confined to just agricultural crops, it continues to be used in the poultry and pig industry for instance, where it is used in feed to increase the weight of both pigs and poultry and the skin colouration of poultry, the manure and droppings of which is then liberally sprayed across agricultural fields, with the arsenic still bound within it (a proportion of arsenic definitely passes straight through the bodily system, not becoming bio-assimilated). Rice, worryingly, is one of the crops most efficiently able to take on board arsenic (because in many instances it is left to stand in wet paddies where it remains in a chemical soup instead of being drained through the soil, with the rice sucking up the arsenic, although jasmine and basmati rice are less prone to do this). This arsenic laced 'fertilizer' has even been allowed to be used quite legally on organic rice crops, hence why in many instances there was no difference in arsenic content found in organic or non-organic rice in the Consumer Reports study. As these poultry and pig feeds have been used internationally, the problem is not just confined within the US. The persistence of the arsenic compounds in pesticides that were used in many countries long after the ban and sold to new markets, as pressure in Europe and America closed the market doors to the pharmaceutical corporations for their deadly chemicals, resulted in opening new doors in new territorial markets, continuing the dangers inherent from arsenic in the human food chain. So there it is, arsenic can be found in rice as a direct result of the obviously dangerous practice of spraying deadly toxins liberally across vast swathes of a country since after WWII.

It's not all bad for brown rice

All this rather puts a serious dampener on the alleged health benefits that can be achieved from brown rice. Such dangers with rice have been snapped up by advocates of the Paleo-diet as further confirmation that grains are unfit for human consumption and that their diet is the best and healthiest, which clearly has some weight to it, but it certainly does not lend itself to any justification that humans have never eaten grains, whilst selling the message that we need to be eating a meat rich diet just as our caveman ancestors did to achieve health and homeostasis, which is an erroneous standpoint already mentioned in this book (also just wait until further evidence surfaces about the extent of the poisoning inherent in the meat industry from chemicals and pharmaceuticals, let alone the lack of monitoring, as exposed by the recent horse meat scandal).

The solution to this, if you want to continue eating rice and the last two pages haven't put the fear in you, (because there are varying levels of arsenic in most agricultural produce, just not to the extent found within some rice, even apple juice has been found to have more arsenic in it than rice, where are the cautionary notices to avoid apple juice?) just eat brown rice. If you can't be bothered to soak the brown rice for either a day or two weeks to make gaba rice, at least make sure it's well rinsed before boiling in plenty of water (at least 6 times the volume of water to rice, if not more if your saucepan is big enough) and thoroughly rinse and drain after cooking. Also if possible look at the provenance of the rice, being particularly weary of American rice, although Californian rice has the lowest levels, put your faith in organic rice, preferably from Thailand or Indonesia (Chinese and Indian rice is probably okay in the main but these countries are also big cotton growers and how on earth can you know if the rice comes from what was ten years ago a cotton farm?). Personally, I'll continue eating organic brown rice from India about once a fortnight and eat more organic quinoa (which sadly also comes with problems, as its recent surge in popularity has caused a 300% price rise, pricing out the locals in South America for whom it was a staple, leading to potential starvation troubles as its becomes more fashionable in Europe and North America).

A good way to help clean your body of unwanted toxins, not just arsenic, is to increase glutathione in your body. Plants produce this to cleanse themselves of free-radicals, and so can we. The best way to achieve this is to eat food that makes this glutathione in your body, achieved in the main by three amino acids: cysteine, glutamate and glycine. Cysteine is the hardest to get a good dose of, although this sulphur containing amino acid can be found in eggs, garlic and onions (all the alliums including wild garlic leaves, ransoms, pick them fresh in the spring). Food that can boost your overall glutathione production includes asparagus, avocados, broccoli, brussel sprouts (all the brassicas), peaches, walnuts and watermelon (in alphabetical order not glutathione order). Selenium is also an important co-worker with glutathione and the best source of this is nuts and seeds.

Basically, eat loads of fresh vegetables, garlic, nuts and seeds, just as the caveman did and you will significantly negate the possibility of not just arsenic poisoning but most forms of poisoning, as well as boosting your general health. As an aside, do not think a supplement of glutathione will be an easy answer, clinical trials have shown that the body does not bio-assimilate this in a denatured pill form (just as with most supplements) so make the effort and go for the food types mentioned above.

To ease your mind a little more about consuming rice, especially brown rice in regards to phytic acid and arsenic, there should be little concern as the phytic acid bonds with the arsenic and is safely excreted from the bodily system, this probably accounts for the fact that there is as of yet no epidemiological evidence that suggests that the increased arsenic in rice is causing a dramatic rise in cancers across Asia (see www.curezone.org for more) unlike the diabetes epidemic from increased white rice consumption (which will have an increase in cancer incidence as diabetes is a definite risk factor for cancer and most of the other diseases of civilization).

Of course ignorance is bliss regarding the extent of dangers inherent in the food industry. I haven't wasted the past nine years researching these books to simply increase the stress and put the heeby-jeebies in my readership. The aim was to spread the truth about what has been going on behind our backs and when this is exposed the chance of a safer future should be a little easier to accomplish. As Paracelus said, "the dose makes the poison", so with this in mind, moderation is the key. If your general diet is predominately fresh vegetables with a variety of grains and tubers, a minimum of processed foods and a good selection of nuts, fruit and seeds, with a large mixed salad (preferably not from a bag) as often as possible, you needn't worry too much, if at all, that the food you are eating may be causing you potential illness. The potential of illness is every-where in life, but as Hippocrates said "Food is your medicine" and if your food is as good as you can get, don't let the stress of worrying about your food be yet another negative factor to your health.

The halo dims on Golden Rice

This brings us onto the last case study pertaining to rice and food in this book.

A modern book on food could hardly be written without some mention of the recent agricultural practice regarding the unleashing of genetically modified organisms (GMO) into the food chain. There is no space to look at GM foods in general, as the evidence as of yet is far from conclusive that all GM foods are or will be problematic, however, its roll-out will undoubtedly lead to catastrophic consequences if only a couple of global corporations are allowed to monopolize it, with only short-term profits as their overriding *raison d'etre*. There has been recent news that many countries are banning the growing of GM crops, such as France, Ireland and Russia.

There is no doubt that for most corporations the introduction of GM is profit driven, with no thought given to what may be best for mankind. Just as with the world of health, where the focus is virtually exclusively on pharmaceuticals, there has been a division that has split health between those who trust modern medicine and those that don't – there is no middle ground. Exactly the same circumstance is the case with GMO, where there is an industry led campaign to promote GM as being a people-saver producing more food and types of food with extra nutrients, and then there is the other camp that is against all 'frankenfoods'. Industry no doubt is content with this dualism as they can more happily fight their case with enormous budgets at their disposal. Although the reality is, as with modern medicine where there is a place for some pharmaceuticals, there is a place for some GM crops. The problem is quantifying which ones are the best, most beneficial and safe. Permaculture (meaning not just permanent agriculture, but the whole philosophy of working with nature rather than against it to create a sustainable and non-destructive existence) has to be the ultimate long-term solution, although there is still a place for some monoculture. We have lost all sense of balance and this will never be achieved if one side is only after profits and driven by the modern definition of economy. So let's just have a brief glimpse at a tiny niche of this GM world that directly involves rice, that of the euphemistically entitled 'Golden Rice'.

Golden Rice, a name derived from the golden hue of the grain (which is the colour given to it by the beta-carotene content, a precursor of vitamin A) is a fascinating case study. On the face of it, it is an altruistic enterprise by two scientists, Ingo Potrykus and Peter Beyer, whose only interest is in trying to supply vitamin A to as many people as possible (although their initial intention was to tackle iron deficiency, which sadly failed completely). Figures from 2005 put Vitamin A deficiency affecting 190 million children and 19 million pregnant women in over 122 countries and causing up to two million deaths (670,000 under five year olds) and 500,000 cases of xerophthalmia (blindness) every year. There are already programmes in place to alleviate this deficiency, with vitamin A pills and injections in 43 countries, with UNICEF backing two high-dose supplements per year since 1999, accepted as not the best methods, these are the most viable at present. So this vitamin A deficiency is a well recognised problem and Golden Rice could alleviate some of this suffering. However, as vitamin A is fat soluble (hydrophobic) there needs to be sufficient fat in the diet for the conversion from carotene to vitamin A to take place, which of course presents other problems for those impoverished, even if the newer strains of Golden Rice could deliver a sufficient vitamin A dose in as little as a half a cup serving.

To disagree with this stance of supplying vitamin A to the poorest can easily be viewed as wishing the death of these two million people, but of course it's not as straightforward as that. No one in their right mind could think this a bad idea, but regardless of the actual truth behind the motives of the two scientists (whom I sure just want a solution), there is much trickery and deceit in promoting this pure GM crop, being pillared as a saviour crop, all thanks to the magic of GM. By using this one example, the name of GM is hoping to pull itself out of the mire and be polished clean, white and pure, just like the refined rice that is causing so many incidents of ill-health. The global corporations of Syngenta and Monsanto have of course put their oars in, with Monsanto trying to stir up some rare positive public relations by stating it isn't looking at profits from its involvement in Golden Rice, being prepared to give out licences and seeds to any grower who makes less than $10,000 a year in a vain attempt to show they really do care (certainly not a word easily associated with them, unless it's caring about their profits).

Points against Golden Rice are that it hasn't been tested on animals let alone humans for adverse effects, with a danger that birth defects could be a side-effect (personally I feel this is a bit alarmist but without sufficient tests, who knows?). This all makes a mockery of the draconian Codex Alimentarius, creating one set of rules for the ordinary small business and another set for the multinationals. Think back to what was mentioned about the Codex Alimentarius earlier, where it is becoming more common to make it possible to arrest and close down businesses that make any association between a food item and its nutrients and any health claims attached to them. This is now illegal, so what is this claim about Golden Rice being a possible solution to save millions? This has to be either a drug claim, an illegal one, or quite simply it exposes the truth behind the grip that the food corporations have on WHO and government agencies. It's illegal for a greengrocer to claim that a carrot or kale can save lives from vitamin A deficiency, but a similar claim made by a GM crop which may have the same outcome is perfectly legal. Do you see the clear duplicity in this statement?

Greenpeace are of course opposed to all GM crops and fear quite rightly that an acceptance of Golden Rice will open the door to all other GM crops that will not have any health claims attached to them. This is definitely an avenue of acceptance the multinationals are seeking, such as Monsanto, whom up till now have done little but brought defilement upon our beautiful Mother with their poisons and patents, although of course its not just Monsanto, they just bear the brunt of condemnation being one of the largest and most active corporations. It's hard to think of one positive attribute these companies has brought to any environmental debate apart from their expensive and biased PR and predominately erroneous, pseudo-scientific research.

Vandana Shiva has much to say about GM crops and correctly points out that instead of focusing on such a narrow problem as vitamin A deficiency, the broader picture needs to be looked at, which is the serious deficiency of the availability of a broad range of nutritional foods. If rice can be grown, why not vegetables rich in natural vitamin A such as sweet potatoes, carrots, fruit and green leafy vegetables? If a policy of global permaculture can be instilled then self-sufficiency can be achieved. It is total nonsense, if not a clear injustice, that so many of the countries where we in the west buy our food from can't even feed themselves a bowl of unrefined rice once a day.

The current Golden Rice being grown in trials has genes and enzymes from a couple of bacteria, one from the soil and the other an E-coli, apparently an inert one, but where are the guarantees on this being safe coming from? There also appears to be bits from daffodils, cauliflower, pea and a wild rice also thrown together (from the horse's mouth at goldenrice.org) to boost the beta-carotene content.

Another failing of Golden Rice is that it is S.E Asian children that are predominately deficient in vitamin A, a region where *Oryza indica* is the rice grown, although Golden Rice has been genetically modified with a strain of *Oryza japonica* (all the information available only ever states its *Oryza sativa*, which isn't quite true as that's the same as saying its from rice, the specifics aren't mentioned). So straight away there is the inherent problem of attempting to grow a crop that is not suited to the S.E Asian climate, as *Oryza japonica* has repeatedly failed to be cultivated in most of Thailand and Indonesia, which is why *indica* is grown there. This means that if the scheme is to have any success it will require significant transportation and distribution logistics. Surely, developing a strain that can be grown by the local people who need it would have made far more sense, although there appears to be no mention of this problem from those involved in Golden Rice, I wonder why?

Vitamin A (or at least its pre-cursor, beta carotene) is relatively delicate and there has been little to no studies on the time factor of how long the beta-carotene will remain viable in rice grown some distance away, or how stable it is when cooked. Questions that certainly need answers before the rhetoric and propaganda of saving millions of children is emblazoned quite so triumphantly.

Uganda and Mozambique already have a programme of distributing sweet potatoes that have been conventionally bred to contain more beta-carotene, doubling the vitamin A intake of women and children who are beneficiaries of this programme. This represents an excellent example of working with nature, as sweet potatoes naturally have a good vitamin A content and as such, if this programme were to be expanded it would be almost impossible for it to lead to any long term complications, an assurance that is not possible from Golden Rice. It's also quite revealing that the news of this sweet potato initiative has been silent in our press, whilst the news about Golden Rice has been considerably louder, I wonder why? Another more recent initiative in Uganda has been to increase, via genetically modifying a cooking banana, the vitamin A content of what is a staple for the majority. Research and trials will attest to its potential, whilst the clamour about Golden Rice gets forever quieter. This is hardly surprising when one considers the cost so far of not developing a finished Golden Rice product, which has stretched well beyond $100 million in investment thus far. All this has been going on whilst the Vitamin Angel Alliance have been handing out high potency tablets twice-a-year at a cost of 5c per tablet, meaning that it costs 10c a year to prevent blindness from vitamin A deficiency for one person or child, $1 for ten people and that an expenditure of $100 million on Golden Rice's failure could have saved a billion people. Or at two million deaths a year attributed to this vitamin deficiency, this $100 million would have prevented these particular deficiency deaths for the next 500 years (not including distribution costs). Economics or *oikonomia*, who wins?

Patent pending

Instead of spending tens of millions on 'frankenfoods' or even distributing supplements, why have there been no programmes spending a similar amount on creating permaculture in impoverished and deficient regions? In the same light as the Confucius quote at the beginning of this chapter, the poor and starving can feed themselves *ad infinitum*. This has to be the real solution to those who are so poor that a balanced diet is impossible, to simply give them a foundation where permaculture becomes viable and they can grow a varied allotment, because if they can grow rice, why is it impossible to grow other crops, particularly crops that are considerably easier to grow and more nutritious than rice, which has labour intensiveness and excessive water requirements? Rice is not a whole food in the sense of providing all the essential amino acids, vitamins and minerals. This truly would be a miracle food, as nothing provides this, although some types of food do come close such as peas and certain seeds such as hemp. So, a diet that consisted of rice and peas would easily sustain a human organism for a lifetime, with only the occasional addition of say a little fish once a month and a deep green leafy vegetable and a fruit once a week. Such a diet would far surpass the average western diet so dominated by processed foods and lacking in fresh food.

What has been made clear by the pursuit of what was undoubtedly a humanitarian goal by Beyer and Potrykus with their Golden Rice is the tangled web that has been created by the world of patents. Ignoring GM concerns (because it is unbelievably complicated when looking at GM and patents), it has been the ability of the multinational seed and agricultural corporations to twist legislation worldwide and completely in their own favor to manipulate and preserve their monopoly on future harvests – this is a major concern. As if getting rice to grow with beta-carotene within its structure wasn't hard enough, the fact that at the end of their experiment they had infringed 70 patents between 32 different corporations, proving a clearly near-impossible situation which to find a solution for. It is the added complication of these patents that will eventually lead to what has to be a revolution in what and how food is grown, where morals and human rights have to win over foreign investment. Before 1994 there was no patent for a GM crop, toady there are hundreds of thousands, most of which overlap. Much has been left to the clever wording of the biotech lawyers, who have patented techniques that could involve any number of species. All that has been achieved is to significantly boost the powers and profits of the lawyers, whilst ignoring the rest of the world's basic necessity to be allowed to grow their own food. This patenting of the world's grain has been dubbed 'bio-piracy', arguably an ongoing process, occurring even before Europeans brought back potatoes from the New World or when wheat was spread across the Old World. No individuals from the parent country grew immensely wealthy from this old biological kidnapping, even if the Native Americans had spent millennia breeding corn or potatoes, there was no money repatriated for their agricultural innovations, just wholesale theft. So where is the precedent that somehow today it becomes 'legal' for corporations to protect their monopolies?

At the end of the day its all bullshit paperwork, used as some form of justification for this modern version of monopolising the world's harvest, a very dangerous game that is guaranteed to end in disaster, because once again this made-up paper world has been constructed on the back of our modern definition of the word 'economics' (money and profit dominated). When *oikonomia* (household management) resurfaces after being held down for as long as six millennia (since the time of Adam), the paper world will burn and only then will justice and equality be re-established (I will cling to this dream of an egalitarian future, as this is the only viable solution if humans are ever going to hitch a lift back onto the path of evolution, not the current descent into devolution that is taking place before our very eyes, conveniently obscured by those filters on our twenty first century spectacles).

Just a very quick final word on what else is going on in the world of GM rice – here's another one that could have disastrous consequences. If putting a strain of E.coli in Golden Rice wasn't dodgy enough, how does human breast milk in rice grab you? It's obviously not breast milk *per se*, that would be just too weird, but rice that has been genetically modified to express lactoferrin (a protein, abundant in breast milk and an antibacterial agent), lysozyme (an enzyme with anti-diarrhoeal properties) and human serum albumin (protein found in blood plasma). Just to throw this one in there, it's a fairly recent development and I don't want to comment beyond just three letters – WTF!!

I wouldn't argue with the Chinese over rice
Modern detractors of rice are quite simply barking up the wrong tree. The only reason the Paleo-diet advocates attack brown rice

is because in their blinkered field of vision all grains are allegedly harmful. Epidemiologically this is absolute nonsense, there is no evidence to show that before the staple grains were refined there was any significant prevalence of the diseases of civilization. The fundamental problem with the grains is due to them having been refined, with the removal of the nutritious aspect, leaving an empty shell, which most definitely is more often than not nothing more than a negative dietary input. To attack brown rice because it has a greater arsenic concentration than the refined white version does not justify the consumption of white rice, although it does send out this distorted message. The danger from arsenic in brown rice is certainly not to be ignored as this is a carcinogen and poison of some repute, however, the danger this poses is not due to brown rice but due rather to modern agricultural practices, notably the agricultural chemical industry. There is no inherent danger in the consumption of brown rice, one only has to consider the amount of people that this grass grain has fed in the past 8,000 years. It would be fair to assume that at some point in those 8,000 years the Chinese have used rice as a staple, with their infinite wisdom and meticulous scientific study, far outstretching that of Europe, they would have at some point flagged their consumption of rice as a potential danger had they encountered problems with it. If white refined rice was the way forward they would have consumed this, surely? This denatured rice only came about from economic considerations as seen through the eyes of European traders, never the indigenous growers of the rice.

There is a consensus of opinion amongst all researchers in the field of health and nutrition that wholegrain types of food definitely hold preventative characterisitics against heart disease, cancers and the diseases of civilization, although somewhat surprisingly when it comes to reviewing the research directly there is little tangible evidence. This runs counterpoint to common sense; if the former is true that wholegrains are undeniably good for you, surely it's obvious that to exclude them would be detrimental. It's exactly the same as stating that nutrients from food are health-promoting and then in the same breath stating that a diet that excludes the majority of nutrients has no effect on health, which is how the stance of the Codex Alimentaruis is being positioned by the concerned corporations. The corporations state that their supplements and nutrients are healthy, whilst manipulating legislation so that exactly the same nutrients from natural food can not claim to have the same health benefits. Clearly there is much consumer confusion and deliberate propaganda being nurtured by these corporations in favouring their artificial products, especially as the natural products from Mother Nature's larder are direct competition and as such pose the biggest threat to their continuing profitability and emerging monopoly. Hence, as is the remit of all corporations to protect their profits, they have to undertake indoctrination to vilify all competition whilst promoting their products and insuring dividend payments to shareholders.

If there is any lesson to be learnt from the previous six chapters it has to be that Mankind has been supremely arrogant and dangerous in ridiculously assuming s/he can do a better job than Mother Nature. If we had only paid more attention to Her and less to our greed we would not find ourselves in the predicament we do today, where even eating a bowl of organic brown rice comes with potentially serious health ramifications attached.

The more we learn of Mother Nature, the more amazing she proves. Even in the world of computers, surely an iconic symbol of our modernity, Mother Nature has devised a considerably better memory and storage facility The world of computers and the shrinking of memory size has always been limited to a world dominated by ones and zeros, which is proving to be inefficient in the new era of gigabytes and terabytes. The new, state of the art computer chips, will all be designed just as Nature has done since the beginning of the cell a billion years ago, as information stored on the DNA helix with its infinite combinations of four letters. When these new computers are finally developed, they will still only be poor mimics of a system that is as old as life itself, not that this will stop the companies selling us the newest, best, as nature designed, v 3:02, solid-state DNA memory, holographic screen and retina activated personal computers.

Ponder this as we finally leave the world of the damaged food chain that modern Man has created and step into what will hopefully be a more cooperative and caring future as we strip away some of the White Lies that pervade our modern existence.

The Seventh Deadly White

White Lies

"White lies always introduce others of a darker complexion"
(William Paley, theologian and moral philosopher)

There is a fine line between what we innocently call a 'white lie'
and an industrial lie on an international level, affecting millions
of people. The truth – as with the nutritious content of the
previous six deadly whites – has been processed, manufactured
and bastardized by economic man and turned into the final
deadly white: a lie.

White lies can loosely be defined as untruths, said in order to
minimize, diminish or prevent upset, harm, embarrassment,
damage or injury. This leaves a lot of leverage in how we define
those terms from 'upset to injury', with such a broad range of
meaning, all dependent upon who is saying the white lie and
who is the recipient. As will be shown, most industrial lies – or
the 'losing', 'misplacing' or 'not publishing' of research results –
easily falls within the definition of what constitutes a white lie. If
research results could damage, minimize or diminish profits,
then in the eyes of industrial protectionism (insuring dividend
payments to shareholders) this white lie is economically permissible. Its crucial to reiterate that the only legal remit of a corporation is to guarantee dividend payments to shareholders and
any mechanism that allows this payment, even if morally,
ethically or environmentally wrong is irrelevant, as long as the
payments (profits) are maintained, this is justification for the
lies.

"It wouldn't be allowed to be put in, if it wasn't safe"
Before getting to some nitty-gritty about industrial lies, let's take
a quick look at some white lies that circulate on a more

individual, family and societal level. One of the biggest white lies we are forever telling ourselves is the delusion that someone, somewhere, is looking after the interests and safety of the consumer, the erroneous assumption that deleterious ingredients would never be allowed into food if detrimental health implications are attached to their consumption. The little inner-voice of conviction that says all has to be okay, "Someone must have checked it" and "It wouldn't be allowed in the food chain if it was dangerous", often placates us, making it fall well within the definition of a white lie, as any greater harm is prevented by the avoidance of both worrying and knowing the truth.

False impression, delusional assumptions and egotism, accounts for the thought that someone somewhere in the government is protecting us from the likes of aspartame, herbicides, sugars and fats. There are many health and safety agencies, whose work is often faultless, with only the public's safety as their overriding objective. The problem with these agencies is that the vast majority of their work is only carried out after public information has been passed to them, making their actions always reactive – they work on public complaints of malpractice and persistent sickness from consumption of a product – they are not working in a preventative manner. Instead, the safety of any food product is left to the companies wishing to sell that very product. As Dr Spock would have said: "It's not logical captain."

This hijacking of the food-chain by the food industry bares many similarities to the scenario of pharmaceuticals taking the health industry hostage, to such an extreme that for most people there is and has never been any notion or alternative route to health other than pills and creams. In the same light, the public assume that whatever the food industry churns out is by its very existence, an item of food. Incredibly we have been manoeuvred into a position where we blindly assume the food industry is the sole provider of good food, just as the health industry is the sole provider of good health.

The American FDA have lost much public respect, with repeated, controversial, duplicitous involvement with the large corporations (there appears to be a revolving door feely available to politicians and policy makers to rotate between employment in the government and directorship of multinationals). The same is the case with the British FSA (Food Safety Agency). The legal and financial ramifications of liability has tied the hands of responsibility. We need to be aware that in reality there is no one protecting people from the evils of the food chain.

The FDA has approved a staggering amount of food and drugs, in many instances with no safety checks except those carried out by the corporation intending to sell the item. A glimpse at the pharmaceutical industry shows that between 2004 and 2008, Pfizer's turnover was in excess of $245billion, whilst sales of Eli Lily's Zyprexa (an anti-psychotic for schizophrenia and bi-polar) topped $36billion. These astronomical figures do not warrant leniency with regards to regulations, but of course they do, with fines for malpractice merely being seen as pocket money and easily factored into such enormous finances. During that same four year period (2004-08) the major pharmaceutical corporations paid out $7 billion in fines, lawsuits and penalties; which amounts to a miniscule business expense, although it clearly shows their methods of conducting business tips the scales of illegality and ethicalness. Where is Hippocrates when you need him? Banana, chocolate, kelp, salmon and figs can work just as well for depression, if not better and certainly come with none of the dangerous side-effects, although to state such a natural solution, is branded by some as lunacy and heresy. Considering that the vast majority of drugs come with very serious side-effects, effecting more than 10% of those taking them, they are not just glib words on the pull-out leaflet in the packet. (This very dangerous world of irrational toxic health pharmaceuticals is looked at in much more detail in Book 2: Pollutants.)

With regards to food, there are exhaustive guidelines, although any scientific backing tends to smooth the entry of a product into the market place. This looks safe on the surface, but of course it is only the larger companies that have the resources to finance scientific studies to prove the safety and legitimacy of any claims. This allows a considerable amount of legal leverage and of course if at the end the legal hammer falls against the large company's claims, the company simply drops the product, pays any fines incurred and moves onto another product and looks for another angle to exploit the confidence of the consumer. Of course the FDA isn't a gangster in a white lab suit, its merely a regulatory body, and its tiny staff means their main job is paper shuffling, reading industrial in-house scientific research and checking that it appears truthful, which considering the extraordinary lengths the corporations go to cover their tracks, the FDA cannot be solely blamed for not always catching the slippery buggers of industry, who usually manage to worm free. The FDA and other regulatory bodies are not privy to the facts that often scientific literature has been manipulated and is biased; they are certainly not complicit when research isn't even put forward, where of course contradictory and potentially damaging research is rarely put forward and often buried.

What message does giving sweets as a treat and a reward give?

Another white lie is the fact that we constantly tell ourselves that the diet we are eating is in the main, okay. Especially pertinent is the white lie where parents feed their children frozen meals, crisps and sweets throughout the day and somehow convince themselves it is causing no harm, even as they get fatter and fatter. There must be a point when every parent sees this, although I guess by this stage other white lies take over to absolve parental responsibility, or it's never seen or considered, deemed a coincidence or a cruel dealing of genes meaning all the family get bigger together. Is it a white lie each time we fob sweets off on kids as a treat? All those millions of tons of sweets produced, most as an almost exclusive poison for kids.

A major concern of this chapter is the question how on earth did the sweet manufacturers manage to shift liability for type 2 diabetes and obesity away from sugar? The poisons inherent in packets of sweets and the addictive ability of sugar and the other additives is comparable to giving a drug addict their desired drug to allow them to go away quietly, leaving us in peace and to stop any fuss. There aren't many adults who would chomp through a whole packet of sweets, but it's alright for a little kid to munch through them. After all its marketed and meant for kids; if the sweets weren't alright someone would have mentioned it in a health agency, or there would have been an advert on telly about it, surely? No, it's kept very quiet to avoid any legal wrangling and expensive lawsuits. Just look at the natural additives that are rapidly creeping into kid's sweets these days: colours from nettles, beetroot and spirulina, replacing the colours from coal tars and Dante's inferno of chemicals, which recent scientific research has been unequivocal in proving to be harmful. This beggars the question that if all those colours, eaten by millions of kids when growing up (like me and all my school mates) have been proven to be carcinogenic and endocrine disrupting from independent research, how many deaths yet to come will they be responsible for?

Who is responsible?

Was it a daily white lie or ignorance and stupidity that led to the recent arrest of the parents of a 15 stone 10 year old, or the removal of a 10 stone 5 year old from his parents? I would never solely blame fat people for being fat, but there has to be a line drawn somewhere. Interviews with the parents of the 15 stone ten year old suggest that the parents genuinely assumed he was just a big chap, emulating the obesity of his parents, as they each shovel down a thick crust pizza in the evening, accompanied with biscuits, crisps and fizzy drink; with a diet consisting in the region of 95%+ processed deadly whites, the parents didn't necessarily knowingly produce obese children, surely there has to be some culpability from the food industry, doesn't there? When did the consumer demand obesity and diabetes as a consequence of cheap food?

These stories that generate significant national press coverage quickly slip out of the public consciousness, why is this? Probably because when anyone with any sense searches for the real accountable parties in matters such as obese kids, the blame predominately falls on the food industry not the parents. If the food industry had had proper regulation, not allowing the lawyers and lobbyists such control, the food chain would be a safer industry. After all, everyone needs to eat, so it's a very secure industry, growing in line with the rise in population, but as clearly shown throughout this book, it's all gone askew as the diet today is the foundational stage for most of the diseases of civilization to take root. The competition element within the food industry should always have been centred on who can supply the best food, not the cheapest. As soon as the cheapest became a target, quality goes out the window.

The same goes for the increasing waistlines and the white lie that it's hereditary, arguing that it's in the family's genes to be on the large size, that it's got little to do with the constant poor diet and lack of exercise. Coincidentally, as soon as these alleged victims of genetics change their diets and do some sustained exercise, miraculously this hereditary disposition to largeness disappears – is that a white lie or self-denial again – or are they the same thing? What is often misunderstood about genetic predispositions is that we have the ability to alter our genes for the worse in as little as one generation. Often the ancestors are blamed, when in fact it was the endocrine disrupting chemicals the individual or the parents encountered that altered the genome; chromosomal damage can take seconds to occur, not the centuries we have been misled to believe.

Also the drink or three every evening and the other drugs being taken, whether prescription, over-the-counter, cannabis or cocaine. We are forever telling ourselves we have it under control, it's not a problem, it's not as bad as so-and-so's consumption. Medical literature has for decades now been warning of the dangers of alcohol, cigarettes and drugs, although its only when the cost of remediation outweighs the taxation gathered from these that anything is officially done about these personal pollutants. All these white lies of self-denial are leading us down a path of ruination in no short measure, especially as these personal pollutants can have drastic consequences for the next generation, as these genetic mutagens act that quickly – that's why they are called endocrine disrupters, they mutate the genome in the same way that a carcinogen causes cancer. A classic white lie we tell ourselves regarding this alcohol and drug abuse are sayings such as: "just one more can't hurt" and that a weekend's abstinence can be termed a de-tox making it okay to continue with the detrimental inputs for the rest of the year. This very term de-tox is a misnomer (and a white lie) as it's never going to work. The only de-tox that could ever work would be a preventative diet, where there is no accumulation of toxicity to begin with. All those fat soluble toxins are not going to be flushed out of your system just because you've bought 500g of blueberries, some Evian, a packet of seeds and green tea with a couple of days abstinence. These are white lies, they are a form of protection, seen as preventing a greater harm, often in this case revolving around peace of mind and avoiding depression.

Calorie confusion

If there is a white lie about our diets, what really doesn't help is that when we want to do something about this adverse diet and try to seek out the healthiest foods, the wording on the packaging in the supermarket makes everything look so lovely, healthy, tasty and fresh, when of course all of these are themselves white lies (well, they're actually stretching the truth until its only a micron thick, whilst liberally coating it in bovine faeces). Determined as you may be to put a stop to an unhealthy diet, unless you have studied the food industry and nutrition, stepping into a supermarket to accomplish this is not as simple a task as initially assumed. Take for instance what may be considered an obvious step in the right direction, swapping your mid-morning bottle of sweetened fizz for a small bottle of juice. A step that has been completely drenched in confusion, not at all helped by the recent press attention to the amount of sugar and calories in juices and smoothies, information which only has a small portion of the truth attached to it. So, whilst making a difficult consumer decision and looking at the vast array of beverages, the allure of a smoothie takes hold, "Buy me, I'm full of fruity goodness" it shouts at you, the Innocent Pomegranate, Blueberry and Acai Smoothie (owned by Coca-cola) wins out, so you decide to see if it's cheaper for a bigger carton which will last all day, a hunch that was correct as it's on offer for only £1.39 for 750ml, cheaper than the 250ml from the chilled lunch section and only 14p more than your normal 500ml bottle of regular coke. Contented with a healthy alternative and your economic prowess in getting 3 times as much at a cheaper price, as well as consuming at least 2 of your 5-a-day, you go for the kill and actually take a look at the ingredients and nutritional bumpf just to check how wonderfully you have done for yourself. This is when you notice the kcals content (the figures are preceded with a k, as 1kcal is actually 1000 calories, but don't worry about that as a calorie is actually a measure of the energy requirements for burning candles, so all a bit nonsensical, as for this book and other literature a kcal and calorie are interchangeable). You are amazed the total kcals for the carton is over 500 (it's actually 532), whilst the coke is only 210kcals. Oh! The wife was moaning about your belly and now it looks as if the healthy choice wasn't so healthy after all, particularly as 532kcals is equal to nearly two and a half Mars Bars, two pints of Guinness (actually 600kcals), a rather large serving of French fries or a Burger King Bacon Double Cheeseburger (with only 477kcals). Proving that the Innocent smoothie wasn't quite so innocent after all. Sadly this is only the beginning of this particular trail of nutritional discovery, because calories don't really count for very much, only being the start of the white lies encountered.

The shocking truth about 'fresh' premium juice

It's always perplexed me how so much fruit can be sourced so cheaply and used in these juices and smoothies, especially as 10 years ago if you wanted a smoothie a health café would have been the best, if not the only option to find one. There's been a niggling little voice in the back of my head saying "Things are not as they seem here", especially factors not just dealing with price and quantity of fruit required, but also how it manages to always taste identical, week in week out, even when not in season (as even Floridian oranges have a season), as well as being able to last so long un-refrigerated, particularly if all the wordage on the labels is to be believed about it being 'pure', 'freshly squeezed', 'never from concentrate', 'natural' etc. I guess by this stage of the book you will not be at all surprised to hear that the advertising words and the truth have been separated for some time now. They are not even on speaking terms.

What happens with juices is not as I ignorantly assumed; that a buyer for the juicing company secures tons of fruit in not perfect condition, seconds as it were, takes these to a giant squeezer and bottles it all up. Erm!! not quite right. The first stage is indeed a vast amount of fruit, all the excess from a farmer's harvest, all the fruit that didn't make it to the shops or sold onto further processing. All this fruit is juiced and at this stage it is 100% natural, it's obviously an orange, apple or mango, as just fruit has been used, hence why the packaging blurb carries these titbits of information about 'freshly squeezed', 'pure', 'natural', and 'only fresh fruit', irrespective of the fact it got squeezed eight months ago, 6,000 miles away and from here on in, things become very much not as nature intended. Because squeezed juice has the inconvenience of going off in a matter of days, so the juice is pasteurized at temperatures reaching 85-95 degrees Celsius, killing off most of the vitamins (vitamin C is a fairly delicate vitamin), flavonoids in the pulp, as well as damaging the minerals, as these nutritious bits have the annoying habit of 'going off'; whilst those enzymes which aid digestion in the gut make juices separate, so these have to go as well. Then it is put in million litre vats where it can sit for up to a year, being siphoned off when required, although to accomplish this all the oxygen has to be removed using a process known as deaeration. What is left is a million litres of clear, flavourless, denatured water with fructose in, which tastes and looks unpalatable. So to turn the fructose 'water' back to juice, those clever food scientists developed flavour packs, where each juice company can have its own signature flavour, which is why every carton of Tropicana (owned by Pepsi Co Inc.) or any other brand tastes identical each time, wherever in the world you drink it.

It's not all bad news, as a proportion of these flavour packs will contain actual fruit flavours, oils produced from the waste, skins etc., although some ingredients such as the colourings and preservatives are definitely not natural, but we aren't going to find out what they are, as flavour packs' ingredients don't need to be and are never mentioned on the ingredients panel, falling within the very handy term of 'trade secrets'. A major concern here is that the flavour packs by reusing the skins for flavor are also including all the agricultural chemicals that have become concentrated in the skins, all those cancer causing, endocrine disrupting chemicals, all pass from the peel to the flavour pack and into your gut where they are free to cause havoc as another free-radical. Nice. So if you're going to buy a carton of juice, seriously consider spending a few pence more on an organic one. By the time any juice carton reaches the supermarket shelf there is no 'fresh' or 'alive' bits in it, which is why it doesn't need to be refrigerated and is further protected by the Teflon or BPA lined carton, causing what kind of damage only Gaia knows, as there have been no tests on the safety of these flavour packs or containers.

The only reason the consumer pays more for premium, not from concentrate juices is because it costs more to store and transport than frozen concentrates. Concentrated juices are also pasteurized, then dried and frozen (where its fructose content is a staggering 65%) and when reconstituted with water their own flavour pack is added. Undoubtedly the juice makers had some form of agreement to artificially keep the prices higher for 'premium' juices as a perfect way to give the impression it is a better product than the cheaper concentrated version, when on a nutritional basis, both are very similar. A bit like when Sunny Delight was introduced to the public amid a whirl of advertising; a mixture of water, concentrated juice, colourings and vegetable oil, which the makers insisted was put in the chilled section to give the allusion of it being fresh. Heavily marketed, it sold by the truck load for a few years until the truth caught up with it, with many press articles slating it, although the point is, it was still bought in huge numbers by the susceptible, indoctrinated consumer (it is still available today, although now with different ingredients).

Natural chemicals such as ethyl butyrate, the decanals or terpene compounds are a major constituent of the natural flavor chemicals found in real, whole oranges, although when isolated and put back (these chemicals could just as likely have come from a laboratory/factory, it is made industrially by reacting butyric acid with ethanol) they have lost all the other bits, such as the enzymes and fibre that aids digestion. Tests on juices found that this ethyl butyrate content was up to seven times that found in real oranges (considering ethyl butyrate is a known skin, eye and respiratory irritant, is used as a plasticizer for cellulose, is flammable and considered a hazardous material when transported). 700% more than the natural amount is not going to bestow any health qualities. It can also be found in many citrus flavoured products whether pineapple, mango, peach, plum, cherry even bubble gum.

Some flavour packs also include a pulp-dissolving enzyme (pectinase) to obtain a consistent mix. While talking of pulp, any idea what the bits in a carton of orange juice are? I can't find any evidence that it is what we innocently assume it to be, those tiny little juice sacs within each segment of an orange, called juice vesicles, another name for pulp. There is absolutely no guarantee that what is added to juice 'with bits' in it are these juice vesicles. The ingredient profile states that there is no fibre in either the 'smooth' or 'with bits' orange juice, which doesn't make any sense if it was the pulp. The pith and pulp contain not only fibre but also micro-nutrients (phytonutrients), so even a blended drink of whole oranges outweighs a freshly squeezed juice, although both are better than a store bought one. Flavonoids are found in the white part, working in conjunction with vitamin C (obviously not when it's been removed). When the whole fruit is eaten, the fructose is bound within fibres and other plant matter, meaning that a significant proportion is carried to the large intestinal tract where it is fermented by gut biota (a useful prebiotic). This requires no sudden insulin surge, and when broken down insulin's use may still be unnecessary, depending on the item of food eaten. If the sugar from the plant is inulin or oligofructose then these will be released and converted to glucose with no insulin requirements. Fruit juice, not one you've squeezed yourself, will require insulin to break it down as well as the kidneys doing some of the conversion, thus putting a strain on the metabolism of the diabetic and becoming a risk factor in causing diabetes in the first place.

To top it all off, after years of propaganda through advertising and exaggerating the fact that the most prevalent vitamin associated with oranges is vitamin C, the juice industry has spent a lot of time, money and effort in making sure the public knew of this, as this was an excellent way of getting into the mind of the consumer that their produce was healthy. In actual fact an orange has less vitamin C than broccoli, kale or sorrel (which has potentially more vitamin C than any other plant from Mother Nature's larder), and to make matters worse, once it's been processed, most of this vitamin C is destroyed. Any claimed vitamin C content is usually false, as ascorbic or citric acid is put in the flavour packs and this is far from being vitamin C, it's merely what protects vitamin C in nature. As reality and advertising are so far apart it makes no difference whether its ascorbic acid or vitamin C (except your body knows the difference) – they'll call it vitamin C until such time as they are told to stop, which isn't going to happen soon. The vitamin C and other nutrient analysis is carried out when the oranges are still oranges, the producers most definitely would not want the nutrient profile of their juice to be advertised, as this would show there is next to no nutrient content. (Orange juice has been focused on here only because the information about the American method was relatively easy to research, exactly the same process is undergone for all juices, with China producing a phenomenal quantity of apple juice, although their production methods are far more secretive although certainly carried out along similar lines.)

Remember, all this deception involves what we innocuously assumed to be a perfectly healthy and safe product: juice. I hope that makes you realise that for food products with already a poor reputation as being bad for you, imagine how really bad they actually are for you?

This brings us back around to all the recent media uproar being caused by the fact that these juices and smoothies are calorie-rich, with a litre of these juices and smoothies containing as much as a 1,000 calories. However, it's always been a very well-known fact, certainly not a secret or cover up by the fruit industry, that fruit is relatively high in calories, unlike the sugar industry, whose entire history is shady to say the least. The sugar industry is simply swerving the responsibility of its obvious contribution to obesity and other diseases, whilst highlighting this consumption has increased in the sector of juices and smoothies (direct competition for their market shares of beverages, although of course they now own many of their competitors as well these days). This increase in fruit juice purchasing can be statistically manipulated to make it appear there is indeed an association with the increase in consumption of juice and an increase in obesity levels. That's the only reason it's become news today, because the juices and smoothies have been marketed so well as being a healthy component of diet, this excessive consumption is now having health, particularly weight implications, resulting in confusing the consumer even further about what to eat and where to turn for safe nutritional information. To clarify this position as it's important to get it right, if you do no exercise that's going to be your problem, what you chuck into your body afterwards by way of food is only going to add to this problem, particularly if you, as most people do, eat a surfeit of processed foods. If you went for a jog or a cycle, came home and juiced up an orange, apple, banana and chucked in a little kale and a teaspoon of flaxseed oil, good on you, this has nothing to do with the consumer confusion being caused by the parent who gives their child a glass of concentrated juice with a processed frozen meal. The juice may well have more calories than the food and as the child is doing little exercise there could be weight-gain ramifications.

Five-a-day conundrums

What makes this more of a white lie, if not just a scam, is the fact that along with this pretence of freshness associated with supposed fresh, 'not from concentrate' juices, manufacturers can further substantiate the healthiness of their year-old muck by labelling it as one of your five-a-day, which is complete nutritional bollocks. How can an insipid, denatured glass of juice truly constitute one of your five-a-day to create health? It never will. Quite how those supposed health agencies looking after our safety allowed this to happen can again only be down to pressure exerted by the lobbyists and lawyers of the food industry. The initial five-a-day message was only ever intended to include fresh whole vegetables and fruit, with the best guide being only one or two portions of fruit and three or four of vegetables. This five-a-day was already a compromise, as health experts had argued for eight-a-day, which is nearer the levels associated with guaranteeing a full essential nutrient spectrum, figures nations such as France and Sweden use as their guidelines. A rough idea as to what content constitutes a portion (one of the five-a-day) is roughly a cup full or about 80g to 100g of fruit or vegetables (depending on the weight of the food, as watercress is obviously much lighter than sweet potato or a banana, but far more nutrient dense). All this rationality has been thrown out the window by the food industry, where it has been allowed to put forth some crazy boasts about their products containing one of these five-a-day, such as fruit winders, which are a modern version of the old fashioned fruit leathers, where concentrated fruit pulp was dried and made into a consistency not dissimilar to leather. Traditional 'leathers' included hawthorns and rosehips, the modern ones contain, sugar, aspartame, HFCS and some heavily processed fruit. A packet of these is only ever going to be a negative dietary addition. Many supermarket smoothies even claim to offer two of your five-a-day; with the one in my hand saying 330ml will provide three of your five-a-day, which is not only impossible, it's a lie. How can a pasteurised drink made of grape and apple juice with pumpkin (25% of each), with the rest being peach and apple puree, ever be considered as providing 60% of your daily nutrients? How was this dangerous, misleading message ever allowed to be emblazoned on packaging. Someone needs to take 100g each of fresh pumpkin, apples and grapes, determine the nutrient content and compare this to the nutrient content of 300ml of the supermarket smoothie, informing the appropriate agencies, as this is a complete shambles.

This whole five-a-day message was dreamt up in 1991 by a consortium of fruit and vegetable companies and the U.S. National Cancer Institute. They had good initial intentions, as it was clear the general public were not eating a good-enough diet, it's just that this helpful message has been unsurprisingly picked up by the food industry and turned into a white lie in the shallow hope it will help them sell more of their processed rubbish. Stick to only real, whole vegetables and fruit, organic where applicable and financially viable, throw all the processed food made from the Deadly Whites away and stop worrying about calories and your five-a-day (and of course get active).

The marketing of the five-a-day message should always have focused on fresh vegetable consumption, as vegetables are richer in a broad range of nutrients and are considerably cheaper than the same weight of much fruit. For some reason the fruit industry focused on it's products, where suddenly every month there appears to be a new super fruit, constantly swaying the consumer to assume fruit is the best food source, which is incorrect. There is ample medical literature clearly stating consumption of too much fructose is a danger, as when metabolising fructose the liver plays a role and if the potential energy from the fructose consumption is not required the liver converts this unused fructose into fat, which in olden days would have been an ideal storage system for future energy requirements as glycogen is easily made from fat deposits. Today of course these energy requirements are rarely needed as modern humans are becoming forever sedentary, hence the fat just continues to be laid down and never converted via ketosis into glycogen for energy. This is where juices fall off the line of good health, as all they offer is fructose and this is more often than not converted to fat by the liver as its energy potential is unrealised.

So, once again the dangerous health implication associated with fructose consumption is not the fructose itself but the lack of physical exertion by lazy modern humans. Fructose has often been bandied about by nutritionists and dieticians as being a good form of sugar as it doesn't require as much insulin for the conversion to energy (with its associated lower GI, as the last paragraph said, the liver deals with a proportion of this breakdown of fructose), although of course excessive consumption becomes a problem. Sugar being half sucrose and half fructose means that this fat deposit can be avoided but of course the extra strain is encountered by the pancreas in producing more insulin to convert this glucose into glycogen and potential energy, where this extra insulin dependence actually becomes a direct risk factor in the development of diabetes. It is confusing and I trust that the last couple of paragraphs weren't too perplexing. Moderation is the key, although I appreciate even understanding what constitutes a moderate amount has been deliberately made confusing by the food and health industries, whose only remit is to make the consumer buy and become dependant on as many of their products as they can possibly get down our throats via their brain-washing.

Juice it yourself or eat the fruit whole and ignore all the guff being presently spouted by the sugar industry to discredit a competitor in their quest to grasp as much as possible of the soft drinks market. Modern juice from the supermarket is also a denatured, processed product, bearing little nutritional resemblance to its actual fruit self (which as we have seen, the very nutritional potential of which has been severely compromised by the near sterile soils intensive agriculture has left us with). If it was bought from a supermarket and has a best before date of more than a week in the future, it is not going to be as healthy as the packaging and advertisers lead you to assume it may be. There is no comparison between making a fresh smoothie at home or a store bought one. Stick with eating some fresh fruit everyday and try your hardest to eat a little less meat and a little more fresh vegetables, as fresh vegetables are the best source of nutrients. If in time your meals can become more vegetable orientated, your health will also benefit.

Back to diabetes, because the truth has to be told

Diabetes has been mentioned a few times already in this chapter (and a lot more throughout the book), so let's elaborate upon this disease for a couple of pages, as the white lie that surrounds this medical condition has had a significant impact upon the health of millions, if not billions. Diabetes is looked at in considerable detail in Book 3 'Diseases of Civilization' of this series, although because you're reading this particular book and it is of such importance and so large has been the deceit surrounding this disease, it just has to be mentioned here, as it is definitely an important element in understanding the aetiology of many of the diseases of civilization.

It was in 1949 that the US medical associations collaborated with one another and quite conceivably with the fledgling pharmaceutical industry also, making this not only a conspiracy, but one of the biggest scandals ever to come from the health and food sectors, which is saying something, seeing as these industries are forever mired in controversy. Up until the 1930s, diabetes (defined as an imbalance in the blood sugar levels) when left unchecked for a length of time (anything from a year to twenty years, depending on the individual and the disease) presented itself as a set of symptomatic illnesses, ranging from cancer, heart and kidney disease, depression or obesity and depending on which symptom prevailed, the patient would be treated by a specialist in this particular field. What's important here, is the fact that already by the 1930s it was well understood that it was diabetes that caused these diseases, diseases which today are of course the biggest killers of industrialized mankind, shrouded for the most part in an air of mystery. In the 1930s, the decision to split these diseases into their individual symptomatic conditions was made, whether initially done with good intentions has in time become irrelevant, because today there is no recognition by the medical industry that it is indeed diabetes that is the cause of these diseases and this is the white lie, because if the medical institutions really have no knowledge of this, then I really am a 30,000 year old caveman! I would contend that it has always been known, just kept quiet as a trade secret, in exactly the same way that it is nonsense to assume that the dental industry never knew that mercury placed inches from the brain might not be safe.

The financial implications had to have been recognised with diabetes and its wide ranging symptom set of illnesses, as it requires far more staff and finances to run a diabetes ward in caring for those suffering from cancer, heart disease, depression, obesity, pancreatic, liver and kidney problems, amounting to seven wards worth of illnesses, with seven times the funds required. The logic has become blurred and the initial knowledge that all these illnesses stem from the same dietary imbalance has been lost, replaced with mysterious diseases with little understanding as to how they originate and certainly confusion and ignorance about how to cure them, to the extent that many of them simply get labelled as incurable with a whole lifetime's worth of medication required.

Just consider the fact that it is accepted that there is a significant incubation period before these diseases manifest as the incurable diseases they become. This incubation period is, in many instances, no less than the years of eating an inappropriate diet, rich in sugar and the other processed Deadly Whites (all of which escalate blood sugar levels) finally catching up and displaying as cancer, heart disease, depression or obesity. Today, diabetes is seen as a separate disease when in actual fact it is the mother of most diseases. Of course the preponderance of carcinogens in intimate contact with us everyday has gone through the roof since the 1930s, making it easy to view cancer as a separate disease, but still in most instances of cancer, if the individual's bodily system was not constantly plagued with excessive blood sugar levels the cancer would not have proliferated, as this increase in blood sugar is the very fuel cancer cells crave. In individuals whose diet consists mainly of vegetables and whose sugar intake is low, as is their consumption of processed foods, is it a coincidence that cancer incidence amongst such groups is extremely low? Of course it bloody isn't a coincidence, it's the very reason they don't suffer from cancer, simply because the blood sugar levels are as they should be. Which is all I'm going to say about the white lie that circulates about diabetes for now, and if that wasn't a teaser to get you to read the following books in this series, I don't know what would be.

Sugar needs to be mentioned again (and again and again and again)

Sugar might well have already had its own chapter but there is so much more to say about it, so much so that volumes could be filled regarding not only its detrimental qualities but also the lengths the pushers of sugar have gone to preserve their profits. Considering how detrimental sugar is, it has been truly outstanding how much of a Herculian effort has been made by the sugar industry to have kept it out of the public's gaze or even scrutiny with regards to its blindingly obvious correlation to diabetes (the very definition of which disease is an imbalance in the level of blood sugar, of which sugar consumed has to be a significant risk factor). It's straight forward, unlike the confusion with cholesterol or fat, where dietary cholesterol, say from eggs, does not necessarily have a corresponding rise in blood cholesterol or that fats do not necessarily make you fat; with sugar, when its eaten blood sugar goes up (as it goes up with consumption of any of the Deadly Whites). What sugar is causing is exactly as outlined in its dedicated chapter, all those diseases are not exaggerations, scaremongering or suppositions, they are actual diseases that have been attributed to excessive sugar consumption.

So why has sugar been left unmolested to reap these catastrophic diseases?

Well, as mentioned in the Sugar chapter, the industry has meticulously put itself into a position where if any scientific research were to be made public about its obvious deleterious properties, the industry could flood the public's consciousness with exactly the opposite impression, with supposed reputable scientific credentials as well as taking out newspaper adverts, sending out mass mail-outs of press-releases and discrediting any detractors. With their immense capital and profits to protect, there is no end to their meddling.

The tide was beginning to turn against sugar in the 1970s, with heaps of scientific evidence linking its consumption to the initial surge in the diseases of civilization being experienced in those nations with the greatest sugar consumption, primarily America. There had been a similar situation in the 1930s (and for decades before), when sugar was the biggest negative dietary source and was taking the flak for a lot of diseases, although because of sugar's smaller consumption and the fact that processed foods only formed a minority of the overall diet in those days, the diseases had not reached the epidemic proportions of today. Since the end of WWII in America people have been progressively fed an ever-decreasing nutritious diet of processed shit, long before the rest of the world, so predictably their incidence of diseases related to this consumption occurs at least a decade or two before the rest of the world. This coincidence had not gone unnoticed, and during the 1970s sugar had been repeatedly bombarded with negative media stories, meaning that sales were down a couple of percent every year, reaching as much as 5% per year by the mid-70s. The priority for the sugar industry was clearly to halt this downward spiral in consumption of their deadly white, which they achieved with some success, as the spotlight was moved away from sugar, until today that is.

The Sugar Association (representing the American sugar industry) managed to deflect this spotlight by undertaking a substantial and pricey programme of adverts and easily misinterpreted press statements using their own heavily biased, erroneous and flawed scientific reports as proof of sugar's safety. This culminated in 1976 with the FDA, upon review, upholding sugar's GRAS status (Generally Recognised As Safe). So successful was the Sugar Association in turning the public's attention away from their product that in 1976 the Sugar Association also won what is the most coveted award in such matters of marketing and public relations, the 'Award for Excellence in the Forging of Public Opinion'. Their peers gave them due respect for their successful mind control and brainwashing; make no mistake, this is how sugar has remained to be such an ubiquitous poison throughout the food chain, one that we happily and enthusiastically reward our children with for good behaviour, positioning sugar as a good thing, not the cancer causing, heart stopping, fat and diabetes inducing deadly toxin that it actually is.

Let's hope this time around there is no repeat of the insanity of sugar walking away scot-free, as sugar consumption has to be severely reduced. In the past, the sugar industry in America ceaselessly conducted research with the aim of exonerating sugar from any culpability with any associated increased risk factor in such diseases as obesity, diabetes, heart disease and cancer. Endless ad campaigns linked sugar products with sporting prowess and any other achievements it could bung a few grand at to endorse their sugary vileness. The sugar industry attacked its detractors as being the real enemy, effectively programming the public. So successful had the sugar industry's campaign of indoctrination been that by the end of the 1990s the American Diabetes Association and the American Heart Association actually endorsed sugar as being part of a modern balanced diet despite being two of the very diseases sugar is most widely linked as being a causative agent in, diabetes and heart disease. What a victory! Instead of damning sugar to the core, these bastions of the diseases they represent (diabetes and heart) do not even have the temerity to say the truth, that it is sugar contributing to these diseases. What hope is there?

The Sugar Association emerged in 1943 after sugar rationing. Several public information commercials attested to the dangers and uselessness of sugar, which was confirmed by the fact that the national health index peaked during the war for many nations. Was it just another coincidence that these years are the very years sugar consumption was at an international low? Such facts were easily lost in the carnage and excuses that a world war brings. It would be an interesting experiment to conduct, to return to the ration days of little sugar and meat and plenty of home-grown vegetables . . . Although scientifically such an experiment would always be flawed as there are so many other variables that could be argued to be at play when determining health, from the initial health of the participants, the age distribution, the soils, types of food eaten as well as the depressing fact that any modern person already comes soaked and saturated in hundreds of unnatural and dangerous chemicals that would have been absent 70 years ago. However, it doesn't need to be scientific for it to be the truth, particularly if as already mentioned, every decade 25% of scientific fact is disproved. What we need are Natural facts that are not so readily disproved and generally approved as being irrefutable.

With sugar's diminishing public perception a couple of decades after WWII, internal memos from the Sugar Association show that they were fully aware of the potential links between sugar and such diseases as cancer, obesity, diabetes and heart disease in 1962. This reveals there is a lie being perpetrated, even if that lie is only on a moral or health level, the fact that the consequences of ignoring their own concerns have led to the deaths of millions and subjugated millions more (probably billions by the time its use is curtailed) to a similar death from obesity and diabetes and all the other deadly diseases these spawn is inexcusable. Making matters worse for the sugar peddlers of the 1960s was a corresponding rise in the consumption of sugar alternative beverages, sweetened with saccharin and cyclamate. The ensuing battle saw saccharin retain its market position alongside sugar, although cyclamates were thoroughly battered into submission by the Sugar Association (it cost them about $4m in today's money to squash the cyclamates threat and conduct their own flawed experiments involving rats and bladder cancer associations). Ironically, cyclamates could be one of the better alternatives to sugar, alongside the current batch of devils masquerading as sweeteners such as aspartame, neotame, sucralose and HFCS.

Sugar is also cholesterol free (as only animal products have dietary cholesterol), so if the cholesterol rich foods can be repeatedly blamed for high blood cholesterol rates and subsequent heart disease, so much the better. Irrespective of the fact that sugar most definitely causes blood cholesterol to rise was unimportant to the Sugar Association, what was important is that the links with saturated fats and heart disease were more pertinent to advertise than sugar's association with any diseases. Even if this link between many natural saturated fats and heart disease has been scientifically disproved, it should not be a surprise to hear that the promoter of this flawed scientific link, Ancel Keys (who we met in the Fats/Oils chapter), was in the pay of the Sugar Association from just a year after its inception in 1943, being one of the first scientists they drafted in to espouse this phoney science. What a coincidence. Not. It's all a part of the strategic model the polluters employ in attempting to exonerate themselves.

The Sugar Association holds conferences with sympathetic scientists who all agree there is more work required to irrefutably come to any conclusions, positive or negative, which is what they always say, as it's not actually a lie and limits damage to their own credibility. The sugar industry can also block and stop research grants to facilities before negative results transpire about sugars negative role in health. It all chips away at the efficiency of the truth getting out, whilst increasing the pro-sugar stance in the public's perception. Establishing institutes such as the Food and Nutrition Advisory Council (FNAC established in 1977) inhabited by paid-off scientists all willing to swear to the safety of sugar, especially in a balanced diet (words that are a white lie as this 'balanced diet' is a euphemism, it's a disguised acceptance that one aspect is a negative input which needs to be 'balanced' with a positive dietary input). In the course of time such institutions make many reports about the safety of sugar, eclipsing any negative scientific papers from independent research. It was a colleague of Keys', Biermann, who was responsible for shifting the weight of blame away from sugar for heart disease onto saturated fats, financed by the FNAC.

When quizzed about these suspicious coincidences, the Sugar Association explains them away as being historical issues, emphasising that their current operations are run along very different lines (perhaps those lines are pronounced with a silent 'n'?). And so it has become common practice for industry-sponsored scientific reports being used to validate safety of products, even if the scientists are clearly in receipt of industry finances. This use of scientists to validate false claims took a huge leap in 2002 when the FDA introduced a new category of pre-approved product claims, known as 'qualified health claims,' used to boost marketing assertions if a company's product meets certain qualifications, which of course is nothing new. What was pushed through was that the lawyers had argued for a 'no consensus needed', which simply amounted to paying a scientist to endorse and make claims for the product and this was deemed as sufficient evidence, this could then be used on the packaging and the marketing campaigns. Such qualified health claims by paid-up scientists has led to a whole string of untrue health claims attached to many products from yoghurts and cereals to a never-ending succession of super fruit and superfood. This practice has to stop as it is discrediting science more than it deserves.

Aspartame, in a league of its own

Whilst on the subject of sugar and the sweet stuff, with the heavy whiff of bullshit or white lies attached, a couple of examples need a quick mention from the effluence ridden entrails of aspartame and HFCS, before we delve further into the depths of industrial (white) lies.

Everything involving aspartame comes away with a putrid stench of big business and political incorrectness; with no surprise that Monsanto can be found holding centre-stage. As the public was turning against sugar and fats due to the clear rise of civilized diseases, this gave aspartame a strong helping hand into the market. Its entire route to market is filled with independent scientific warnings, whilst still the pseudo-science of the corporations won through. At no stage was there any ignorance about the very real and significant adverse health claims by those attempting to market it and add aspartame to the human food chain. The producers have always known about its danger and all they have done is lead the public on a chase to find the truth behind their strategy of lies. Because of its GRAS status, aspartame is a legal addition to food and as such there has been no long-term study into its safety as it's considered safe. The initial scientific research confirming its alleged safety was carried out in-house, conducted by Richard Doll. The truth will come out, and when it does it will be shown what a significant detrimental ingredient aspartame has been, added to the bubbling cauldron of other dangerous chemicals already awash throughout the modern human. (The Food and Safety Agency in the UK is currently undertaking a long-term study on aspartame to objectively see its true position with regards safety and repeated ingestion.)

Since the early 1980s there has been a rapid rise in the consumption of artificial sweeteners and HFCS, as well as in the consumption of sugar, either in the USA, the UK or in the European Union as a whole. This implies that in aggregate, artificial sweeteners are not acting as sugar substitutes but merely as supplements to sugar consumption. Many of the products containing artificial sweeteners are labelled as 'diet' products, even though there is no reliable evidence to indicate that artificial sweeteners actually help people lose weight. On the contrary, the bulk of the available evidence suggests that in relation to attempted weight loss, artificial sweeteners are at best ineffective and at worst counter-productive. There is, in particular, evidence that artificial sweeteners are appetite stimulants, and while a mouthful of artificially sweetened food or drink may contain fewer calories than their sugar-sweetened equivalents, the consumption of artificial sweeteners may provoke people into going on what might be termed 'a calorie hunt'. One only needs to look at the wording for the patent application for aspartame. There is no mention of it being intended as a diet or calorie-free additive, only stating its purpose is as a diet stimulant, promoting food consumption. Which is where the white lie begins and ends with aspartame (at least in this book, there is much more on aspartame in 'Book 2: Pollutants' to really get the laver frothing up with irritability about this particularly destructive pollutant, masquerading as a sweet saviour).

Next up is HFCS, a sweetener that is at the forefront of controversy, as there is so much thoroughly reputable scientific evidence damning this for its association with obesity. How this occurs has already been explained in the Sugar chapter and briefly earlier in this one (remember? about the liver breaking it down and if not utilized via energy expenditure it is laid down as fat), so just a quick mention about one matter that confines this awful product as a white lie, coming direct from the top executives of the industry at the Corn Refiners Association and their Sweet Surprise advertising campaign regarding their use of the word 'natural'. Shortly after the campaign began airing the Corn Refiner's Association (CRA) petitioned the FDA to legally change the name of High Fructose Corn Syrup to the more natural sounding "corn sugar." Thankfully the FDA declined this and the CRAs president Audrae Erickson (in April 2009) requested that the CRA should not be publicly associated with the ad campaign, saying: "Our sponsorship of this campaign (should) remain confidential". I guess there is little comfort to be had in the fact that at least they are fully aware of the unnaturalness of their HFCS poison, not that this limits their capacity to get it into as many products as possible.

Words are meaningless in a world full of lies

Moving onto more industrial (white) lies, there are far too many to mention as literally every single aspect of the food and health industries are littered with these lies (industrial protectionism), so any of the examples presented in this chapter and book are just skimming the surface of an ocean of effluence and corruption. The fact that memos from as long ago as 1962 from the Sugar

Association clearly point to the fact they produced their deleterious products in the full knowledge that it was extremely likely such foods were causing heart disease and obesity should not solely point the finger of blame at the Sugar Association merely because they have been caught out; the real concern here is that it is all the other industries who have not been caught out, or whistle-blown, who are also fully cognizant of the risk factors of their industries causing the diseases of civilization. Open your eyes to what has taken place, or as Jim Morrison shouted "WAKE UP!" With business there is no trust, honour or allegiance if profits are threatened, they genuinely are at war to maintain profits and keep ignorance rife.

The lies of corporations, which ultimately spread carcinogens and endocrine disrupting chemicals throughout the air, soil and water or food chain can still be treated as a white lie to prevent or diminish damage or injury, whether that's damage to the public perception of the corporation or damage to its profits that are injurious to the corporation. They stretch semantics to such an extent, that even the opposite of what is thought to being said is actually what is being said, such as with the statement 'no added sugar', when many types of what we assume to be a sugar are added, be they natural, fermented or artificial (just not cane or beet derived). This, as we have seen throughout this book, is how the corporate world presents itself in the capitalist world, with blatant lies used to advertise products, false claims of this and that, whilst allegedly making you happier, healthier, thinner and more attractive to the opposite sex.

Industry led research often lays down the benchmark for information about their own industries; unsurprisingly it usually results in conclusions that ameliorate the paymasters, whilst independent research ends with damning results at the other end of the scale. Sometimes industry will deliberately conduct research to counter negative independent research that questions the safety of an industry (it could be argued that this is actually the only reason industry carries out scientific research), with this counter research having significant funding and marketing behind it and which will often be what is headline news, although of course it is not news at all, more like advertising. Further confusing this stance is the fact that those in the position to 'market' their results through the press are often the very same parties. Take for instance the Murdoch empire. Everyone knows they own a significant proportion of the news and media networks, from television stations to newspapers and even film companies. So how does one separate their vested interests when one finds out they also own a considerable portion of the pharmaceutical industry. Just because an illness is repeatedly on the news, how do we actually know with any certainty that this is not just advertising for a drug that they want to sell, wrapped in a deliberately confusing news headline?

Shameful orchestrated flu hysteria

A case in point of a news story creating hysteria has to be the disease-mongery that goes on with so many new diseases from ADHD, obesity to bird and swine flu. If swine flu is repeatedly headline news it is obviously much easier for a company selling alleged vaccines, where even the British Department of Health fell for it hook, line and sinker, paying out an astronomical £424 million on 40 million vaccines of Tamiflu in 2009. The scaremongering was so aggressive the press was daily spouting out that in the winter of 2009 at least 50,000 would die from swine flu in the UK alone, if not considerably more than 300,000, perhaps even a million. This forced the hand of global Health authorities, because if they did nothing they would be seen as the villain. In the end less died of flu that winter than normally die from flu every winter, although globally over £5 billion was spent by health authorities on stockpiles of Tamiflu, whilst Roche the producers and Rumsfeld a major shareholder must have been grinning from ear to ear, leaving the public in fear about who was going to die from this imminent epidemic.

What makes this a white lie (at best) is that Roche always knew Tamiflu was ineffective, paying scientists to give positive results. Its effectiveness was minimal, perhaps reducing the length of sickness from 7 days to 6.3 days. It was unable to prevent any transmission of the virus, while to top it all off the side-effects were often more severe than the flu itself, with many experiencing headaches, nausea, vomiting, psychiatric disturbances and kidney problems. The Labour Health Secretary Andy Burnham promised all under fives will be offered the vaccine, regardless of the side-effects. The fact that Japanese children had committed suicide due to psychiatric problems from the jab didn't rate a mention (perhaps he was in the pay of Roche to). The white lie here, aside from the scaremongering and fear created, was that Roche knew all along that Tamiflu was next to useless, not handing over their data from trials until as late as April 2014, by which time the sell by date for most of the huge stockpiles had elapsed. The scandal here is that Roche broke no laws by withholding the data, which once again beggars the question involving the bigger picture of what truly is the efficiency of the pharmaceutical industry in general? Of course some drugs work, most have serious side-effects, and from the Tamiflu scandal it is clear that many don't do as they say on the label, but this is of little consequence, the marketing works and its sold in massive quantities. The vitamin C available from a handful of sorrel is probably capable of doing a better job than Tamiflu, or for that matter eat some star anise, as this is where Roche obtained the active ingredient found in Tamiflu.

Is all health and illness media driven now?

It is a similar scenario with the nonsense about PUFAs, MUFAs and saturated fats seen in the Fats/Oils chapter. Repeated press stories about heart disease associations can force the hand of health agencies to act and give the green light to any new industrial move to combat it, irrespective of any negative results or any backing from science. They continue with these plans, fine combing any nutritional science in a desperate attempt to find any evidence that can be manipulated to bolster their erroneous health claims. It must have been obvious to the food and fats/oils industry that their claims of health flied in the face of reason, as the evidence suggested health was decreasing with the continual consumption of these fats/oils (just like the independent food scientists said it would years before).

Little snippets of the truth encased in an unhealthy wrapping of marketing and propaganda rarely stand the test of time, whereas the perpetual elephant in the room is always the obvious fact that it is the food chain that is incorrect. There is sense in telling an obese person it is food that has caused the problem, although by this time it is of course much too late. To not to have become obese in the first place would have been the solution, but this sensible logic got lost somewhere in the mechanisms of capitalism and short-term profiteering. Drug companies would rather find a drug to deal with obesity than simply tell people to eat properly and do some exercise. The pharma companies really don't give a toss if 1 or a 100,000 people suffer fatal heart attacks as a side-effect from their fat busting drugs if it means they can sell millions of them. Take for instance the headline I just read whilst going to the toilet: "Breakthrough for obesity, pill that really works" (The I tabloid 9/12/14), when in actual fact all this pill may do is turn white fat cells into brown fat cells which are apparently better and don't cause diabetes or heart disease. Quite where adipose fat causes diabetes is news to me, it's imbalances of blood sugar and insulin that causes diabetes not fat, all the sugar consumed in the process of becoming obese would have been the factor that caused the diabetes, never the adipose fat (as well as some substances such as glucose and aspartame damaging the workings of the pancreas). The article was nonsense and the actual trials were on rats and a linkage between an enzyme (glucokinase) and the desire for consuming glucose. Considering that rats metabolise fats in a very different way to humans, and the fact that it is already common knowledge that chromium lessens the cravings for glucose forming foods, the article screamed 'patent for glucokinase and future profits', because chromium cannot be patented. I should have wiped my arse with the article. It was cruelly raising people's hopes to the wonders of science being able to repair the damage caused by the food industry.

Another quick article that needs to be mentioned, as once again my preferred location for research (the toilet) pays dividends, this time from the May 2015 edition of National Geographic. I've always loved this magazine but have always been weary of its clear Americanisation and bias toward big business. The first eight pages of this edition are an intricate web of adverts from Cargill, whilst each facing page is a supposed article about the changes in the food chain required to feed the world, which surprise-surprise, looks very much as if Cargill have initiated these developments from wheat, rice and oil. They even have the cheek to argue they have improved the health of millions of Indians by fortifying cooking oil free of charge, when of course as we saw in the Fats/Oils chapter this legislative move away from traditional artisan oils has caused havoc, mass malnutrition and a vast increase in the susceptibility to a range of diseases. Most people reading National Geographic actually believe they are reading breaking news, when often it's no more than a maze of corporate propaganda disguised as news. More disturbing is the news that it's just been purchased by Fox News, (73% for something like $725 million) with Murdoch a strong climate change denier, the magazine has now lost any vestige of scientific credentials, particularly when reporting on any business that forms a part of his extensive portfolio. Considering that the first business decision made by the new owners was to sack 180 'fact-finders', allowing any future bullshit to be published unchecked and unchallenged.

A few drops from a sea of wrongness

To emphasise that this shady business ethic of knowingly polluting and poisoning is endemic across all industries, here is just a few tiny extracts from the endless infractions, perjury, lies, obstructions and avoidances from an industry that only needs to perform such ceaseless white lies because the truth is that their entire business has no place in the diet of any sensible culture, with it's consumption being a serious risk factor in the very diseases we see all around us today. Perhaps the following could be seen as a little taster into how it is that these international corporations really do not have any foibles or qualms when it comes down to making money.

I've mentioned Monsanto already, although they are not alone as a corporation spreading pestilence and death. DuPont have done a much better job at this considering they began life as an explosives producer, making 40% of the gunpowder used in WWI, as well as being involved with I.G.Farben who made the Zyklon B gas used in the Nazi extermination camps. DuPont obviously have little in the way of morals or ethics. They feature in the next book in this series, here I just want to make a quick mention of their involvement in the food industry, not food *per se*, but the production of their Teflon used for non-stick frying pans, as well as many food wrappers and lining for cartons etc. It involves the chemical PFOA, used to bond the Teflon to the pan, and their white lie here is that for twenty two years they withheld evidence about the extreme toxicity of this PFOA up until 2005, being fined $16.5 million by the Environmental Protection Agency, the largest administrative penalty ever. The fine was for contamination of waters, although only covering administrative costs. They had also been fined $107 million by local residents in West Virginia where their plant producing PFOA had contami-nated local waters. Considering that PFOA, a known carcinogen, can now be found in most mammalian life worldwide, the fines were clearly woefully inadequate, and to top it off, DuPont have neither admitted liability or apologized. It is unsurprising to find out that the initial reports on the safety of PFOA were conducted by a Monsanto employee, Richard Doll (who we just saw was responsible for his false science in claiming aspartame safe), who was paid $1,500 per day to write erroneous reports refuting any possible links between Agent Orange, PVC, PFOA and other now known carcinogens. Amazingly Doll has never been prosecuted for his lies. To show how small the fines for PFOA were, a year later in 2006 DuPont paid out over a $1billion in compensation to Costa Rica for its fungicide Benlate, which actually did the opposite and encouraged bacterial growth, whilst DuPont's only pro-action was to instruct all employees to destroy all records that implicated Benlate.

What it boils down to could be what has been argued throughout this book, this duel between economics and *oikonomia*. In the modern world of economics, industry assumes it is okay to lie if they are guarding profits, as it is profits that determine how many can be employed and how much taxation is being paid from these wages and profits. This issue of taxation has become embroiled itself in a huge white lie, because industry has claimed that the profits it generates employ and pay taxes, whilst the press repeatedly shows these large corporations aren't even paying business taxes on their profits, the only contribution they are making is employing people who pay taxes from their wages, whilst 'clever' accounting significantly reduces any tax bills. We all know about Amazon and Apple and scores of other corporations all avoiding corporation taxes by locating HQs offshore in countries with extremely low tax rates, notably Luxembourg, whose former Prime Minister is now head of the European Commission. This system has been working for the enormous accountancy firms unabated for decades. How on earth do you assume that PriceCooperWaterhouse (PwC) the largest, followed by Deloitte and KPMG and the rest have gotten so fabulously wealthy themselves? (British MPs are currently looking into PwC, not for ethical reasons mind you, merely because these companies should be paying more to bolster the Westminster and British coffers). Corporations and accountants have devised a strategy to shift a huge proportion of the tax liability elsewhere and thus avoid paying tax, this can only be deemed as conspiring. Protection of their profits from the truth is in their eyes merely a white lie. If natural law held sway these corporations would not exist, as in Gaia's eyes these polluting and sickness causing corporations are a desecration to all planetary life.

Again I state that this book is concerned with only one thing and that is a search for the truth, and in this respect a lie is a lie and there is no justification for it being uttered, especially if the white lies that have been espoused thus far have culminated in the health catastrophe we are currently experiencing. If the truth had been allowed to surface from the start the current predicament would not have been reached. The truth has always been available, without having to travel as far back as the caveman or Hippocrates, many of our current ills have been correctly predicted from before our current economic model of capitalism kicked in after WWII. There have been many mentions of those doctors and Nobel Prize winners from the late 1920s and 1930s who clearly foresaw that the path that was being set in their time would arrive at this *cul de sac* called Devolution, just down from Disease Drive.

Food shockers

Time is running out for this particular book, so please bare with me whilst just a few more white lies are highlighted, specifically centred on the food industry – apologies for any glaring omissions, as there are so many (white lies and omissions).

Since the 1980s prepared chickens have had water and saline

solution added to them, up to 30% by weight, although that's not all. For decades the vast majority of our 'fresh' chicken has been infused with a whole bunch of other substances, including beef and pork waste. That's bad news for Hindus and Muslims choosing a chicken dish, as beef and pork are forbidden by their respective religions. It can still be called 'natural' if the added ingredients come from a natural source, which as we've seen throughout this book, this natural tag can be very loosely applied. The meat industry has to be one of biggest fibbers and concealers, or at least it's the sector that gets most frequently caught out for its transgressions.

The meat industry also uses a 'glue' to join bits of off-cuts together to give the impression it's a single piece of meat, using what is called transglutaminase, which isn't among the substances required to be mentioned in the table of ingredients. You'll have little chance of knowing it's there unless you're an expert at interpreting the seams in your meat. This process not only sells you a tapestry of scraps for the price of prime meat, but it also leaves you with a 'steak' that might well have come from a dozen different cows, making it virtually impossible to trace the source of your food poisoning, the chances of which are increased tenfold due to the uneven consistency of what you're trying to fry up. This meat glue works just as well on chicken and seafood and as transglutaminase comes from cow and pig's blood this is bad news once again for any Muslims, Jews or Hindus.

As for that lovely deep pink salmon fillet, giving the impression of a wild salmon swimming upstream, avoiding the claws of a bear with an Alaskan vista in the background. Erm!! Well that's most unlikely, because the vast majority of salmon in the supermarket comes from big ponds, so full of fish they get little chance to move and develop much muscle, with grey meat soaked in antibiotics. Those friendly folk at Hoffman La-Roche have developed a pantone range of pinks to choose from that is added to the feed pellets, known as the SalmoFan. Of course it's not just salmon that is dyed artificially to produce a wholesome hearty colour, chickens are dyed a golden colour with a mix of dyes and marigold petals, steaks are dyed a deeper blood red (with colours suspected of being carcinogenic) and its certainly not exclusively meats that are dyed. Breads have molasses added to make them appear browner and healthier, whilst cheeses, especially cheddars are dyed orangey to give them a homogenous even colouration, giving the false impression of cows enjoying deep lush pastures, although it's only done because cheddars if not dyed come in a range of pallid, anaemic off-whites.

Dying meats and other commodities is probably to be expected to a certain extent, but what about something a little more unexpected, such as olive oil? We've already seen the semantics used to confuse consumers about the term 'cold-pressed', well it gets even worse. In many instances what's in the bottle isn't even olive oil, or at least it's been heavily diluted and it's not just the small producers. Bertoli have been implicated in this scandal, one that has been orchestrated by no less than the Italian mafia for quite a while now. It's been going on for so long now that even the supposed food connoisseurs can't tell the difference between a diluted version and a pure 100% one, often assuming the real Mckoy to be the imposter. I can't vouch for the genuineness of olive oils in the UK, but in the U.S the problem is rife and very real, with some mafia families possibly making more from the counterfeit olive oil industry than they do from cocaine, which doesn't quite fit with the gangster image does it?

Perhaps the Yakuza and other Asian gangster firms are involved in another food enterprise that bares little resemblance to their hard man image, that of honey. It's always amazed me how much honey there is on the market, as each bee makes no more than a teaspoon in a lifetime and there is millions of tons of the stuff on supermarket shelves throughout England, let alone the whole world. Bootleg Chinese honey is a major constituent of much of this honey and it will have had all of the pollen filtered out to make its origin impossible to gauge. Often it will have had other cheaper sweeteners added such as HFCS and the industry must be aware of this fraud because there simply are not enough bees in the world to make all the honey on the market (not that I've personally counted them all!). The FDA clearly states that for a label to claim the contents are honey there has to be pollen within the product, yet most of the 'honey' when tested contained none.

As we saw in the last chapter, arsenic is widespread in the world of rice products and as of yet there has been no long-term research into how this known carcinogen affects cancer rates, which is not only scary but it also demonstrates that there could be some major industry cover-up as its not hard to imagine that a known carcinogen causes cancer! Has the lack of long term research been somehow influenced by the fact that in the U.S the rice industry is worth $34 billion and worldwide its worth nearer a trillion dollars? Which is bad enough, but there is a snippet of good news regarding this crisis of arsenic (found in rice because of the multi-trillion dollar agricultural chemical industry) if you want to call it good news and that is the simple fact that it is out in the open. The lid has been lifted on this particular can-of-worms, although the real worry, and where the white lie resides, is when one ponders on what the heck is going on with all the other food crops and agricultural chemicals that have not had their lids lifted to peer inside and expose the sordid world of carcinogens, endocrine and developmental disrupters. If we see the news behind arsenic now, what is behind the news, what is out there that we do not know about as of yet? Considering that every single pesticide is definitely a toxin, what is next to break the news?

Finally onto cellulose which is best imagined as the skeletal structure of a plant from which the rest is formed. Its indigestible fibre is a good thing to consume as fibre is well known as aiding digestion, transit of faeces through the digestive tract and colon and helps to soak up undesirable matter through its course. The problem with cellulose is that the form found in food is more often than not derived from waste wood pulp and more recently from recycled paper pulp. Cellulose from eating broccoli or potato is of course what we would consider healthy and natural, when it's from wood pulp, been boiled with various chemicals to extract the cellulose it is anything but natural. This is the form cellulose takes when found in most products in the food chain, although it can still be labelled as natural and even organic. By adding cellulose the product can hold more water (one of the cheapest ingredients to bulk it out), as well as more air, as well as providing a creamy texture and increasing the fibre content, whilst being naturally low-fat. It's also very low in calories, another great reason to stick as much in as possible in supposed diet and health foods. McDonalds was caught out years ago because the main ingredient in its milkshakes wasn't milk, as one would expect, but cellulose from paper pulp, so they had to change the ingredient quantities or change the name to 'paper-shake'. Unsurprisingly they changed the proportions and subsequently customers complained that the milkshake was no longer as good or creamy as before – you just can't win sometimes can you?

The jury is out as to whether this form of cellulose is a health risk, the problem is that its not quite what one expects to find in such a broad range of goods, whether organic, health or processed from ready grated cheese, bakery goods such as bagels to sauces, syrups and spreads. It is found under many names but usually with the word cellulose attached. The best advice would be to just eat more whole foods and your intake of natural cellulose will increase also.

Conscious capitalism please . . .

I'm probably being far too diplomatic by putting much of this chapter down as white lies, as in fact criminal proceedings should be brought against these companies, such as Monsanto, Dow, Bayer, DuPont and GSK, not proceedings to fine them as this makes no difference – they need to be shut down. If the products they make are truly required then they shall continue to be made, so no one loses their jobs. These corporations have for too long done as they please and then pay a fine if required, if and when they get caught. Such position aren't blatantly white lies, and to be honest, I believe that criminal undertakings by industry are in short flagrant violations of regulations, ethics, morality and natural law. The white lies occur when the guilty companies console themselves that what they do is no more contemptible than any other company, and this is the crux of the problem; they are right, they are no worse, all of them are as bad as each other, so its unfair to ever single out one company when it is all of them doing it. This is why in the future we would be much better off without these industries, and we have the unique opportunity to learn from this terrible mistake and do what we know needs to be done to turn the tide of destruction, otherwise it's just madness that we have not learnt from all the mistakes already made. The very definition of insanity is repeating the same mistakes and expecting a different outcome each time.

At long last we can move onto some positivity with this book, with the prospect of a brighter future from the next chapter. The change will be imperceptible at first, then in years to come, hindsight will allow us to see that we were indeed living through revolutionary times. This time is right here, right now. Bring it on.

Conclusion and Solutions

"All truth passes through three stages.

First, it is ridiculed.

Second, it is violently opposed.

Third, it is accepted as being self-evident."

(Arthur Schopenhauer, German philosopher 1788-1860)

"There is a nutritional basis for modern physical, mental and moral degeneration."

(Weston Price 'Nutrition and Physical Degeneration' 1939)

This book thus far has been predominately a reportage of the terrible state of the food chain, which is dominated by the deadly whites, interspersed with snippets of possible solutions. This was the intention of the book, however, it is somewhat negative to simply highlight how bad the world is without offering some more concrete solutions. For this, I'm delighted to state that there is a definite answer. It's easy to understand and also to follow and appears a little later. It has already been mentioned throughout the book, although it is so simple it may have slipped the reader's notice.

Stepping out of the dark

It is my conviction that we already know the truth about what is causing the state of ill health, which is becoming forever more blatant and noticeable, as more friends and family become sick with a disease of civilization. When I talk to people there is a general consensus about what this truth is. We know the way forward, but for some reason we always manage to take two steps backwards after taking one forward. When we come together or watch a television programme, documentary or film, the collective consciousness fills us with a sense of being and correctness. This feeling is usually only temporary as we withdraw back to our own personal lives, whether that's surrounded by our family or alone in our own space. We taste the truth, agree that the path is achievable, but somehow it flitters away as everyday worries and concerns take over. There is a spirit of revolution within every one of us, but upon reflection this is superseded by a general apathy and malaise – the thought that life isn't so bad overwhelms and the spark of change is all too easily extinguished. We need to keep the fires burning because this is the only way change and revolution can happen.

This book is my little flame, a lighter held up aloft saying 'here it is'. At the moment my lighter is not alone, there are other small flames, although in between these small circles of light there is much darkness. With time more flames will be lit and the area of darkness will gradually recede as there is a definite slow and gradual illumination occurring, although for many it feels as if we are alone in the darkness not being able to see other people's flames. People have deliberately been separated because the workings of the government and industry can only be achieved if we are kept in the dark.

Tuning back into Gaia

We need to reconnect with the planet and make the critical connection that all life on our planet has with the soil. It is this alone that provides the essential nutrients to guarantee the possibility of health from our food. It doesn't take long when looked at from this perspective to realise that we have snapped the connection and with it the door has been opened to the diseases of civilization, not only the cause of them, also their remediation. It has of course become more complicated than that thanks to the proliferation of other cancer causing, genome destroying chemicals that are omnipresent in our world. However, underlying these variables is the constant truth that it is only nutrients that provide life and health, nothing else (the 50 essential nutrients can be found in the appendices).

Mother Earth, she who the Greeks called Gaia, is in fact dying, and if you aren't aware of this then its time to truly wake up. The cancers ripping through the human race is merely a reflection of the cancer we have caused in Gaia. Ultimately there is little to nothing in the soils, the constant chemical barrage has broken the immune system of the earth and with it the immune systems of those dependent upon it.

In need of balance and harmonization, humans need to tune back into Gaia's frequency. We need to feel a sense of purpose and oneness with the planet, because this will aid with reconnecting with ourselves, with other humans, with other living things and with the entire planet. We have become disconnected, lost in our selfish pursuit of an erroneous economy, dominated as we all know by money. Sounding wishy-washy with hippy overtones there is no other way to explain it, as thousands have said in the past, the answer is love. Which it is indeed, although if you don't eat properly, your love isn't going to go very far.

A simple way to begin this process of reconnection is to begin to forage, or if you do already, extend your knowledge to include new species and try to take a friend with you who has never foraged before. If you can't get out to the country, there is still an abundance to be found in the urban landscape. There is a saying (I don't know its provenance) – that the plants of greatest value to humans are those very plants growing so readily alongside us. Whether this is a part of Gaia's plan or a coincidence is immaterial, the saying is true. It won't take long to find some nettles, pinch out the tops and remove the top leaves (breathing in whilst picking prevents getting stung, which has something to do with the pores of the skin closing as we breath in, making us fully air tight). Two good washed handfuls will make an ideal and superlatively nutritious soup, with some garlic (pick some wild garlic leaves, ramsons, from April to May) and wild oregano as flavour and nutrient additions. For a simple pesto, blend down some nettles, add them to ground seeds and season – delicious. Or pick a couple of nice big dandelion leaves (preferably before it flowers, although this is not essential), wash them, chop them fine and add to a salad or sandwich. Blackberries – easy. Get creative, get 'Food For Free' by R. Mabey and slip back into a time when we all foraged, sharing Mother Earth with everyone and praising Her for providing. Take a bus journey once a month on a sunny day to a beautiful foraging area in our lovely country, from sea to river or woods. Creating new food, being partly self-sufficient, exploring and doing it with a friend can only be good for the soul and provide excellent nutrition as well as partly restoring our connection with the planet. As this connection becomes more firmly entrenched, detrimental, un-environmental and unhealthy lifestyles will be so jarring with the new mind-set; a natural transition will take place toward this more connected perspective.

By engaging in some foraging, if you truly haven't done any before, it will be good for you, as it is certainly a challenge and one with achievable goals. It is also a fantastic conversational topic, one that can go on for some time with much wisdom to be shared by so many people more than happy to do so. It is a potential to broaden ones horizons and spend more time in nature, which may not be for everyone, but for some it is all that is needed. You will never know unless you give it a go.

Soil for the soul

Where are the nutrients coming from, to either help with health or to re-establish health when ill? Vitamin supplement tablets have repeatedly been shown not to provide health, with our white lie that a pill will suffice only making matters worse. Soil, soil and soil, give it some thought, consider the soil of today and then consider the soil of 40,000 years ago (this is the focus of Book 4 in this series, as without healthy soil there would never have been much by way of evolution). There is little comparison.

The soil of today is exhausted, whilst the aggressive use of agricultural chemicals has compounded the problem, making it toxic to all life-forms. For over 60 years this senseless chemical barrage has coated the surface of our amazing planet with a deadly poison, which we have been indoctrinated into believing promotes life and fecundity, when of course all it has really done has landed us in the current predicament of cancers caused by known carcinogens in the pesticides, as well as demineralization, not to mention the loss of hedgerows and loss of species, from voles to moles, badgers, birds to bees and butterflies. The countryside has truly been obliterated and ripped apart with only NPK (Nitrogen, Phosphorus and Potassium) fertilizer and numerous deadly chemicals, many derived from biological warfare weapons intended to maim humans, put back in.

Today we ignorantly assume that the pinnacle of health would be eating organic food, with little consideration given to the soil, the true life and health giver. Agricultural programmes for future survival need to start focusing on this regeneration of the soil, although no one in control of our destiny (the government, preoccupied with controlling our minds) has any comprehension of the vital importance of this aspect, as well as there being no focus on any long-term goals. It falls well beyond any vision of economics, but of course as repeated throughout this book, it falls well within the remit of *oikonomia*.

Where else would a diet of processed foods with all nutrients removed ultimately lead but to sickness? For most people the only conceivable source of food is plastic packaged with a sell by date from a supermarket, which is madness. As soon as people begin to really understand food it will be easier to see that the demineralized, plastic-packaged, processed food has indeed been the catalyst for many diseases, then changes will be made.

Only healthy soil provides healthy plants, providing health to all that eat them – this is so simple a point that it must have gone over the heads of those allegedly intelligent people making the decisions about whether to allow these poor substitutes for food into the food chain. As a consequence malnutrition is common, which is not a lack of food, as we are eating more than ever, but a diet that is lacking in any nutritional content. We are not obtaining sufficient natural mineralization from the soil to guarantee efficient biological mechanisms to prevent and fight off disease.

We have gotten to a point today where a large percentage of the earth's soils have been weakened, and we need to step away from the possibility of a short-term profit to be made from this programme of re-establishing healthy soils. There is no short-term monetary profitability possible from this, only long-term security and health, which is clearly worth much more. Although of course with our present economic system, health will always lose out to wealth. *Oikonomia* has to prevail and we have to drop the current economic system. Long-term plans also need to be made that incorporate self-sufficiency for the public, from water to electricity as well as local communities being able to feed and cloth themselves.

A nation can only be as healthy as the earth it stands on

Is it asking too much for a country to regenerate its soil? How can a new terminal at an airport, or a new rail-line be more important than this? The first thing that needs to be done is to re-mineralize the soil of the country, because there is no argument that the people can only be as healthy as the soil, with the soil in Britain being some way off its best. There are in excess of 2 million potential farmers already in the country (the unemployed); if a proportion of these are formally employed, housed and fed, with the brief for their work being so simple as soil improvement, then we could be a long way toward the solution. This would have profound future benefits, immeasurable in today's economic sense. Millions of acres can be converted into super-fertile, mineral-replete soil, with the full compliment of worms and mycorrhiza, returning the soil to a living interconnected super-structure, easily capable of fending off adverse bacterium and pathogens, negating the need for toxic, carcinogenic, endocrine disrupting chemicals – as well as re-establishing the network of farming communities that once linked Britain, putting some human life back into the countryside. A simple beginning would be to increase available allotment areas outside of towns and villages, this would improve the soil fertility and productivity, particularly as many retired custodians of allotments possess extraordinary local horticultural knowledge, which could be utilised to educate and extend the range of extremely fecund small-holdings significantly.

There are already many methods to improve soil fertility naturally and more efficiently, as well as of course, chemical-free. The easiest method is to do nothing. Leave the fields alone, let all the vegetative growth mulch back into the soil. Or introduce sheep, goats or cattle to graze on the meadow, fertilizing as they munch and shit. More active and effective re-mineralizing can be achieved by replicating how the soils got a super-boost of minerals from the melting ice at the end of the last ice age. All the billions of tons of rock, scraped free by the gnawing ice, washed downstream when the ice melted, spreading sediment to make super fertile, vast alluvial floodplains, home to super-rich plants (this also provided the ideal conditions for the first city-states to emerge from these glacial sediment rich river valleys millennia ago). It may seem laborious, although with a rock crusher it is possible for two people to re-mineralize with rock dust 100s of acres a year. We also need to restart fertilizing the soil with seaweed. Millions of tons of seaweed grows and is washed up around Britain organically (and depending on the water quality, it is relatively clean as well as being free), the only cost is collecting and distributing it. These simple ideas (not to mention the better ideas from people far more learned than I in such matters pertaining to pedology) will allow the harvesting of nutrient rich foods, feeding nutrient rich, disease-free citizens. Is that expecting too much? Mankind needs to stop thinking outside of the Nature box, arrogantly assuming we are above such concerns. Attempting to create a better ecosystem for food supplies than the one created by Nature over millions of years, is and has, gotten us into all sorts of bother. The further we venture down this dislocation with more GMO foods, mutated meats and bionic beets the further we will be from pulling ourselves back to reality and ultimately, survival.

Such large scale soil improvement scheme would cost £bn's, with the relocation of people and distribution of minerals and educational information required, but consider this; the current nuclear weapons programme costs well in excess of £100bn. Now, I can't speak for Putin or ISIS, or have any idea what's in the mind of any leader with nuclear arms and a big army at their disposal, but I do consider it fairly old-fashioned to somehow be concerned that Britain is going to be attacked by a foe, meaning that nuclear weapons have to be deployed to somehow abate the attack. That's very unlikely, and if it were to occur, I'm sure we could borrow a couple of bombs from the French or Americans, if that would make any difference. Whilst the money saved on not updating weapons of mass destruction could be spent on making Britain a nation of healthy soil once again, with crops that are nutritious and health promoting, saving future money on health and concerns about food security and supply. This could be all done at a fraction of the cost of updating our genocidal, apocalyptic nuclear arsenal. The rest of the savings could then be spent on health, welfare and real education (such as how to live, teaching about health, food, cooking, society and being social, identifying fauna and flora as well as playing games and sports).

It's only natural

We also need to move away from the current agriculture model where the land is placed under aggressive and toxic servitude. This needs to be replaced with permaculture, creating an ecosystem that is permanent, complete and self-sustaining, where pests are controlled by natural predators and where soils are created and enhanced with manure from grazing animals and plant waste. It's the logical next step and one tier up from organic, close to what some know as bio-diverse (search the internet for information about permaculture around the world today). This extremely productive and sustainable method of agriculture can be easily initiated alongside the soil improvement scheme and the increase in smallholdings. Britain could become a shining example of how it is possible to become as close to self-sufficient as possible as a result of such massive public programmes.

This is not rocket science, it is no more basic than it being one of the pre-requisites of being not just a human but any living thing on this planet. All life forms' sole purpose is to find the most nutritious source of food it can, then go about procreating and living in a respectful, harmonious and peaceful way, all of which we are failing at abysmally.

It's encoded in our DNA. So let's get the first part of the solution started as soon as possible: this country has easily enough land to feed its inhabitants, directly and from trading any surplus. Stop eating so much meat, eat more vegetables and start incorporating insects into your diet as a protein replacement for those entrenched in the dogma that protein can only come from a living, breathing animal. If a proportion of the extra vegetables eaten includes wild foraged plants such as nettles and dande-lions, not only are these around 15 to 18% protein, they are a far more easily digested and utilisable source of protein, as well as containing a plethora of other life-sustaining and enriching minerals. This also helps, as we just saw, to re-establish the critical link we once had with nature. If we can do this, the connections shared by all humans become self evident and all the extremism and isolationism endemic in religion will dissolve away, leaving only the shared precepts, which are conveniently all based around love and sharing.

Change the means of distribution of farmed produce

We need to start to buy more produce from farmer's markets, giving them a fairer price for their produce. Lose the middle-men and encourage them to begin to compete with one another, not over price but in quality, flavour and nutrients (this was the failing of the entire food industry, always looking at the cheapest, not the healthiest). The current generation of farmers also need to be re-educated, because far too many of them have been indoctrinated by the agricultural and chemical companies into believing that the only way to farm is to use their deadly products. The only information most farmers have about agricultural has come from the seed and chemical companies themselves, from their salesmen, trade-shows and trade-magazines. The truth or solution will never be found this way.

Organic farmers do what they do, not because they are wrong, but because they have had their eyes opened to what needs or should be done. Not all of them of course, as some organic farmers only turned to organics because the crops can achieve a higher price at market, which they can't be blamed for, as the supermarkets perpetually attempt to obtain everything at a rock bottom price, beating any residual determination by the farmers to produce goods with quality attached to them. If the supermarkets had competed on quality and not price there would have been an increase in general quality, done so at competitive prices, a coup for the consumer, as opposed to today where the crap is not quite so cheap, whilst quality is harder to find and expensive.

Many farmers today have little idea about pest control, weeds and even the soil, continuing the false dogma, that it is an impossible task to cope with weeds without poisons, which is a serious concern. There needs to be educational programmes for these farmers to teach them about companion planting and about the importance of establishing a fertile soil to increase productivity. These people are supposed to work with nature, instead they are doing the very opposite, poisoning the soil and local inhabitants, humans as well as all other animals.

What will motivate most farmers will be, apart from legislation, greater productivity, better prices and more profits. If this is achieved then more and more will make the switch. It's not a short-term solution, it's a long-term one and to achieve this patience and subsidies need to be made available to actualize any programmes. As it is today, the farmers are most definitely a part of the problem by continuing to use poisons. It is a simple step to make them a part of the solution and to do this they need to be coerced away from the mega-corporations who monopolize the seeds and chemicals and re-establish their role as guardians of the soil. These guardians have merely become pawns in the hapless pursuit of profits by the massive international agricultural corporations.

Definitely time for the ®Evolution

There is a lot of talk of revolution at the moment with the likes of Russell Brand, who hopefully will continue to mature as a public orator and servant, as well as an excellent ascorbic comedian. Also amongst others, Hollywood star Matt Damon with his water campaign and some very interesting speeches. Where this revolution needs to take place, at least where its beginnings originate, is within the heads of the general public. If it takes people like Mr Brand to vocalize aspects of the revolution all the better, as most people would rather listen to him (and others such as Jamie Oliver, with his excellent campaigns for better school meals and sugar awareness) than they would to David Cameron, our supposed leader (as I write this last edit, re-elected, which can only mean the bin for any environmental and green plans and initiatives for the next five years).

It costs nothing to think, all it takes is a little time, and as all of our time gets fuller and fuller, simple thought has become a luxury. Where this revolution of thought needs to be ignited is pertaining to matters about our whole existence and what makes us happy and healthy. Thought has to be concerned with your personal health, how your next actions can contribute or adversely affect your health. It is the first instinctual thought that any animal has concerning what is best for itself. This is not selfish necessarily, as what is best for most people is social time with friends and family, activities shared and goals achieved together.

Food eaten should be done with the knowledge about what it is, where it's from, what it does and why it's eaten, because if you are made aware of such matters to do with food, the bad food becomes less attractive. This is exactly the intention of this book, to make processed foods made from the deadly whites as unattractive as possible. It's madness to be eating so much detrimental food, especially when we have so much good food to choose from, so why do we keep making the same erroneous choices?

Well that has been answered throughout this book, it wasn't our choice to be eating the food we do today, just like agriculture, urbanism, religion and capitalism were not our choices, they weren't naturally gifted from Gaia, they were marketed, brainwashed, coerced and forced upon us by those with greed and power in their eyes. Without going into details, the best first step anybody can make in achieving better health would be to eliminate as much processed food from the diet. Too many people say that their ailments are too far gone for diet to make much difference, which is said even when in many instances it was the deleterious diet that caused the ailment to become so profound. Why would it be inappropriate to at least entertain the possibility that what was a causative agent could be just as Hippocrates said, your medicine? Eating a better diet, one suited to you personally is never going to be bad advice, although most people at best attempt a day of change, arguing it's too difficult to give up all the luxuries like chocolate, ice cream and alcohol. This is not only weak willed, it's wrong. How can falling sick from the consumption of these ever be associated with a luxury; surely health and happiness should be the only luxuries on our minds.

Oikonomia time?

As long as the main aspiration and supposed path to happiness is a new 50" flat-screen, iPhone6, pair of shoes or a new BMW, nothing is going to change. The first question that should spring to mind when considering a path to happiness has to be one directed toward health and longevity, whether your actual health or the health of the relationship you have with your partner, family, friends and community. A major part of this has got to do with food, with its health promoting ability and sense of community it can establish; not how much money can be made out of it.

This transition to health from wealth will allow a natural evolution to *oikonomia*. The world needs a new you, not a new car, tv or ready meal. It's happening anyway, the information age is freely available to most of the world and the message is slowly spreading and coalescing into a global unification of people power. Take off your twenty first century spectacles and see the world for what it is. Be happy and free from fear and learn to enjoy a well made vegetarian roast or pie, ditch the processed rubbish and the revolution will have begun. Everything else will simply fall into place as the natural order re-establishes itself.

There is no question that the initial rumblings of a food revolution is taking shape. The general public is slowly awakening to the unarguable logic that health and weight are dependent upon what is being eaten and that the current diet is not as good as it could be. Less meat is being eaten and an increase in different vegetables is becoming more common, albeit far too slowly. What is encouraging is the fact that finally there is the realisation that our personal health has to be achieved by ourselves. It's about time we stopped looking elsewhere for answers and being dependent upon others for the solution. We are the problem and the solution, whilst a major part of the solution and the problem can be found in the daily shopping basket and trolley.

We can only hope that in a couple of generations we can look back at the period from 1950 to 2015 with disgust and incredulity that we were so stupid to reek such havoc and Armageddon against every biological entity on this beautiful planet. There is no sense in growing foods using deadly cancer causing and endocrine disrupting chemicals, processing all the nutrients out of foods making it little more than a poison; washing and soaking ourselves in deadly poisons; brushing teeth with drain cleaner and fixing them with mercury; using fossil fuels; poisoning the water and air; burning down the rainforest; as well as allowing individual greed and power to dominate countries and industries. We have been coerced into a ridiculously precarious position by the rule of economics, this has to end and *oikonomia* needs to rule again.

The poor are getting poorer whilst the rich are getting richer

The message needs to be repeatedly told until it sinks in. Reading it once or hearing it once and agreeing with it is only a start, because when that message of revolution is not being said we return to the world of being constantly bombarded with the indoctrination of capitalist marketing, and this is why even when we know the answer, if we are not being told all the time to change, the fear and worry of paranoia sets in and we assume its okay to allow those in charge to continue to be in control. This is nonsense and they need to be usurped. In our supposed democracy the majority are in total agreement that the politicians and industrialists are not to be trusted. The politicians are the very people who have the most to lose, so they are the ones most against change, as all they are doing is upholding the capitalist system – with a different system they will no longer be required. The ruling families of this country are the very same families who initiated the slave trade, and through a clever use of semantics (forever telling us we live in a free, democratic society, where we chose them, even though little more than half even vote and less than half of these voted for the current Tories, that's less than one in four getting what they want in the current democratic system) and smoke screens they have continued this slave trade right up until today. There has to be a breaking point, we are forever being told we are currently living in austere times, although paradoxically it is only the poor who are getting poorer, whilst the rich are getting richer. This has to end.

The system isn't programmed to allow itself to be usurped

Industry might well have irreparably damaged a large proportion of the current generation alive today, although this will have to be seen as a consequence of the change about to happen, because if we continue blindly down the current path, the next generation will be a little more damaged and it will be a little harder to restore the genome back onto the path of evolution. Eugenics may well be the only answer soon, where only those with a healthy genome (and bank account) can procreate, otherwise we will continue to dilute the healthy aspect out of the human race. To lose a generation or two will be nothing like as catastrophic as losing the entire species, which is exactly what will happen within three generations if there is no change to both our cultural existence, as well as the soils and foods eaten (and of course our attitude to one another and the planet). It is the very system itself that is wrong. It is this system that upholds the capitalist, consumerist system and so it is the system that has to change, as opposed to tinkering with little bits within it. The political system needs not only an overhaul, it needs to be replaced, as does the education system, legal system and the health system. Systemic revolution!

The selfish consumerist lifestyle we have at present is unsustainable. Instead of looking back in 50 years and saying "I told you so" when it will be too late, let's start to make that change today and begin to focus on our health and where we will be in a few years time. As soon as more and more people realise that the world today is only geared to benefit a miniscule fraction of the people, which are those super wealthy families, those 50 or so families who control most of the planet's wealth. This divide between the rich and the poor is starting to be emblazoned across the media more frequently. Inequality is beginning to stretch the seams of reason and it will not be long before the poor start a revolution of their own, although this will be one of violence, and violence will only beget violence. If we can increase peace then it will be this peace and love that will be the overriding force of change.

There is more than enough land in England to house and feed everyone with prosperity, it's just that we need to alter the perception of prosperity, shifting it to a position where health and happiness rule. We are so wealthy in the west we don't even know it, but this wealth needs to be converted to health, and this can only be achieved in the long run if true equality becomes the norm. Obviously the rich will desperately cling onto their wealth, although if we reject money then over-night all that wealth becomes meaningless. The true revolution begins when the soil is replenished and the addictions to sugar and money are jettisoned. Perhaps we need a catastrophe to occur for us to really see where the future lies. If electricity were to suddenly fail, if a solar flare or plasma ejection from the sun wipes out electricity, where will we be then? Such an occurrence would start a revolution, but that's not how it should occur, we need to stop being reactive and start being preventative.

The simple answer

The six Deadly Food Whites from this book can easily be avoided, with a simple solution, which is to consume whole foods. If the consumer can achieve this, a switch that needn't be wholesale, it can easily be incremental: as more whole food is added to the diet less processed ones are consumed, and as less processed food is consumed the food industry will have to pay attention because their only responsibility is to make profits and if the only way they can continue to make profits is by offering less processed food and more whole food, so be it, this will be consumer power and democracy in full force. Governments would back such a plan because as more whole food is consumed there will be a decrease in the diseases of civilization, which will have the knock on effect of there being less resources and finances required for the health service. Less money spent on health will mean less money needed to be taken from the public, meaning more money in the pocket of the public. Net result will therefore be a richer and healthier public, everyone will be a winner and such a plan can be so easily instigated by such a simple course as eating better. As health becomes the priority for more people then this will have a knock-on effect throughout society. It's a no-brainer surely, and it would be nothing short of a revolution because it is such a radical change that no other term better describes it.

The paragraph above surely holds within it the true making of a revolution, one so simple and achievable, using nothing more than what is already available. With the soils regenerated and more whole food eaten with a greater nutritious content it will put Britain in a position it has not held since the beginning of the Industrial Revolution. With a healthier, happier and wealthier populace the decision becomes ours as to what the next step is, no longer pawns for the industrialists but kings and queens of our own destiny – the future can look bright.

It has gotten to the ridiculous position today where companies such as Walkers Crisps, Mars, Coke and Nestle have a say in our future health and nutrition, with them being on all advisory boards and sponsoring publication of research. If this continues there is never going to be any drift toward a healthier and disease freer future. If we don't buy their products then they will start to listen and change what they put in their products. Governments can apply heavy taxation to deleterious food as these come with expensive future price tags in the form of the years of toxic drug treatment to suppress the diseases of civilization they cause. Processed food producers should never have been allowed to get themselves into any position of power or influence. It's exactly the same as believing that Shell and Esso, who now control many institutions dealing with climate change and environmental renewables, have an answer that is both truly environmental and of any longevity. Of course they don't. The public need to exert pressure on the system, as the system is dependent upon the citizens.

The answer is simple and it can be summed up in a short sentence: stop eating processed foods and do more exercise. It truly is that simple, and the importance of exercise must not be underestimated – even if its just standing up for longer or walking up the stairs, this will have a major impact after time.

The brainwashing by the food industry (and of course all other industries engaging in the very same weapons of mass psychological distraction) has been fairly complete, their only problem is that the Information Revolution, with the readily accessed free-flow of information that is possible about any subject, will make misinformation harder to propagate when the propagandists no longer control the means of information. This Information Revolution will hopefully keep the doors open, allowing the real ®Evolution to take place, the one involving money and health and the reinstating of *oikonomia*.

I love this quote so much it deserves to not only to be in the Introduction it also needs to be repeated here as a gentle reminder of what Jean-Jacques Rousseau stated 250 years ago, as it hits the nail firmly on its head:

"The greater part of our ills are of our own making, and we might have avoided them, nearly all, by adhering to that simple manner of life that nature prescribed."

Not wanting to end with someone else's words, I think its pertinent to end this book with no words from anyone but a thought from yourself, as it's important that the link is made between your health and the health of the soil that sustains us. If you weren't aware of the connection, now is the time for such a thought.

Thanks for joining me on this journey so far. Next stop 'Pollutants'.

Appendix

i) 50 essential nutrients
ii) Todays diet Vs caveman
iii) E Numbers
iv) Hippocratic Oath
v) Country GDPs Vs Corporation Revenues
i) 50 Essential Nutrients

These are considered 'Essential' because the body cannot produce these nutrients that are required for health, it is therefore essential they are consumed. The best way of sourcing them will always have been an intuitively driven goal. It goes without saying at this stage of the book, that the nutrient content is solely determined by the soil, which means that a certain item of food only has a potential to be an excellent source if it is grown in mineral rich soils, which sadly is a rarity these days. Do not worry about the finer details about these essential nutrients. If your diet is varied, involves eating a lot of green leaves, colourful salads and plates of home-cooked healthy food, with or without a little quality meat thrown in as well and snacks of nuts and seeds, there should be little concern, as you are already eating a good dose of all of these nutrients.

Water – arguably the best source would be a stream bubbling up after the water has spent some time filtering through various rocks leaving various trace elements within the water. As long as of course, these trace elements are not radioactive minerals, arsenic, lead or other dangerous elements in high concentrations. However, your tap water filtered through a normal Brita filter will more than suffice. With a diet consisting of predominately vegetables, the daily water requirement can be met from these alone as vegetables are anything from 80 to 90% plus water, depending on ones individual temperature and energy expenditure.

Oxygen – clean air, likewise clean water, will become a political and territorial lynch pin in the coming decades, as they become scarcer resources. Remember though, air is actually about 78% nitrogen and only 20% oxygen (any more and it would be flammable) and just under 2% of other gases, notably argon. Breath in deep in the middle of woodland, that's got to be the best source of clean fresh oxygen you could ever wish for.

Light – is determined by the sunshine and the human position in it enabling hormones to function effectively. Vitamin D is most frequently associated with this, although this counts as another nutrient discussed later. Light can also be seen as the type of bulb used indoors, with a spectrum of lumens and colours attached.

Fibre – as with carbohydrates below, fibre is a secondary product of any food items eaten. Processed foods have little or no fibre, so simply eating a wholefood diet will inevitably increase fibre intake.

Carbohydrates – for traditions sake I have stuck with this one, although it is a biological source of energy so it is best to include it, although as already mentioned all food has an element of carbs just as all food has a protein content, with well sourced whole foods always being best. What's important is that the modern diet is made of predominately processed carbohydrates, which is an enormous shift from any preceding diet of the past 40 plus millennia. Even what may be seen as an awful medieval diet of perhaps stale bread and gruel (a barley stew, with other roots and veg thrown in) offers considerably more nutritional value than a bowl of choco-pops, artificially sweetened squash, crisps, white bread cheese sandwich, cereal bar, soda, chocolate bar, chips, beans, burger and a bowl of ice-cream (a daily diet followed by many millions across the industrial world).

Protein as the following Amino Acids – there are 21 amino acids (one other pyrrolysine is not used by humans), although the following ten are not able to be made by the human body, hence why these are considered essential:

Leucine – utilized primarily by muscle and adipose tissue as well as the liver. The best sources for it are soybeans, peanuts, beef, nuts, fish, pulses, oat, poultry and eggs. It is also known as E641, used as a flavour enhancer.

Isoleucine – the -iso prefix indicates that it is an isomer of leucine, this means they have the same number of atoms of each element but are arranged in a different way, meaning they don't necessarily share properties. It is used for the conversion of energy for both ketogenic and glucogenic. Both leucine and isoleucine require biotin (vitamin B7) for biological utilisation. Good sources include, eggs, soy protein, fish, seaweed, cheese and chicken.

Lysine – used as a building block for all protein in the body, it builds muscle, plays a vital role in calcium absorption and the production of hormones, enzymes and antibodies. Best sources can be found in a variety of fish, pulses, beef, seeds, quinoa, raw milk and eggs. Has some success in fighting cold sores (*Herpes simplex*) and could help with osteoporosis.

Threonine – used to create the non-essential amino acids glycine and serine for the production of collagen and muscle tissue. Threonine promotes normal growth and maintains the proper protein balance, as well as supporting the cardiovascular, nervous and immune systems. Meat is the best source, although lentils and sesame seeds have a good amount.

Tryptophan – is a precursor for serotonin (which makes melatonin) and aids in the production of niacin (vitamin B3). Best sources are cocoa, oats, fish, seeds, banana, peanuts, spirulina, meats, raw milk, eggs and quinoa. Research is looking at how tryptophan may aid depression, reduce aggression and insomnia.

Methionine – supports liver functioning as well as regulating the natural antioxidant amino acid glutathione, which neutralizes toxins in the liver. Methionine also aids in the production of the amino acids taurine and cysteine. As with the other amino acids it is best sourced from nuts, beans, eggs, fish, garlic and onions (for the sulphur), lentils, meat, seeds and yoghurt. Co-factors (helpers) are vitamin B6 and B12.

Valine – works alongside leucine and isoleucine to promote normal growth, tissue repair, regulating blood sugar levels and providing energy. It also stimulates the central nervous system and proper mental functioning. Found in beans, nuts, legumes, meats, dairy and soy products.

Phenylalanine – the body needs phenylalanine, it crosses the blood brain barrier to make epinephrine, dopamine and norepinephrine, neurotransmitters that control how we perceive and interact with the world. This underlines the danger poised by aspartame (made from 50% phenylalanine, methanol and aspartic acid) as this too can pass direct to the brain causing havoc – just wait for future research to clarify this. There isn't such a strong movement to ban aspartame because we're being difficult and wrong, it's a pernicious and deadly food additive that has to be removed from the food chain. Phenylalanine also aids in the production of adrenaline and thyroid hormones. Best sourced from nuts, legumes, soy products, dairy and meats and definitely not aspartame.

Histidine – argued by some as non-essential (initially only considered essential for infants), although as natural levels can easily run too low it is often classed as essential. It maintains healthy tissues and importantly the myelin sheath that protects nerves, guaranteeing proper transmission of signalling from the brain and various parts of the body. Histidine also gets converted to histamine, essential for the immune system and also sexual arousal. Too much has links with mental health issues, although a balanced predominately fresh food diet will provide a balanced amount of all amino acids. Best sourced from meat, dairy, rice, wheat and rye.

Arginine – babies cannot make this so it is considered essential only for them, although levels can run low, especially when a wound is healing. It detoxifies the liver, strengthens the immune system, regulates hormones and blood sugar. Found in good quantities from meats, dairy, grains, flours, nuts, seeds and soy products.

Cysteine – semi-essential as with arginine above, it is converted from methionine and shares properties with this essential amino acid, notably the production of glutathione with its immune and expulsion properties. It is found in the same types of food as methionine, as well as red peppers, brassicas (broccoli and sprouts etc.), lentils, meats and dairy.

Other amino acids such as glutamine, glycine, proline, serine, tyrosine and asparagine are in some instances, such as ill health and recovery, considered semi-essential. Their sources are all similar and that's all that needs to be said here in the essential appendix.

(I would not recommend supplementing any individual amino acids because there is a delicate balance, with any short-term gains undoubtedly undone in the long-run, it is always best to source organic nuts, seeds, meat, dairy and grains and simply eat more quality food to boost overall levels. However, for some medical conditions it may be appropriate, such advice will have to be sourced from a trusted medical professional.)

The human body cannot make any minerals, so the extent of the list could in fact be more substantial depending on future research determining the essentialness of various trace elements/minerals, especially all those phyto and micro nutrients.

Calcium – vital for healthy teeth and bones as well as being crucial for nerves, heart and muscle contraction and the blood. Can only be assimilated if magnesium is also present, ingested in ratio with phosphorus with a healthy parathyroid. Best source by a long way are nettles, peppermint and parsley, sesame seeds and grass-fed dairy.

Chloride – is an essential electrolyte, maintaining bodily acid levels, regulating movement in and out of cells and transmission of nerve impulses and a component of some proteins and the manufacture of hydrochloric acid for gastric juices. With excessive salt intake chloride is persistently out of balance, this is bad news for the kidneys and osmosis from the cellular level up. For homeostasis, chloride, potassium and sodium need to be consumed in ratio with each other. With a low salt diet, chloride can be found in most vegetables, rye, tomatoes, lettuces, celery, seaweeds and most aquatic foods.

Chromium – is another mineral which is commonly deficient in out diet as well as one often dangerously neglected, as its health benefits are huge. Chromium controls insulin and normalizes blood sugar levels (as well as removing cravings for sweets and alcohol), it lowers LDL and raises HDL (the 'good' cholesterol'), lowers blood pressure and boosts levels of DHEA, a hormone associated with longevity and ageing. Best dietary source is broccoli, grapes, mushrooms, asparagus, green beans, potatoes, organ meats, nuts, bananas, many spices impart a small amount such as pepper and even red wine.

Cobalt – is the key constituent of cobalamin, otherwise known as vitamin B12, which is where more information can be found.

Copper – important in bone growth and strength, as well as being responsible for connective tissue and myelin sheath production. Best sources are spirulina, sesame seeds, cocoa, sunflower and hemp seeds.

Iodine – antiseptic, antibiotic and probably an anti-carcinogen. It is essential in thyroid hormone production, foetal and later development, as well as tissue and muscle functions. It is best sourced from organic kelp (not from near Fukushima!) and fish.

Iron – essential in the production of red blood cells, DNA, RNA, enzymes and vitamin A. Vitamin C aids its absorption and it needs to be consumed in ratio with zinc. Surprisingly, best source is chickweed, raspberry leaf, dandelion leaf, peppermint and nettles, all being miles in front of seeds and meats.

Magnesium – important in the proper functioning of nerves, heart and muscles. Works in conjunction with calcium, best consumed in a 3:2 (Ca:Mg) ratio, as well as vitamins B1, B3, C and D. Our diet is often deficient in it. The best sources are liquorice, nettles, peppermint, chickweed, cocoa, pumpkin and sesame seeds and brazil nuts.

Manganese – regulates blood sugar levels and insulin production as well as thyroid hormones. The best source by some distance is raspberry leaf, then chickweed, hemp oil, nettles and hazelnuts.

Molybdenum – forms compounds with many organic molecules, such as carbohydrates and amino acids as well as over 50 enzymes mostly in bacteria ensuring proper digestion and nutrient delivery. It helps the body utilise iron (so its deficiency is commonly the cause of anaemia, erroneously assumed to be caused by an iron deficiency). Molybdenum is found in dark green leafy vegetables, raw milk, liver, beans, peas and cereal grains.

Phosphorus – indispensable for teeth and bones. Helps absorb nutrients from foods and subsequent energy release to cells. Often the excessive consumption from fizzy drinks (phosphates) prevents calcium utilisation. Its best source is pumpkin seeds, peppermint, cocoa, nettles and chickweed (again), dandelions, dates and peas.

Potassium – works in conjunction with sodium in maintaining fluid and electrolyte balance in cells and tissues. Removes waste from cells. Needs to be consumed in a 1:1 ratio with sodium, which is of course excessively consumed so potassium's role is hindered. Best sources are parsley, sun dried tomatoes, peppermint and here it is again, chickweed (bet you've never even eaten it before), unrefined stevia, nettles, cocoa (which does not mean chocolate!), spirulina, pistachio nuts, almonds, banana and avocado.

Selenium – works with iodine in thyroid hormone production. As an anti-oxidant it protects against free radicals, also making it an anti-carcinogen. It assists the roles of vitamins B3, C and E and zinc. Deficiency of it is very common. Its best source by a country mile is Brazil nuts, then other nuts, tuna, crab and sunflower seeds.

Sodium – plays a vital role along with potassium for transmission of nerve impulses, regulating blood volume, pressure, acidity and osmotic equilibrium. Due to salt's excessive consumption this delicate and vital homeostatic balance is rarely as it should be for optimum health. However, by eliminating sodium completely many serious deficiency symptoms can manifest. Avoid salt and eat food with naturally occurring sodium (not preserved in a saline solution) such as broccoli, artichoke, carrot, celery, sweet potato, organ meats, kelp and other aquatic foods.

Sulphur (Sulfur is also the correct spelling) – found in its organic form in the vitamins biotin (B7) and thiamine (B1), as well as many enzymes and antioxidant molecules such as glutathione, also a component of amino acids (esp. cysteine and methione) and other proteins such as keratin (found in skin and hair). Eggs, alliums (garlic, onions and leeks) are excellent sources of dietary sulphur as are the cruciferous vegetables (broccoli, cauliflower, cabbage), kale, fish, poultry, nuts and legumes.

Zinc – vital for the reproductive, nervous and immune systems, brain health as well as a component of enzymes, DNA and RNA, all being crucial for growth. Needs to be consumed in ratio with iron and manganese, another one that our diet is commonly deficient in. Its best source are oysters, followed by sesame, pumpkin and sunflower seeds, cocoa, hemp oil, nettles, chickweed and lamb.

Vitamins

Vitamin A (retinol and beta-carotene) – a powerful antioxidant. Associated with cell division and the health of bone, skin, urinary tract, digestive and respiratory systems. Regulates the thyroid gland and is protected by vitamin E. Retinol is from animals and is toxic at high levels, from as little as 150g. Beef liver is the richest source for retinol. Beta-carotenes are sourced from vegetables, with spirulina (an algae) being the best source, followed by wheatgrass, peppermint, carrots, nettles, raspberry leaf and broccoli and are not toxic at any level.

Vitamin B1 (thiamine) – vital for the metabolism of foods, conversion of energy from fats and carbohydrates, as well as the bio-assimilation of proteins. Helps to prevent the build-up of toxins. Best sources are spirulina, sunflower, hemp and sesame seeds, pork, nettles and dandelions.

Vitamin B2 (riboflavin) – bio-assimilates the energy from foods, maintains the skin and acidity levels. Essential for the production of vitamins B3 and B6. Its best dietary source is peppermint, spirulina, hemp seeds, comfrey, almond, crab, nettles, sunflower seeds, mushrooms, peas, mackerel and lamb.

Vitamin B3 (niacin) – also involved in the bio-assimilation of energy from food, as well as maintaining the brain and skin and regulating blood sugar levels. Best source is raspberry leaves, peanuts, spirulina, peppermint, comfrey, chickweed, nettles, sunflower seeds and peas.

Vitamin B5 (pantothenic acid) – breaks down proteins into amino acids as well as being critical for the production of anti-stress hormones and haemoglobin. Spirulina is once again the best source, followed by shitake mushrooms, sun-dried tomatoes, eggs, sunflower seeds, broccoli and other mushrooms.

Vitamin B6 (pyridoxine) – essential for the production and balance of hormones. It is a well-known anti-depressant as well as aiding the upkeep of the immune system. It is best sourced from pistachios, sunflower and sesame seeds, banana, rabbit, hemp seeds and kale.

Vitamin B7 (biotin) – also known as vitamin H (from the German for 'hair and skin', '*haar and haut*'), involved in the synthesis of fatty acids and the amino acids isoleucine and valine, necessary for cell growth and the various metabolic reactions involving the transfer of carbon dioxide. It is not strictly essential at all as the intestinal bacteria produces biotin but I thought it interesting to put here, being a forgotten vitamin along with B8 below (there are also other B vitamins such as B15 and B17 which will be looked at in later books in this series). Best dietary sources for biotin include peanuts, green leafy vegetables, liver and some berries.

Vitamin B8 (inositol) – as with B7 it is not essential as it is produced from glucose in the kidneys in usually sufficient quantities (other vitamins are also produced in the body but in inadequate quantities for optimum health). Inositol is used in the breakdown of fats, assembly of cytoskeleton (intracellular matrix) and gene expression (which generates the macromole-cular machinery for life). Best sources are fruit, particularly canteloupe melons and oranges, beans, grains and nuts (although inositol can be found in two forms as a bioavailable lecithin and its unavailable phytate form, more common in seeds and grains).

Vitamin B9 (folic acid) – crucial for cell division, hence why it is seen as essential for pregnant women, although it's essential for everyone and is sadly commonly deficient in our diets. The best source by a long way is parsley, followed by sunflower seeds, spinach, kelp, lentils, asparagus and sesame seeds.

Vitamin B12 (cobalamin) – plays a key role in normal functioning of the brain, nervous system and the formation of blood. It is a strange vitamin as only bacteria have the available enzymes for its synthesis, it is also the only metal-containing vitamin (cobalt), although consumption of cobalt does not help synthesis as it requires bacteria for this. Deficiency in it is far more common amongst vegans as its most reliable source is animal products including eggs and dairy, even some insects. However, not all vegans suffer from deficiency symptoms (including anaemia, fatigue, psychosis, neurological damage and poor memory) as it can be found in fermented products such as tofu, possibly spirulina and chlorella (some studies suggest in these two it is found in an unavailable form), marmite (in yeast) and comfrey has been shown to have some. There is even the possibility that human gut bacteria can produce some (more research required to prove this) which would blow the arguments out of the water about humans never being vegetarian because of B12's essentialness, although as seen there are other ways of ingesting the required miniscule amount.

Vitamin C (ascorbic acid) – is actually a complex with ascorbic acid merely being its protecting case, the vitamin itself is much more than ascorbic acid. It is the body's most powerful antioxidant and antibiotic, strengthening the immune system. Used for iron absorption and the production of hormones. It is surprisingly commonly deficient in an average diet and could play a future role in cancer and CVD prevention. The best natural source (as ascorbic acid is often industrially produced) is vitamin C extract from acerola cherries by some distance, followed by rosehip, guava, blackcurrants, pumpkin seeds, parsley, nettles, kiwi fruit, broccoli and oranges.

Vitamin D (D2 ergocalciferol, D3 cholecalciferol) – requires enzymatic conversion (hydroxylation) in the liver and kidneys into calcitriol when ingested, or of course the skin synthesizes enough with about 30 minutes exposure to the sun. Strictly speaking it is more of a hormone than a vitamin. It's most common form of deficiency is rickets, characterized by soft, weak and bendy bones (often bowed legs). Fortification in food allegedly helped to reduce rickets (studies are inconclusive however) although it has been reported that as many as half of the children in a study in Southampton showed onset rickets with the root cause being children staying indoors much more and playing consoles. The increase in meat and dairy intake during the twentieth century could be a factor in rickets incidence decreasing, although dietary sources are rare (skin of fish and animals a good source), such as fatty fish, alfalfa, eggs and mushrooms.

Vitamin E (d-alpha tocopherol) – another antioxidant, working best in conjunction with vitamins A, C and B complex. It promotes healthy blood and organs. Its best sources are sunflower seeds, comfrey leaves, hemp oil, almonds, peanuts, sweet potato, spirulina, hemp seeds, dandelions, spinach, and salmon.

Vitamin K (phylloquinone) – is essential for blood coagulation and the binding of calcium in bone and other tissues (often injected into babies at birth). The best source is green leafy vegetables as they are involved in photosynthesis, especially dandelion leaves, kale, spinach, greens, broccoli, lettuce and asparagus, kiwifruit and grapes, also goose liver, cheeses and eggs.

(These vitamins are either fat or water-soluble. Vitamins B and C are water soluble, meaning they can be utilized in water and generally will be excreted in urine if excessively consumed. Vitamins A, D, E and K are fat soluble, meaning they require ingestion with fats to be best utilized but they are also readily absorbed in body fat if excessive, and this can cause problems, although as they are stored in fat they can be converted from there, so the water soluble ones are the ones requiring a daily input.)

The following Fats are most definitely essential, even going by the name Essential Fatty acids (EFAs) and eaten way out of balance, severely jeopardizing any possibility of biological utilization and the potential benefits.

Linolenic Acid (Omega3), is not used directly by the body, it is converted to the acids of eicosapentaenoic acid (EPA) and docosahexaenoic acid (DHA); as well as several others all of varying chain lengths. Because these can be sourced directly from fish, aquatic life is advertised as being the best and only source for these, when in fact the best source is organic seeds such as linseeds, hemp and chia seeds, as the human body converts the omega3 to the long chained polyunsaturated fatty acids EPA and DHA efficiently, without the worry of ingesting fat-soluble pollutants and deadly metals such as mercury, long known to be associated with fish. Omega3 is found in small amounts in many other foods from kiwi fruit to nuts, deep green vegetables from kale to purslane and broccoli, kelp, meats and in eggs, if the chickens have been fed seeds and insects it is enhanced. Omega3 is best utilized when it is consumed in a beneficial ratio with Omega6 (between 1:1 to 1:2), although as Omega6 is present in vegetable oils and is omnipresent throughout the modern food chain, it is eaten way beyond the beneficial ratio, eaten more like 1:10 to 1:30, which many doctors and those looking at these oils associate as a direct risk factor for many of the diseases of civilization. Too much Omega6 also hampers conversion of the Omega3.

Linoleic Acid (Omega6), again is not used directly by the body, it is converted to the long chained polyunsaturated fatty acids gamma-linolenic acid (GLA), dihomo-gamma-linolenic acid (DGLA) and arachidonic acid (AA). As just mentioned, it is excessively consumed as well as being found in large quantities in vegetable oils, it can also be found in a wide range of foods, from nuts, poultry and grains, with evening primrose oil being perhaps the best source for GLA. Because it is consumed excessively (from vegetable oils and processed foods) with associated health risks, Omega6 is viewed in our dualistic world as being the bad fatty acid with Omega3 being the good guy, which is too simplistic and wrong. When consumed in ratio with Omega3, Omega6 is a positive, essential, dietary input. That said, there have been medical links that indicate that certain Omega6s, when consumed excessively, significantly increase the risk of arthritis, inflammation and certain cancers.

Amongst many other nutrients, three currently stand out

Bioflavonoids - over 5000 naturally occurring flavonoids have been recognised from plants. Some familiar ones include anthoxanthins, quercitrin, flavanone, anthocyanidins, polyphenols, flavanol, flavans and isoflavanes. There has been only a little current research on these, results so far indicate that they have positive results in relation to cardiovascular disease, inflammation and cancer as well as having antibacterial properties. Being a part of the colour of plants they can be found in all plants (I bet future studies will demonstrate that a healthy diet is one concerned with colour counting not calorie counting), with berries having excellent quantities, as does parsley, onions, black and green tea, bananas, citrus fruits, cocoa and many, many more.

Choline – is water-soluble and is often grouped with the B vitamins. Choline has been shown to support a foetus's developing nervous system (making it a co-factor with vitamins B9 and B12), is an anti-inflammatory and it's deficiency may play a role in neurological disorders, atherosclerosis, liver and muscle damage, as well as certain cancers. Good dietary sources include seeds, nuts, cruciferous vegetables, rice, spinach, eggs, tofu, fish, organ meats and grapefruit.

Co-enzyme Q10 – is fat soluble and very similar to a vitamin (E in particular), functioning in every cell of the body to synthesize energy and acts as an antioxidant. It possibly inhibits the effectiveness of warfarin and is adversely affected in its roles by statins and beta-blockers. Good dietary sources are meat and fish, avocado, vegetable oils (soy, olive and grapeseed), nuts, seeds, parsley and spinach.

There are also a huge group of chemicals known as phyto-chemicals/nutrients that will with more research also unlock another door to the potential health benefits that plants offer. Some better known ones are lycopene (tomato, grapefruit, carrots), zeaxanthin (spinach, kale, greens, eggs, red pepper), lutein (spinach, greens, brassicas, avocado, lettuce), saponins (beans, legumes, grains), limonene (oils of citrus, cherries, mint, garlic, rosemary, ginger, basil), phytosterols (nuts, seeds, grains and oils), all the bioflavonoids above and literally 1000s of others.

I really hope that after seeing the best sources (with ingestion of 100g) for the minerals and vitamins it becomes clearer why our ancestors enjoyed a life predominately free from the diseases of civilization. If not, have another look through them. Many of the foods are forage-able, with seeds coming out on top, whilst modern meat predominately only registers with the amino acids and processed foods, the staples of the modern diet don't even register on the lists because they contain the minimum of nutrients. We need to remineralize before catastrophe sets in any further.

ii) Caveman diet vs Modern diet

It is fair and scientific to assume that the diet of the caveman, anytime from 100,000 to 4,000 years ago would in many instances resemble that of a foraged diet of today and is certainly compa-rable to a modern hunter-gatherer's diet and that of many tribal societies'. If climatic, environmental and topographical features are similar, there is every reason to surmise that the diet would also be similar, irrespective of the time.

Ethnographic comparisons from modern day hunter-gatherers are also applicable, as well as the growing body of archaeological evidence uncovering the vast extent of the former plants that were utilized by our ancestors. The picture needs to be redrawn of the erroneous stereotype of our ancestors being carnivorous thugs, as a reality of omnivorous, harmonious forest folk, is a much truer and fairer picture, especially as it is the foraged plants that possess the most nutrients. The dietary list to follow below for the caveman is a foraged diet still possible to be foraged today in southern England (and much of Europe).

Seasons vary for the caveman diet and it makes sense to assume that our European ancestors would have had a dynamic existence, moving from camp to camp, some of which would have been many weeks travel apart. The picture of our movements is falsely based on our ancestors following the migratory grazers, as erroneous assumption and cultural indoctrination has led us to believe that grazing animals were our main food. They weren't, we merely moved with the varying seasons for flowering plants and grasses. There would be no point remaining anywhere if there was no forage-able food available, that's bleeding obvious, that's why the animals moved and that's why our ancestors moved. That's our twenty first century spectacles obscuring the truth again!

Much confusion has been caused by the recent Paleo-diet fad, with many fanatic followers all fervently believing they are eating the same food as we did 10,000 years ago and indeed the whole of evolution, gorging themselves on a high protein, predominately meat diet daily. In the past (and from recent ethnographic evidence) all tribes and hunter-gatherers do indeed gorge themselves on large mammals from time to time, this is indisputable. However, what is omitted from the Paleo-diet is the scientific archaeological bit about what the diet would really have consisted of. A wild diet is of course completely dependant upon the climate, with large mammals contributing to the diet, although for most climatic regions, especially the warmer ones, insects, bugs, grubs and worms would have contributed the bulk of what can be termed as meat, with small rodents being the commonest recognisable 'meat' eaten, with a young or medium sized deer being the largest prey commonly hunted.

The actual nutritious content of the food eaten is nigh on impossible to ascertain. There is very little if any nutrient profile analysis of wild foraged foods and those that are available for modern food types come with absolutely no guarantee that the figures are relevant, with the variations of actual content having a vast range, as well as of course the fact that the soils would have been astronomically more mineral rich than today's barren, sterile crumb. With this in mind, the following is only an outline of the massive gulf between the food types we would have evolved on and contemporary, demineralized foods and the possible correlation with the gigantic leap in the diseases of civilization. Coincidence or obvious correlation? You decide.

Typical modern, daily food regime:

Breakfast – coffee, milk, sugar; white toast, margarine, jam; cornflakes, milk, sugar.

Mid-morning snack – cereal bar; apple; coffee, milk, sugar.

Lunch – white bread sandwich, cheese, iceberg lettuce, cucumber, mayonnaise; coffee, milk, sugar.

Afternoon snack – tea, milk, sugar; packet of crisps.

Pint of beer.

Dinner – white pasta, tinned tomatoes, tinned tuna, onion, garlic, dried mixed herbs; white baguette, butter, garlic; slice of apple pie, vanilla ice-cream; pint of beer.

There is little variation in this diet from day to day, the pasta will be swapped with a pizza, a Chinese or Indian take-away as a treat, dinners will vary the most from day-to-day, although a total of 10 different dishes will be eaten on average throughout the year. Items throughout the rest of the day will be swapped, a pasty instead of a sandwich for instance, ice-cream for the pie, chocolate bar instead of crisps. Some days will of course also contain a side salad (usually from a bag), a portion of vegetables (boiled). With a whole world of food and cuisines available, it is amazing how unadventurous and bland the modern palette has become, even if we assume we are pushing the boundaries with a fiery curry.

Typical daily diet of a tribesperson or modern hunter-gatherer:

Here we need to lose all our modern concepts about how we ate in the past. Breakfast, lunch and dinner are modern constructs forced upon us to make our lives fit within a feudal then capitalist system. The wild food collectors of the past would have grazed all day long as they foraged and performed necessary tasks from repairing clothes and shelters to preparing food. Those grazed on foods would have included any of the following if living within a similar climatic zone as that experienced in parts of Britain today:

A huge selection of green leaf vegetables, from chickweed (which as shown above in the Essential 50 nutrients, is superlative in a broad spectrum of health giving nutrients as are all of the others in the list below), watercress, bittercress, winter-cress, marjoram, pennywort, ivy-leaved toadflax, wild cabbage, stinging nettles, white and red dead-nettle, cow-parsley, lady's smock, cleavers, scurvy grass, wild garlic, hedge garlic, alexanders, lamb's lettuce, sea kale, sea beet, sea purslane, samphire, bistort, bog myrtle, sorrel, dandelion, sweet cicely, rape, black mustard, wild cabbage, comfrey, butterburr, ground elder, hogweed, clover, thyme, parsley, broom, horseradish, Good King Henry, Jack-by-the-hedge, fat-hen, mint, chervil, pennyroyal mint, apple mint, mallow, goosefoot, mugwort, burdock, tansy, coltsfoot and sow thistle.

Leaves from loads of trees, especially when young such as hawthorn, oak, lime, mulberry, walnut, birch and beech and many more; it is best to get an identifier and pick when just emerged in spring to summer. Leaves are an almost completely neglected source of food, wrongly assumed to be inedible, when in fact they have a fantastic range of vitamins and minerals (dependent on the soil they grow in of course).

Flowers from plants to trees such as basil, bean, broccoli, chamomile, chervil, primrose, elderflower, rowan, linden, sweet violet, mint, sunflower, snap-dragons, marigold and nasturtium, to name just a few, usually only eaten a few at a time, they do have unrivalled beta-carotene content, as it's in the colour. As with all food, moderation is the key as they can be toxic if eaten in large quantities.

Fruits and berries from blackberry, elder, hawthorn, crab apples, sloes, wild cherry, wild strawberry, raspberry, bilberry, cowberry, crowberry, cloudberry, cranberry, gooseberry, redcurrant, medlar, rosehip and rowan.

Roots and tubers from fennel, parsley, pignut, dandelion, horseradish and silverweed, all somewhat smaller than the larger tubers such as potatoes and yams etc., whose provenance is from far more exotic locales than Britain.

Nuts from hazel, acorns, beech, chestnut and walnut, are an abundant and reliable source of food, remaining fresh for months, would have once represented significant staples for many people, just as mongongo nuts are so prolific they provide the majority of the diet for the !Kung and other foragers of wild foods in S & SE Africa.

Seeds from wild grasses (oat, wheat, barley etc), fat-hen, chervil, Good King Henry, poppy, nettles and whole array of plants, particularly those already mentioned.

Mushrooms such as chanterelles, field mushrooms, horse mushroom, Jew's ear, chicken of the woods, russulas, cauliflower fungus, beefsteak fungus, morel, parasol, blewits, puff-ball, ceps, boletus', oyster and St George's mushroom are a few of the better tasting ones although many more are still edible. Mushrooms are so abundant it would be a folly to ignore them, for both their calorific and nutritional, not to mention their alter-dimensional potential.

Seaweeds such as kelp, laver, sweet oarweed, sea lettuce, dulse, carragheen and with enough boiling, just about any seaweed found off the coast of Britain. Man-made dangerous chemicals and spillages have meant that the sea and consequently the seaweed is often contaminated today (hardly surprising when one considers that seaweed is an excellent food to eat for its unrivalled ability to pull toxins out of the body).

Wow! That's a significantly diverse natural larder already and that's only what's on the vegan menu. Just check out all the other food types available that would have been regularly ingested by our omnivorous ancestors –

Bugs, crawlers and wrigglers from bee larvae, cockroach, cockchafer, dragonfly (a slightly disturbing delicacy in Bali, unless I'm alone in my admiration of this particular insect), earthworms, fly pupae, cricket, grasshopper, caterpillars, louse, midge and woodlice to name just a few. Constantly snacked on, crunched on, crushed into pastes, providing some very fine and essential fatty acids. Over half the world already has entomophagy (eating insects) as a part of their culinary cultural cuisine, soon to be adopted by the rest of the world.

Fish were in astronomical numbers only a century or two ago. With the same range as today from herring, carp, cod, minnows, bream, rudd, chub, ling, loach, catfish, pike, slickheads, salmon, trout, charr, sturgeon, eels, hake, pollock, monkfish, mullet, John Dory, turbot, sole, dab, plaice, flounder, halibut, haddock, gurnard, perch, pomfret, seabass, mullet, wrasse, goby, mackerel, tuna, sailfish and many more from the seas, lakes and rivers.

A small selection of crustaceans and molluscs (shellfish) from crabs, lobster, clams, mussels, prawns, oysters, crayfish, seasnails, whelks, periwinkles and limpets, would have provided superb nutrition, as they do today for those living near to the sea and inland waters.

Meat from seals, dolphins, whales, deer, rabbit, birds, rodents, aurochs (massive and ferocious testosterone surging bulls) and basically anything that moved was fair game, although the other types of food from above would have been the main component of the food eaten, just as they are for the miniscule amount of hunter-gatherers who are fortunate to live in their preferred location, instead of being marginalised and compromised, if not annihilated.

Any number of the above and a plethora of similar species, varieties and types would have been eaten when in season and in view. This is the diet of old, not the stereotype our cultural indoctrination has implanted in us, with our ancestors barely surviving, in near frozen wastelands, near to starvation until the men bring back the rewards from their dangerous hunt. What utter nonsense. They all foraged, eating the local fauna and flora.

All of the above food would knock modern food out of the water for nutritious content. I can't emphasis enough that the diet of the past and the diet of today are not comparable. The quality and quantity of vitamins and minerals from rich soils and seas all unpolluted just blows my mind, especially when we stupidly assume the food we eat today is good. It's not, it is rubbish and in most instances, it's toxic.

An important difference between the modern diet and the timeless foraged diet is the fact that the hunter-gatherer diet has a relatively balanced proportion of fats, high in beneficial fats, derived from nuts and seeds as well as a myriad of small insects, grubs and rodents and a very low amount of carbohydrate rich foods, unlike the diet of today, solely dominated by processed carbohydrate-rich foods. It is these highly refined, processed, almost pure carbs, which have rightly come in for much flack throughout this book due to their very detrimental attributes. It is these carbohydrate rich foods that are the main difference between the diets, irrespective of what the actual food consumed is.

You haven't just read almost the entire book for me to refute any of what has gone before, as it clearly is this diet dominated by the Deadly Whites that is the largest difference between modern life and traditional life. Hence there is little surprise that this massive change in diet has resulted in it being a significant risk factor in the diseases of civilization. Ignore ridiculous arguments about lifespan and that cancer, heart disease etc. are degenerative so only occur in later life after a significant incubation period (this does account for some but how on earth can this account for an increasingly younger demographic who are falling sick?). As already mentioned in this book, the modern diet is the cause of such incubation period and it is because of this flawed diet that the door to the diseases of civilization has been opened. Yes, many tribal people do die before the age of 75, very few or any however, die the same deaths as us in the west, and for those that live to a similar age as those of us in the west, none succumb to dementia, cancer and heart disease.

A very important point to raise here is that it is only since contact with outsiders (that'd be us, traders and nosey anthropologists) that has seen the hunter-gatherers and tribal populations being decimated by infectious diseases, dramatically reducing their average life expectancies. Because of this 'contact' anomaly, it is unscientific to paint all traditional life with a modern disease ridden brush. I'm not implying a golden age before white man's contact with 'savages' as it's obvious the past was a potentially very violent world, where a large proportion of deaths would have come in the shape of an end of a spear or club. This aspect of past societies is not the premise of this series of books, a subject well covered by many books. The first three books of this series are only looking at modern man and why it is we are so susceptible to the diseases of civilization. Murder today accounts for a miniscule amount of deaths, whereas cancer and heart disease (and iatrogenics) account for most deaths, so the fact that our ancestors might have met an untimely death from a spear is irrelevant, as that speared victim would not have died from cancer if left to live till old age, we on the other hand do, and it has

Appendix

absolutely nothing to do with the preponderance or avoidance of a clubbing or spearing.

As seen in the 50 essential nutrients above, it is those plants still available in the wild that provide the best nutritious content. We are not eating those plants anymore and we are not getting those nutrients anymore but we are getting a whole bunch of deadly diseases now. Coincidence or a contributory factor for the illnesses?

iii) E – Numbers

Avoid as many of the following as possible, if you really do care about you and your families health and future. Where possible I have included its status according to the regulatory bodies of the UK and US. E100- E199 are generally colours. E200-E299 are preservatives. E300-E399 are antioxidants and acidity regulators. E400-E499 are thickeners, emulsifiers and stabilisers. E500-E599 are acidity regulators and anti-caking agents. E600-E699 are flavour enhancers. E700-E799 are antibiotics. E900-E999 are miscellaneous. E1000-E1999 are new and additional.

The following abbreviations are used where research has linked the E number to Asthma - A, Cancer - C, or Hyperactivity - H.

Harmful E Numbers

E102 Tartrazine (Yellow 5) A C H Dangerous Unpermitted in EU (Colouring)
E103 Chrysoine resorcinol A C H Banned since 1984 (Colouring)
E104 Quinoline Yellow A C H Dangerous (Colouring)
E105 Fast Yellow AB Forbidden (Colouring)
E107 Yellow 2G A C H Dangerous (Colouring)
E110 Sunset Yellow (Yellow 6) A C H Dangerous (Colouring)
E111 Orange GGN Forbidden (Colouring)
E120 Carmines/ Cochineal A H Dangerous (Colouring)

E121 Citrus Red 2 Forbidden (Colouring)

E122 Azorubine/ Carmoisine A C H (Colouring)

E123 Amaranth (Red 2) A C H Extremely dangerous Forbidden (Colouring)

E124 Ponceau 4 R (Brilliant scarlet) A C H Dangerous Unpermitted in US (Colouring)

E125 Ponceau SX Forbidden (Colouring)

E126 Ponceau 6R Forbidden (Colouring)

E127 Erythrosine (Red 3) A C H Dangerous Unpermitted (Colouring)

E128 Red 2G A C H Forbidden (Colouring)

E129 Allura Red A C H (Colouring)

E130 Indanthrene Blue Forbidden (Colouring)

E131 Patent Blue 5 A C H Dangerous (Colouring)

E132 Indigo Carmine (Blue 2) A C H Dangerous (Colouring)

E133 Brilliant Blue A C H (Colouring)

E142 Green S A C H Unpermitted in EU (Colouring)

E143 Fast Green A (Colouring)

E150 Caramel H (Colouring)

E151 Brilliant Black A C H (Colouring)

E152 Black 7984 Forbidden (Colouring)

E154 Brown FIC/ Kipper Brown A C H Unpermitted (Colouring)

E155 Chocolate Brown A C H (Colouring)

E160b Annatto/ Bixin A H Dangerous (Colouring)

E173 Aluminium C Unpermitted (Colouring)

E180 Pigment Rubine A C H Unpermitted (Colouring)

E181 Tannin Forbidden (Colouring)

E200-E203 Potassium and Calcium Sorbates, Sorbic Acid A C H (Preservative)

E210 Benzoic Acid A C H Unpermitted in UK (Preservative)

E211 Sodium Benzoate A C H (Preservative)

E212 Potassium Benzoate A C (Preservative)

E213 Calcium Benzoate A C (Preservative)

E214 Ethylparaben (Ethyl para-hydroxybenzoate) A C Dangerous (Preservative)

E215 Sodium Ethyl para-hydroxybenzoate C (Preservative)

E216 Propylparaben (Propyl para-hydroxybenzoate) A Forbidden (Preservative)

E217 Sodium Propyl para-hydroxybenzoate A C Forbidden (Preservative)

E220 Sulphur Dioxide A H (Preservative)

E221 Sodium Sulphite A (Preservative)

E222 Sodium Bisulphite A (Preservative)

E223 Sodium Metabisulphite A (Preservative)

E224 Potassium Metabisulphite A (Preservative)

E225 Potassium Sulphite A (Preservative)

E226 Calcium Sulphite A (Preservative)

E227 Calcium Hydrogen Sulphite A (Preservative)

E228 Potassium Bisulphite A H (Preservative)

E230 Biphenyl/ Diphenyl C Dangerous (Preservative)

E231 Orthophenyl Phenol C Dangerous (Preservative)

E232 Sodium Orthophenyl Phenol Dangerous (Preservative)

E236 Formic Acid C (Preservative)

E239 Hexamine (Hexamethylene Tetramine) C Dangerous (Preservative)

E240 Formaldehyde Forbidden (Preservative)

E249 Potassium Nitrate A C (Preservative)

E250 Sodium Nitrite A C H (Preservative)

E251 Sodium Nitrate C H (Preservative)

E252 Potassium Nitrate C H (Preservative)

E260 Acetic Acid A (Preservative)

E280-E283 Calcium/ Potassium/ Sodium Propionates A H (Preservative)

E310 Propyl Gallate A C Dangerous (Synthetic antioxidant)

E311 Octyl Gallate A Dangerous (Synthetic antioxidant)

E312 Dodecyl Gallate A Dangerous (Synthetic antioxidant)

E313 Ethyl Gallate Dangerous (Synthetic antioxidant)
E319 Tert Butylhydroquinone (TBHQ) A H (Antioxidant)
E320 Butylated Hydroxyanisole (BHA) A C H (Antioxidant)
E321 Butylated Hydroxytoluene (BHT) A C H (Antioxidant)
E343 Mono/ Dimagnesium Phosphate Under consideration (Anti-caking agent)
E388 Thiodipropionic Acid Unpermitted
E389 Dilauryl Thiodipropionate Unpermitted

E407 Carrageenan A C (Thickener and stabiliser)
E413 Tragacanth A (Thickener and emulsifier)
E414 Acacia Gum A (Stabiliser)
E416 Karaya Gum A (Food thickener and stabiliser)
E421 Mannitol H (Sweetener and anti-caking)
E424 Curdlan Unpermitted
E425 Konjac Gum/ Glucomannane Unpermitted in EU (Emulsifier)
E430 Polyxyethylene Stearate C (Emulsifier)
E432-E436 Polysorbates/ Monostearate C (Emulsifier)
E441 Gelatine A (Gelling agent)
E466 Sodium Carboxymethyl Cellulose C Under consideration

E507 Hydrochloric Acid C (Used in gelatin production)
E512 Stannous Chloride Unpermitted
E518 Magnesium Sulphate C (Tofu coagulant)
E536 Potassium Ferrocyanide A (Anti-caking agent)
E537 Ferrous Hexacyanomanganate Unpermitted
E553-E553b Talc C (Anti-caking agent)
E557 Zinc Silicate Unpermitted

E620-E625 Monosodium Glutamate (MSG)/ Glutamates A C H (Flavour enhancer)
E627 Disodium Guanylate A H (Flavour enhancer)
E631 Disodium Inosinate 5 A (Flavour enhancer)

E635 Disodium Ribonucleotides 5 A (Flavour enhancer)

E903 Carnauba Wax C (Chewing gums, Glazing agent)
E905a,b,c Paraffin, Vaseline, White Mineral Oil C (Glazing agent,
   Lubricant in chewing gum)
E912 Montan Wax Unpermitted (Glazing agent)
E914 Oxidised Polyethylene Wax Unpermitted (Glazing agent)
E916 Calcium Iodate Unpermitted
E917 Potassium Iodate Unpermitted
E918 Nitrogen Oxides Unpermitted
E919 Nitrogen Chloride Unpermitted
E922 Potassium Persulfate Unpermitted (Improving agent)
E923 Ammonium Persulfate Unpermitted (Improving agent)
E924b Calcium Bromate Unpermitted (Improving agent)
E925 Chlorine C Unpermitted (Preservative, Bleach)
E926 Chlorine Dioxide C Unpermitted (Improving agent, Bleach)
E929 Acetone Peroxide Unpermitted
E950 Potassium Acesulfame C (Sweetener)
E951 Aspartame A C H (Sweetener)
E952 Cyclamate/ Cyclamic Acid C (Sweetener)
E954 Saccharine C (Sweetener)
E961 Neotame A C H (Sweetener)

E1202 Insoluble Polyvinylpyrrolidone C (Stabiliser, Clarifying
   agent in wine and beer)
E1403 Bleached Starch A (Thickener, Stabiliser).

The list is not stating that by consuming a particular substance
with any of the above in it you will suffer from asthma, hyperactivity or cancer. What it does indicate, is that an asthmatic should
be warned when consuming a foodstuff which has a chemical
added with an A attached to it. This is because there have been
instances and reportage of that particular chemical causing an
asthma attack. There is also research and results that have linked

certain chemicals as being possible root causes of asthma as well. As with hyperactivity, H, a person, often a child, who is prone to hyperactivity could well have this triggered by consumption of this chemical if it is in the ingredients of his/her food. As with asthma some of the chemicals are implicated as being the initial causal factor in the manifestation of the hyperactive condition. For cancer, C, often the research results have come from laboratory experiments on animals, results of which directly link certain chemicals to the growth of tumours and cancers in these laboratory animals, such as rats and primates.

Surely, it is more than a coincidence, this monumental increase in the consumption of the above chemicals and the rise in cancers, asthmatics, obesity, Alzheimer's, ADD, ADHD and the general disorder amongst people, especially it seems in the young. There must be some kind of a link. These chemicals were definitely not present during the time of our pre-agricultural cousins or prevalent amongst tribes today.

Read through the list again, noting the ones with an A C H beside them, these are the multi-disciplined all-rounders, avoid these. Check the ingredients on some sweets or processed food, there is bound to be at least one if not more with the A C H links. What is shocking is the amount of unpermitted and dangerous E numbers that are still in food items for sale, simply avoiding any prohibition as they are not produced in the EU, or any other number and manner of ways around the bans, legally or illegally. Fines are little disincentive as in most cases they are often minimal for any contraventions, if a conviction occurs.

Just consider what you are actually doing to your body, immune system and health in the long term, by consuming an astronomical quantity of chemicals, estimated to be in the region of more than four kilogram of E numbers every year in the UK, more if you drink diet-drinks daily or have a sweet-tooth. You'd be dead long before you could get through that four kilogram of chemical in one sitting, eating it neat, not that such experiments have been conducted, well they probably have been but that's another story; after only a couple of teaspoons (10g) of most of these E numbers you'd be in serious trouble, toxic shock would hit in at about 40g and coma and or death by 100g.

These chemicals are not a part of the food chain. How have they ended up in drinks and treats for our children? Fed to us from as early as a year old. An incredible 15% of two year olds obtain half of their daily calorific intake from soft drinks!

iv) Hippocratic Oath

"I swear by Apollo, the physician, by Æsculapius, Hygeia, and Panacea, and I take to witness all the gods, all the goddesses, to keep according to my ability and my judgement the following Oath:

"To consider dear to me as my parents him who taught me this art; to live in common with him and if necessary to share my goods with him; to look upon his children as my own brothers, to teach them this art if they so desire without fee or written promise; to impart to my sons and the sons of the master who taught me and the disciples who have enrolled themselves and have agreed to the rules of the profession, but to these alone, the precepts and the instruction. I will prescribe regimen for the good of my patients according to my ability and my judgement and never do harm to anyone. To please no one will I prescribe a deadly drug, nor give advice which may cause his death. Nor will I give a woman a pessary to procure abortion. But I will preserve the purity of my life and my art. I will not cut for stone, even for patients in whom the disease is manifest; I will leave this operation to be performed by practitioners (specialists in the art). In every house where I come I will enter only for the good of my patients, keeping myself far from all intentional ill-doing and all seduction, and especially from the pleasures of love with women or with men, be they free or slaves. All that may come to my knowledge in the exercise of my profession or outside of my profession or in daily commerce with men, which ought not to be spread abroad. I will keep secret and will never reveal. If I keep this oath faithfully, may I enjoy my life and practice my art, respected by all men and in all times; but if I swerve from it or violate it, may the reverse be my lot."

The modern version below is not quite so strict and it certainly doesn't imply that it is okay to repetitively prescribe drugs that are causing side-effects requiring more drugs, with no end in sight for the initial ailment. This version was adopted by the World Medical Association in 1948, known as The Declaration of Geneva –

I solemnly pledge to consecrate my life to the service of humanity;

I will give to my teachers the respect and gratitude that is their due;

I will practice my profession with conscience and dignity;

The health of my patient will be my first consideration;

I will respect the secrets that are confided in me, even after the patient has died;

I will maintain the utmost respect for human life;

I will not use my medical knowledge to violate human rights and civil liberties, even under threat;

I make these promises solemnly, freely and upon my honour. I solemnly pledge to consecrate my life to the service of humanity;

I will maintain by all the means in my power, the honour and the noble traditions of the medical profession;

My colleagues will be my sisters and brothers;

I will not permit considerations of age, disease or disability, creed, ethnic origin, gender, nationality, political affiliation, race, sexual orientation, social standing or any other factor to intervene between my duty and my patient;

I make these promises solemnly, freely and upon my honour.

Appendix

How many uphold this?

In fact, so hypocritical (a word, rather slanderously derived from Hippocrates) has it been to swear any form of allegiance and then become little more than a pharmaceutical dispensary, with little healing taking place, whilst just eliminating the symptoms; the oath is being phased out at many institutions. This is not to take anything away from Hippocrates, who was a most intellectual chap, the phasing out is obviously a reflection on the fact that the modern medical institutions feel their members cannot come close to upholding what was once considered the very precepts of medicine.

v) GDP of countries compared to the revenues of the largest companies

The figures for GDPs are taken from the IMF report of GDPs from 2014; revenues are from Wikipedia and Forbes.

Bare in mind the revenues from the companies will also be part of the sum for GDPs where their HQs are based and taxes paid.

Revenues are not necessarily the overall size of the company. I could have chosen a list that represented the value of assets held, profits or many other indices, which may, for better or worse, give an indication of the size of the companies within their industry. As an indicator to the differences, Land Securities where a good friend works, is about the 790th largest company in the world asset wise with $22.5bn, although with revenues of only (I say 'only' as a comparative word) $1.2bn it would languish nearer 5,000[th].

The list does not pretend to be definitive, however world GDPs are ranked. The largest companies are included within each area of pollutants covered in this series of books, as well as the largest other companies as a reference, as well as of course the 10 largest, who are predominately gas & oil producers, apart from the first, Wal-mart. There have been many omissions; only top ones from each industrial sector have been included as well as the better known ones with some British bias.

It is only intended to be comparatively interesting and thought provoking.

WORLD $77.3 trillion
EU $18.5 trillion
1. USA $17.4 trillion
2. China $10.4 trillion
3. Japan $4.6 trillion
4. Germany $3.9 trillion
5. United Kingdom $2.9 trillion
6. France $2.8 trillion
7. Brazil $2.4 trillion
8. Italy $2.1 trillion
9. India $2 trillion
10. Russia $1.9 trillion
11. Canada $1.8 trillion
12. Australia $1.4 trillion
13. South Korea $1.4 trillion
14. Spain $1.4 trillion
15. Mexico $1.3 trillion
16. Indonesia $888 billion
17. Netherlands $866 billion
18. Turkey $806 billion
19. Saudi Arabia $752 billion
20. Switzerland $712 billion
21. Nigeria $573 billion
24. Argentina $540 billion
27. Norway $500 billion
WALMART $476 billion
Royal Dutch SHELL $451 billion
SINOPEC $445 billion
28. Austria $437 billion

29. Iran $404 billion
30. UAE $402 billion
EXXONMOBIL $394 billion
31. Colombia $385 billion
BP $379 billion
32. Thailand $374 billion
34. Denmark $341 billion
STATE GRID CHINA $338 billion
CHINA PETROLEUM $328 billion
35. Malaysia $327 billion
36, Singapore $308 billion
VITOL $307 billion
37. Israel $304 billion
VOLKSWAGEN $263 billion
41. Chile $258 billion
TOTAL $253 billion
42. Pakistan $250 billion
TOYOTA $249 billion
43. Ireland $246 billion
GLENCORE/XSTRATA $239 billion
44. Greece $238 billion
CHEVRON $220 billion
SAMSUNG $216 billion
47. Algeria $214 billion
CHEVRON $212 billion
APPLE $182 billion
53. New Zealand $181 billion
BERKSHIRE HATH'Y $182 billion
54. Ukraine $178 billion
CHINA RAIL $172 billion
PHILLIPS 66 $171 billion
56. Vietnam $171 billion
E.ON $163 billion
57. Bangladesh $162 billion

GAZPROM $160 billion
DAIMLER $157 billion
GENERAL MOTORS $155 billion
ICBC $149 billion
FORD MOTOR $146 billion
GENERAL ELECTRIC $143 billion
McKESSON $137 billion
CARGILL $134 billion
TRAFIGURA $133 billion
58. Hungary $132 billion
ALLIANZ $131 billion
AT&T $128 billion
59. Angola $124 billion
UNITED HEALTH $122 billion
AXA $122 billion
CHINA Construction Bank $121 billion
VERIZON $120 billion
60. Morocco $113 billion
HEWLETT PACKARD $111 billion
TESCO $107 billion
JP MORGAN CHASE $106 billion
BASF $103 billion
CARREFOUR $101 billion
NESTLE $100 billion
IBM $100 billion
EDF $100 billion
SIEMENS $100 billion
61. Slovakia $96 billion
CITIGROUP $94 billion
62. Ecuador $94 billion
WELLS FARGO $89 billion
PROCTER & GAMBLE $85 billion
PRUDENTIAL $82 billion
HSBC HOLDINGS $80 billion

SONY $78 billion
63. Oman $77 billion
PANASONIC $77 billion
AMAZON $74 billion
64. Azerbaijan $74 billion
JOHNSON & JOHNSON $71 billion
68. Sri Lanka $67 billion
PEPSICO $66 billion
VODAFONE $65 billion
70. Dominican Republic $61 billion
GOOGLE $60 billion
71. Luxembourg $60 billion
NOVARTIS $58 billion
DOW CHEMICAL $57 billion
72. Croatia $57 billion
PFIZER $53 billion
78. Bulgaria $53 billion
SANTANDER $52 billion
ROCHE $50 billion
79. Costa Rica $49 billion
COCA COLA $46 billion
WALT DISNEY $46 billion
86. Serbia $42 billion
GLAXOSMITHKLINE $41 billion
GOLDMAN SACHS $40 billion
88. Panama $40 billion
ERICSSON $35 billion
ING GROUP $34 billion
91. Tanzania $33 billion
21stCENTURY FOX $32 billion
95. Bolivia $31 billion
HALLIBURTON $29 billion
MCDONALD'S $28 billion
BT $28 billion

NIKE $27 billion

99. Trinidad & Tobago $28 billion

ASTRAZENECA $26 billion

101. Estonia $25 billion

ROLLS-ROYCE $24 billion

102. El Salvador $24 billion

NATIONAL GRID $23 billion

104. Cyprus $22 billion

H&M $20 billion

108. Honduras $19 billion

DIAGEO $18 billion

109. Bosnia&Herzegovina $18 billion

112. Papua New Guinea $16 billion

EBAY $16 billion

MONSANTO $15 billion

119. Jamaica $14 billion

VIACOM $13 billion

126. Burkina Faso $12 billion

VISA $12 billion

129. Nicaragua $11 billion

SMURFITKAPPA $10 billion

138. The Bahamas $8 billion

SANDISK $6 billion

145. Guinea $6 billion

NEXT $6 billion

148. Sierra Leone $5 billion

PRADA $5 billion

HERBALIFE $5 billion

ADOBE SYSTEMS $4 billion

149. Montenegro $4 billion

ITV $4 billion

154. Malawi $4 billion

NETFLIX $4 billion

153. Fiji $4 billion

MICHAEL KORS $3 billion
157. Guyana $3 billion
SHIMANO $3 billion
158. Burundi $3 billion
GARMIN $2 billion
161. Bhutan $2 billion
LAND SECURITIES $1 billion
171. Solomon Islands $1 billion
173. Guinea-Bissau $845 million
TWITTER $700 million
187. Tuvalu $38 million

What the numbers clearly indicate is that the company revenues hugely outweigh some countries' revenues, and if a few were to collaborate, as no doubt is already the case, who knows what kind of leverage they could apply to benefit themselves, such as the extraordinary non-payment of taxes such massive companies enjoy.

Bibliography

The following books have had varying degrees of relevance and influence whilst I've been writing and researching this book over the past nine years. There is of course a whole lifetime's worth of reading, with much of the book coming from the deepest recesses of my mind, so the few mentioned below are the ones that I managed to jot down in the past few years only (in no particular order):

A Calendar of Gardeners Lore – S. Campbell (Century Publishing 1983)

Whole Foods Companion – D. Onstad (Chelsea Green Publishing, 1996). A vital compendium of all whole foods, folklore and nutrient breakdowns.

A Taste of History – P. Brears (British Museum Press 1997)

Nutrition for Life – Hark & Deen (Dorling Kindersley 2005)

Healing with Whole Foods – P. Pitchford (North Atlantic Books 2002)

Overfed but Undernourished – Dr.C. Wood (Tower Books 1971)

Nutrition and Physical Degeneration: A Comparison of Primitive and Modern diet and their effects – Dr W Price (Harper Brothers, 1939). A true hero and visionary.

The New Shorter Oxford English Dictionary (Oxford University Press 1993). My favourite book(s), it is like delving into a wonderland of words. It makes you feel clever just looking for a word in it.

Dorland's Illustrated Medical Dictionary (W.B. Saunders Company 1974). Bigger than a standard dictionary (although not the huge one above) and full of medical words and descriptions. It's the secret language they teach to doctors.

Food, Inc. – P.Pringle (Simon & Schuster 2003)

Food, Inc. – Ed.K.Weber (Participant Media 2009), no explanation given as to why it's the identical name to Pringle's book, this is the literary accompaniment to a film of the same name. Great film, and both are great books.

Sweet Poison – J. Starr Hull (Vision Paperbacks 1999), Janet's struggle with overcoming a disease caused by aspartame.

Pure, White and Deadly – J. Yudkin (Penguin 1988)

Aspartame Disease: An Ignored Epidemic – H. Roberts (Sunshine Sentinel 2001). I would like to see it called 'Rumsfeld's Disease', as explained in Book 2: Pollutants.

Health in the 21st Century – R. Horne (Harper Collins 1992)

Plants for People – A. Lewington (Eden Project Books 2003)

Stone Age Diet – L. Chaitow (Macdonald Optima 1987). Made me write this book.

The New Oxford Book of Food Plants – Vaughan & Geissler (Oxford University Press 1997)

Coping with Food Intolerances – D. Thom (Sterling Publishing Company 2002)

Silent Fields – R. Lovegrove (Oxford University Press 2007)

Silent Spring – R. Carson (Penguin 1962)

The Biogenic Diet – Leslie Kenton (Century Hutchinson 1986)

We Want Real Food – G. Harvey (Constable 2006). So easy to read, which makes it all the more scary.

The Healing Power of Nature Foods – S. Smith (HayHouse 2007)

Foodwise – W. Cook (Clairview 2003)

Timeless Secrets of Health and Rejuvenation – A. Moritz (Ener-chi Wellness Press 2005)

E for Additives – M. Hanssen (Thorsons 1984)

The Nature Doctor – Alfred Vogel (Mainstream Publishing 2003). The Don.

You Are What You Eat – Hartvig & Rowley (Piatkus 2003)

The Omnivore's Dilemma – M. Pollan (Bloomsbury 2006)

Not On The Label – F. Lawrence (Penguin 2004)

Omnivore – L. Watson (Corgi 1973)

Secret Ingredients – Cox & Brusseau (Bantam 1997)

Complete Herbal – T. Bruverton (Quercus 2011). This is a rewrite of Culpepper's *English Physician* of 1653

The Grand Salad – M. Mason (Peacock Vane 1984). This is a rewrite of Evelyn's *Acetaria* of 1699

The Optimum Nutrition Bible – P. Holford (Piatkus 2001)

The Complete Guide to Herbs – Ed. J. Holtom (Rodale Press 1979)

Pandora's Seed – S. Wells (Penguin 2011)

The China Study – T. Campbell (Benbella Books 2006)

Fats that Heal, Fats that Kill – U. Erasmus (Alive Books 1993)

Food For Free – R. Mabey (Collins 1972). Along with R. Philips, the authorities on wild foods

New Herbal – Ed. R. Mabey (Penguin 1991). The HerbFather

So Shall We Reap – C. Tudge (Penguin 2004)

Hidden Dangers In What We Eat and Drink – J. de Vries (Mainstream 2003)

Vegetarianism – D. Dombrowski (Thorsons 1984)

Chemistry Essentials for Dummies – J. Moore (John Wiley & Sons 2010)

Biology for Dummies – D. Siegfried (Wiley Publishing 2001)

Molecular & Cell Biology for Dummies – R. Kratz (John Wiley & Sons 2009). No ones a dummy who reads these.

The Human Body Book – S. Parker (Dorling Kindersley 2011). Each picture tells a thousand words and most are real medical photographs using modern techniques.

Your Life In Your Hands – J. Plant (Virgin Books 2007)

The Botany of Desire – M. Pollan (Bloomsbury Publishing 2002)

The Bircher-Benner Health Guide – R.Bircher (Unwin 1978)

Bad Science – B. Goldacre (Fourth estate 2009). One of those books that everyone kept saying I had to read, so I didn't want to and just like Breaking Bad, when my stubbornness subsided, I loved it.

The following websites have often been the launch pad to other numerous texts from other publications by often just flitting through the links pages. Some of these sites provided nothing more than just some hope that the truth is out there or that they are just interesting, light hearted and worth a quick visit. (Thanks to the wonderful staff at Uckfield library in times of no internet, everyone should support their local library.)

www.wikipedia.com – often a first port of call, undeniably useful

www.britannica.com – should have got in there before wiki, still amazingly informative

www.hubpages.com – loads of interesting articles

www.discovermagazine.com – science for the curious

www.allcountries.org – for the love of lists and facts about everything

www.newworldencyclopedia.org – a moralistic wiki

www.answers.com – you got a question?

www.wisegeek.com – ask a question, you may get the answer you want

www.worldometers.info – just watch those meters rise

www.nationmaster.com – everything about everywhere

www.nutritiondata.com – the only way to look at food

www.druglibrary.org – information not a borrowing service!

www.goodplanet.org – interesting and cool stuff for a better future

www.fao.org and www.faostat.fao.org – all about global food supplies

www.unclephilsbooks.co.uk – support all local independent booksellers

www.nutrition.org.uk – British Nutrition Foundation

www.foodtimeline.org – we all love a good timeline

www.forbes.com – who has what amongst the top <1%

www.who.int – World Health Organization

www.environmentalchemistry.com – loads of articles to read, very interesting

www.rain-tree.com – all about the Amazon Rainforest

www.sizes.com – lists and sizes for everything

www.unitconversion.org – conversion is their name

www.dietandfitnesstoday.com – health, diet and fitness

www.the-vitamin-and-supplement-guide.com – extensive

www.grinningplanet.com – some not so funny serious issues

www.pan-europe.info – pesticide action network, keeping you informed

www.sixwise.com – they say 'epiphanies for your empowerment', cool stuff

www.foodreference.com – loads about food

www.stevia.net – lots of talk and info about stevia

www.irri.org – rice research

www.thetruthaboutstuff.com – mainly stuff about aspartame

www.carrotmuseum.co.uk – some people love carrots

www.sproutpeople.com – and some love sprouts, these for 23 years

www.killerplants.com – no it's not a B-Movie!

www.selfsufficientish.com – self sufficiency for the urban environment

www.mealographer.com – check on the nutrition content of your diet

www.prota.org – Plant Resources Of Tropical Africa

www.mamashealth.com – full of clear advice and help about health

www.downwithbasics.com – tons of interesting, ethical and moral articles

www.organicconsumers.org – excellent range of topics and campaigns

www.sovereignty.org.uk – activism to eco living from Alistair McConnachie

www.viva.org.uk – campaigning for vegetarianism and veganism

www.danmedbul.dk – Danish Medical Journal

www.naturodoc.com – naturopathic information and advice

www.statistics.gov.uk – 'lies, lies and statistics', kind of interesting though www.infoplease.com – loads of info to digest here

www.mentalhealth.com

www.mentalhealth.org – the name of the last two says it all

www.cancer.org – info about cancer, mainstream, some interesting facts

www.wri.org – World Resources Institute

www.earthtimes.org – amazing articles about our amazing planet

www.sciencedaily.com – top science news

www.suite.io – stories from the heart and soul

www.veganpeace.com – striving towards peacefully sharing our planet

www.whfoods.com – awesome database for nutrient analysis and more

www.phytochemicals.info – all about those teeny-weeny plant nutrients

www.treehugger.com – driving sustainability mainstream

www.soilerosion.net – the names on the tin for this one

www.uk.oneworld.net – global empathy in action

www.quackwatch.com – keeping an eye on health fraud from the industry

www.thelivingweb.net – creative ways to live frugally

www.pan-uk.org – Pesticide Action Network, worth a look at their work

www.babymilkaction.org – in case you thought formula milk was the best start to life

www.nestlecritics.org – what the largest food corporation is actually up to

www.tree-harvest.com – The Culinary Caveman's suppliers of hearty herbs and more

www.aspartamekills.com – or 'Genetic Roulette', feeling lucky?

www.forksoverknives.com – making health taste good

www.mercola.com – makes some bold claims, we love you Dr Mercola www.glutenfreesociety.org – everything there is to know about gluten

www.wellnessmama.com – simple answers for healthier families

www.theculinarycaveman.co.uk – shameless self-promotion

www.davidsandersgraphics.co.uk – made the awesome site above

www.emilysanders.co.uk – did the gorgeous product design

www.curezone.org – health forums galore

www.earthisland.org – strengthening the environmental movement

www.saltnews.com – the world of gourmet salt

www.nutriology.com – great research site for ailments and nutrients

www.botanical-online.com – all about plants, really interesting

www.naturalnews.com – America's truth news bureau

www.carnicominstitute.org – working for the benefit of humanity

www.theonion.com – tears in my eyes, peeling with laughter

www.the dailymash.co.uk – so stupid, it must be true

www.cracked.com – always good to end with some light heart-edness.

EARTH

BOOKS

Earth Books are practical, scientific and philosophical
publications about our relationship with the environment.
Earth Books explore sustainable ways of living; including green
parenting, gardening, cooking and natural building. They also
look at ecology, conservation and aspects of environmental
science, including green energy. An understanding of the
interdependence of all living things is central to Earth Books,
and therefore consideration of our relationship with other
animals is important. Animal welfare is explored. The purpose
of Earth Books is to deepen our understanding of the
environment and our role within it. The books featured under
this imprint will both present thought-provoking questions and
offer practical solutions.